Culture, Health and Sexuality

The last 20 years have seen major growth in multi-disciplinary work in the area of sexuality, culture and health. What was once a set of specialist concerns has been steadily mainstreamed. Alongside this, a broader interest has developed in social and cultural factors relating to sexuality and sexual health, from family planning and STI management to gender and intimate partner violence and the technologisation of sex.

This book offers a research-based overview of key topics relevant to social and cultural perspectives on sexuality and sexual health. Beginning with an extended introduction and divided into six sections, it looks at culture, sex and gender, sexual diversity, sex work, migration, and sexual violence. Each section opens with an editorial discussion which places the theme, and the chapters that follow, in a contemporary context. Six additional substantive chapters can be accessed online at www.routledge.com/cw/aggleton

Including cutting-edge conceptual and empirical material from around the world, this is a key resource for students in, and across, a variety of disciplines in the social and health sciences. It is especially suitable for readers in sexuality studies, gender studies, development studies, anthropology and sociology as well as those with public health and social work backgrounds.

Peter Aggleton is Scientia Professor of Education and Health in the Centre for Social Research in Health at UNSW Australia. He is an Adjunct Professor in the Australian Research Centre in Sex, Health and Society at La Trobe University, Australia, and holds visiting professorial positions at the UCL Institute of Education in London and at the University of Sussex, UK.

Richard Parker is Professor of Sociomedical Sciences and Anthropology, and Director of the Center for the Study of Culture, Politics and Health at Columbia University, New York, USA, where he is also a member of the Committee on Global Thought.

Felicity Thomas is a Senior Research Fellow in the European Centre for Environment and Human Health, at the University of Exeter Medical School, UK.

Culture, Health and Sexuality

An introduction

Edited by Peter Aggleton,
Richard Parker and
Felicity Thomas

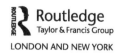
Routledge
Taylor & Francis Group

LONDON AND NEW YORK

First published 2015
by Routledge
2 Park Square, Milton Park, Abingdon, Oxon OX14 4RN

and by Routledge
711 Third Avenue, New York, NY 10017

Routledge is an imprint of the Taylor & Francis Group, an informa business

© 2015 P. Aggleton, R. Parker and F. Thomas

British Library Cataloguing-in-Publication Data
A catalogue record for this book is available from the British Library

Library of Congress Cataloging in Publication Data
Culture, health and sexuality (Aggleton)
Culture, health and sexuality : an introduction / edited by Peter Aggleton, Richard Parker and Felicity Thomas.
p. ; cm. -- (Sexuality, culture and health)
Includes bibliographical references and index. 1. Sex. 2. Sexual health. 3. Culture. I. Aggleton, Peter, editor. II. Parker, Richard G. (Richard Guy), 1956-, editor. III. Thomas, Felicity, editor. IV. Title. V. Series: Sexuality, culture and health series.
[DNLM: 1. Sexuality. 2. Cultural Characteristics. 3. Sexual Behavior. 4. Socioeconomic Factors.]
HQ23.C85 2015
306.7--dc23
2014041459

ISBN: 978-1-138-01558-6 (hbk)
ISBN: 978-1-138-01559-3 (pbk)
ISBN: 978-1-315-79425-9 (ebk)

Typeset in Goudy
by GreenGate Publishing Services, Tonbridge, Kent

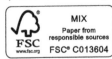

Printed and bound by CPI Group (UK) Ltd, Croydon, CR0 4YY

Contents

List of illustrations   viii
List of contributors   ix
Acknowledgements and permissions   xi

1   From sex to sexuality: sexual cultures and sexual selves   1
    PETER AGGLETON, RICHARD PARKER AND FELICITY THOMAS

SECTION 1
Culture and context   7

2   Sexuality, culture and society: shifting paradigms in sexuality research   9
    RICHARD PARKER

3   Women's work, worry and fear: the portrayal of sexuality and sexual
    health in US magazines for teenage and middle-aged women, 2000–2007   23
    JUANNE CLARKE

4   Cultural politics and masculinities: multiple partners in historical
    perspective in KwaZulu-Natal   37
    MARK HUNTER

SECTION 2
Sex and gender   53

5   HIV prevention and low-income Chilean women: machismo,
    marianismo and HIV misconceptions   55
    ROSINA CIANELLI, LILIAN FERRER AND BEVERLY J. MCELMURRY

6   'What does it take to be a man? What is a real man?': ideologies of
    masculinity and HIV sexual risk among Black heterosexual men   65
    LISA BOWLEG, MICHELLE TETI, JENNE S. MASSIE, ADITI PATEL, DAVID J. MALEBRANCHE AND
    JEANNE M. TSCHANN

7   'I just need to be flashy on campus': female students and transactional
    sex at a university in Zimbabwe   80
    TSITSI B. MASVAWURE

SECTION 3
Sexual diversity and practice   95

8   Constructions of lesbian, gay, bisexual and queer identities among
    young people in contemporary Australia   97
    PAUL WILLIS

9   'It's really a hard life': love, gender and HIV risk among
    male-to-female transgender persons   112
    RITA M. MELENDEZ AND ROGÉRIO PINTO

10 Black lesbian gender and sexual culture: celebration and resistance   125
    BIANCA D.M. WILSON

SECTION 4
Sex work   141

11 Structure and agency: reflections from an exploratory study of
    Vancouver indoor sex workers   143
    VICKY BUNGAY, MICHAEL HALPIN, CHRIS ATCHISON AND CAITLIN JOHNSTON

12 Social context, sexual risk perceptions and stigma: HIV vulnerability
    among male sex workers in Mombasa, Kenya   158
    JERRY OKAL, STANLEY LUCHTERS, SCOTT GEIBEL, MATTHEW F. CHERSICH, DANIEL LANGO
    AND MARLEEN TEMMERMAN

13 Diversity of commercial sex among men and male-born trans people
    in three Peruvian cities   173
    CÉSAR RODOLFO NUREÑA, MARIO ZÚÑIGA, JOSEPH ZUNT, CAROLINA MEJÍA,
    SILVIA MONTANO AND JORGE SÁNCHEZ

SECTION 5
Sexual violence   187

14 Hidden violence is silent rape: sexual and gender-based violence in
    refugees, asylum seekers and undocumented migrants in Belgium
    and the Netherlands   189
    INES KEYGNAERT, NICOLE VETTENBURG AND MARLEEN TEMMERMAN

15 Avoiding shame: young LGBT people, homophobia and
    self-destructive behaviours   207
    ELIZABETH MCDERMOTT, KATRINA ROEN AND JONATHAN SCOURFIELD

16 Barriers to post-exposure prophylaxis (PEP) completion after rape:
    a South African qualitative study   221
    NAEEMAH ABRAHAMS AND RACHEL JEWKES

SECTION 6
Mobility and migration   **235**

17 Youth, sin and sex in Nigeria: Christianity and HIV/AIDS-related
    beliefs and behaviour among rural–urban migrants   237
    DANIEL JORDAN SMITH

18 'Mobile men with money': the sociocultural and politico-economic
    context of 'high-risk' behaviour among wealthy businessmen and
    government officials in urban China   248
    ELANAH URETSKY

19 Race, space, place: notes on the racialisation and spatialisation of
    commercial sex work in Dubai, UAE   261
    PARDIS MAHDAVI

    Index   273

Illustrations

Figures

4.1 Griffiths Motsieloa, a well-known musician in the 1940s   44
4.2 A postcard given away in July 2003 with popular magazine *Drum*   47
4.3 Love Life, South Africa's largest intervention campaign   48
9.1 Stigma and discrimination lead to increased risk of unsafe behaviour   122

Tables

3.1 Circulation rates, median age and household income of magazine audiences   26
5.1 Number and percentage of women responding 'True' to questions of relevance to HIV-related discrimination and stigma   58
6.1 Demographic characteristics of focus group (FG) participants   67
8.1 Participants' pseudonym, age, gender and self-description of sexuality   102
10.1 Focus group participants   129
13.1 Forms and characteristics of sex work in three cities in Peru   177
14.1 SGBV determinants, socio-ecologically clustered   190
14.2 Sociodemographic profile of respondents   193
14.3 Characteristics of victims and perpetrators   195
14.4 Nature of SGBV cases   196

Contributors

The primary affiliations of contributors are as follows.

Naeemah Abrahams, Gender and Health Research Unit, South African Medical Research Council, Cape Town, South Africa.

Peter Aggleton, Centre for Social Research in Health, UNSW Australia.

Chris Atchison, Department of Sociology, University of Victoria, Canada.

Lisa Bowleg, Department of Psychology, The George Washington University, USA.

Vicky Bungay, School of Nursing, University of British Columbia, Canada.

Matthew F. Chersich, Centre for Health Policy, University of the Witwatersrand, South Africa.

Rosina Cianelli, School of Nursing and Health Studies, University of Miami, Florida, USA.

Juanne Clarke, Department of Sociology, Wilfrid Laurier University, Canada.

Lilian Ferrer, Escuela de Enfermeria, Pontificia Universidad Católica, Chile.

Scott Geibel, Population Council, Nairobi, Kenya.

Michael Halpin, Department of Sociology, University of Wisconsin, Madison, USA.

Mark Hunter, Department of Human Geography, University of Toronto Scarborough, Canada, and the University of KwaZulu-Natal, South Africa.

Rachel Jewkes, Gender and Health Research Unit, South African Medical Research Council, South Africa.

Caitlin Johnston, Faculty of Health Science, Simon Fraser University, Canada.

Ines Keygnaert, International Centre for Reproductive Health, Ghent University, Belgium.

Daniel Lango, International Centre for Reproductive Health, Mombasa, Kenya.

Stanley Luchters, Centre for International Health, Burnet Institute, VIC, Australia.

Pardis Mahdavi, Department of Anthropology, Pomona College, USA.

David J. Malebranche, Student Health Services, University of Pennsylvania, USA.

Jenne S. Massie, Department of Psychology, The George Washington University, USA.

Tsitsi B. Masvawure, Independent Researcher, USA.

Elizabeth McDermott, Faculty of Health and Medicine, Lancaster University, UK.

Beverly J. McElmurry (1937–2010), College of Nursing, University of Illinois at Chicago, Illinois, USA.

Carolina Mejía, Carolina Population Center, University of North Carolina at Chapel Hill, USA.

Rita M. Melendez, Sexuality Studies, San Francisco State University, USA.

Silvia Montano, US Naval Medical Research Center Detachment, Hospital Naval, Lima, Peru.

César Rodolfo Nureña, Escuela de Antropología, Facultad de Ciencias Sociales, Universidad Nacional Mayor de San Marcos, Peru.

Jerry Okal, Population Council, Nairobi, Kenya.

Richard Parker, Center for the Study of Culture, Politics and Health, Mailman School of Public Health, Columbia University, New York, USA.

Aditi Patel, College of Medicine, University of Florida, USA.

Rogério Pinto, Columbia University School of Social Work, New York, USA.

Katrina Roen, Department of Psychology, University of Oslo, Norway.

Jorge Sánchez, Asociación Civil Impacta Salud y Educación, Lima, Peru.

Jonathan Scourfield, School of Social Sciences, Cardiff University, UK.

Daniel Jordan Smith, Department of Anthropology, Brown University, USA.

Marleen Temmerman, Department of Reproductive Health and Research, World Health Organization, Geneva, Switzerland.

Michelle Teti, School of Health Professions, University of Missouri, USA.

Felicity Thomas, European Centre for Environment and Human Health, University of Exeter, UK.

Jeanne M. Tschann, Department of Psychiatry, University of California, San Francisco, USA.

Elanah Uretsky, Departments of Global Health, Anthropology and Elliott School of International Affairs, The George Washington University, USA.

Nicole Vettenburg, Department of Social Welfare Studies, Ghent University, Belgium.

Paul Willis, Department of Public Health, Policy and Social Sciences, Swansea University, UK.

Bianca D.M. Wilson, School of Law, The Williams Institute, University of California, Los Angeles, USA.

Mario Zúñiga, Escuela de Antropología, Facultad de Ciencias Sociales, Universidad Nacional Mayor de San Marcos, Peru.

Joseph Zunt, Department of Global Health, School of Medicine/School of Public Health, University of Washington, USA.

Acknowledgements and permissions

We would like to thank Fiona Thirlwell for her support in developing this book and, in particular, for liaising with contributors and preparing the manuscript for publication.

We thank Taylor & Francis for permission to reproduce the following material in edited and, where relevant, slightly updated form.

Sexuality, culture and society: shifting paradigms in sexuality research (2009) by Parker, R. *Culture, Health & Sexuality* 11(3): 251–266.

Women's work, worry and fear: the portrayal of sexuality and sexual health in US magazines for teenage and middle-aged women, 2000–2007 (2009) by Clarke, J. *Culture, Health & Sexuality* 11(4): 415–429.

Cultural politics and masculinities: multiple-partners in historical perspective in KwaZulu-Natal (2005) by Hunter, M. *Culture, Health & Sexuality* 7(4): 389–403.

HIV prevention and low-income Chilean women: machismo, marianismo and HIV misconceptions (2008) by Cianelli, R., Ferrer, L. and McElmurry, B.J. *Culture, Health & Sexuality* 10(3): 297–306.

'What does it take to be a man? What is a real man?' Ideologies of masculinity and HIV sexual risk among Black heterosexual men (2011) by Bowleg, L., Teti, M., Massie, J., Patel, A., Malebranche, D. and Tschann, J. *Culture, Health & Sexuality* 13(5): 545–559.

'I just need to be flashy on campus': female students and transactional sex at a university in Zimbabwe (2010) by Masavawure, T. *Culture, Health & Sexuality* 12(8): 857–870.

Constructions of lesbian, gay, bisexual and queer identities among young people in contemporary Australia (2012) by Willis, P. *Culture, Health & Sexuality* 14(10): 1213–1227.

'It's really a hard life': love, gender and HIV risk among male-to-female transgender persons (2007) by Melendez, R.M. and Pinto, R. *Culture, Health & Sexuality* 9(3): 233–245.

Black lesbian gender and sexual culture: celebration and resistance (2009) by Wilson, B.D.M. *Culture, Health & Sexuality* 11(3): 297–313.

Structure and agency: reflections from an exploratory study of Vancouver indoor sex workers (2011) by Bungay, V., Halpin, M., Atchison, C. and Johnston, C. *Culture, Health & Sexuality* 13(1): 15–29.

Social context, sexual risk perceptions and stigma: HIV vulnerability among male sex workers in Mombasa, Kenya (2009) by Okal, J., Luchters, S., Geibel, S., Chersich, M.F., Lango, D. and Temmerman, M. *Culture, Health & Sexuality* 11(8): 811–826.

Diversity of commercial sex among men and male-born trans people in three Peruvian cities (2011) by Nureña, C.R., Zúñiga, M., Zunt, M., Mejía, M., Montano, S. and Sánchez, J.L. *Culture, Health & Sexuality* 13(10): 1207–1221.

Hidden violence is silent rape: sexual and gender-based violence in refugees, asylum seekers and undocumented migrants in Belgium and the Netherlands (2012) by Keygnaert, I., Vettenburg, N. and Temmerman, M. *Culture, Health & Sexuality* 14(5): 505–520.

Avoiding shame: young LGBT people, homophobia and self-destructive behaviours (2008) by McDermott, E., Roen, K. and Scourfield, J. *Culture, Health & Sexuality* 10(8): 815–829.

Barriers to the post exposure prophylaxis (PEP) completion after rape: a South African qualitative study (2010) by Abrahams, N. and Jewkes, R. *Culture, Health & Sexuality* 12(5): 471–484.

Youth, sin and sex in Nigeria: Christianity and HIV/AIDS-related beliefs and behaviour among rural–urban migrants (2004) by Smith, D.J. *Culture, Health & Sexuality* 6(5): 425–437.

Mobile men with money: the socio-cultural and politico-economic context of 'high risk' behaviour among wealthy businessmen and government officials in urban China (2008) by Uretsky, E. *Culture, Health & Sexuality* 10(8): 801–814.

Race, space, place: notes on the racialisation and spatialisation of commercial sex work in Dubai, UAE (2010) by Mahdavi, P. *Culture, Health & Sexuality* 12(8): 943–954.

Chapter 1

From sex to sexuality

Sexual cultures and sexual selves

*Peter Aggleton, Richard Parker and
Felicity Thomas*

The last three decades have witnessed major changes in the way in which sex, sexuality and sexual relationships are understood.

Up until the 1960s, and in Western contexts at least, sex was understood largely as something that could not easily be talked about. When it was, the focus was usually on sexual 'deviance', or sexual pathology and abnormality. Books on sex and sexual behaviour were hard to find, and when they could be located, they were either encased in plain brown covers or had to be unlocked from the librarian's cupboards, or obtained through specialist mail-order suppliers. Magazines with sexual content were likewise placed on the 'top shelf' or were available 'under the counter' in newsagents and stores, being viewed as a 'specialist' interest, and not relevant to the majority.

In the 1960s, changing attitudes towards marriage, fidelity and same-sex relations, together with the advent of the contraceptive pill, changed much of this. For the first time in generations, sex could be talked about relatively openly: at least late at night on television, and among the growing liberal elites. Free love, flower power, and a rejection of the 'sexual puritanism' of the past characterised the 1960s, giving rise in complex and often contradictory ways to the feminist, gay and lesbian, and men's movements – signalling as they did the 'right' to varying forms of sexual expression – that reached their ascendancy in North America, Europe, Australia and New Zealand in the 1970s and 1980s.

In parallel, and on the international stage, growing anxiety about global population growth, demographic transition, and economic and social development facilitated an opening up of discussion of sex (or reproduction at least) and its consequences, particularly in the poorer nations of the world. A certain legitimacy became attached to research into the determinants of sexual behaviour and sexual behaviour change, at least when it was couched in terms of knowledge, attitudes and their behavioural correlates. Demography provided a new means by which certain aspects of the sexual could be thought about. But the frame remained largely normative, with marriage, 'regular unions' and family planning occupying much of the available discursive space.

For those seeking any detail on human sexual behaviours and practices, the only available options were those provided by sexology (with its focus on sexual difficulties, pathologies and abnormalities), anthropology (with its concern to understand esoteric sexual practices and rituals among 'primitive' people in far-off places), and criminology (with its interest in sexual deviance and particularly in practices that broke the law). But in each of these fields, the dominant framing was constrained by a concern for the 'Other' – the person with the problem, the community with the unusual practice, and the sexual deviant and their (most usually 'his') desires – and not for what lay closer to home. This was a far from satisfactory state of affairs.

Into this arena came AIDS, and the community activism that characterised the earliest days of the epidemic. In part triggered by the unwillingness of politicians, the media and mainstream society to engage with the challenges posed by the epidemic, and in part informed by the 'epidemic of signification' (Treichler 1987) that accompanied a combination of physical and social *dis*-ease for which science had no cure, space was opened up for critical reflection and debate. Where mainstream public health, health promotion and health education had feared to tread, a variety of counter-publics took their place, offering framings of the aetiology and progress of the epidemic that were profoundly located in the social.

Society's unwillingness to recognise gender and sexual minorities, people who inject drugs, sex workers and other 'outsiders within' was correctly identified as rendering some groups more systematically vulnerable to HIV than others. Lack of good quality health education, lack of adequate service provision, and lack of government respect caused gay men quite literally to invent safer sex in the form of condom use (Berkowitz and Callen 1983; Berkowitz 2003). People who inject drugs and their allies in drugs education and outreach projects around the world worked together to develop the safer drug use practices, such as the non-sharing of injection equipment and the use of clean needles and syringes that we have with us today (Riley and O'Hare 2000). Sex workers all over the world were among the first to recognise the importance of safe sex practices both with clients and with regular partners (Chateauvert 2014). These, and allied practices, were not the creation of virologists, doctors, public health experts or social scientists. Instead, they were the result of action from the grassroots, in the face of widespread intransigence and denial, as affected individuals and communities took matters into their own hands.

The origins of a distinct (and distinctive) perspective

But how were such actions and their successors resourced conceptually and intellectually? What forms of knowledge and understanding underpinned their operation, and where did such ideas come from in the first place? At least in part, the answer to this question can be found in the growth of cross-disciplinary and interdisciplinary social scientific enquiry characteristic of the 1980s and 1990s. The limitations of 'single perspective' accounts of the kind offered by disciplines such as anthropology, demography, psychology and sociology were increasingly evident. All too often, research within these fields simply added incrementally to existing understanding, with little real-world benefit. Called for were explanations that crossed disciplinary boundaries, recognising *simultaneously* the importance of personal meanings, social contexts, local cultures and more pervasive social structures relating to age, class, disability, gender, race/ethnicity and sexuality, as factors influencing health-related vulnerability.

Crucial too was a more positive approach to sex, sexuality and sexual relationships: one that recognised the rich diversity of ways in which people can express themselves sexually, in ways that are consensual and respectful of others. The coming together of advocacy and insight from second wave feminism (with its concern for the family, the workplace, sexuality, reproductive rights and de facto inequalities) and lesbian and gay activism (with their focus on the right to inclusion, recognition and respect for sexual minorities) provided fertile ground for the growth of demands: first for sexual health, and later for sexual and reproductive health and rights. The World Health Organization's first expert group meeting on sexual health took place in 1975, and described sexual health as involving 'the integration of the somatic, emotional, intellectual and social aspects of sexual being in ways that are positively enriching and that enhance personality, communication and love' (WHO 1975). It was key in laying the foundations for a more positive understanding of human sexual relationships than had hitherto been possible.

The advent of HIV and AIDS provided further impetus to this trajectory, especially when it became evident that the epidemic was impacting upon the Global South in ways that exploited existing inequalities (Mann and Carballo 1989). Perhaps for the first time it became legitimate to enquire into the sexual from other than a negatively nuanced perspective in the countries of Africa, Asia and Latin America. While this proved challenging initially, especially in contexts that tried to deny the existence of homosexuality, prostitution and sex outside of marriage, with advocacy, opposition and resistance things began to change. In Latin America, particularly, concern for greater openness and democracy in countries such as Brazil, which was throwing off the difficult legacy of military dictatorship, gave rise to vibrant forms of HIV-related activism alongside new demands for sexual and reproductive health and rights.

Key empirical foundations

In 1992–1993, the Social and Behavioural Studies and Support Unit of the World Health Organization's former Global Programme on AIDS commissioned a ground-breaking series of studies focusing on what were then described as 'contextual factors' influencing risk-related sexual behaviour among young people, and household and community responses to HIV (Dowsett and Aggleton 1999). Conducted in diverse countries across Africa, Asia and Latin America, these studies sought to explore some of the local meanings associated with sex and sexuality, together with the individual and community-level practices to which these gave rise. Perhaps for the first time, young people were allowed to speak for themselves about sexual relationships, sexual meanings and sexual practices in the context of HIV. Certainly for the first time, close-focus study at community level highlighted the positive as well as the negative responses arising in the context of HIV and AIDS.

At about the same time, in the early 1990s, a number of private foundations, led by the Ford Foundation, but also including the John D. and Catherine T. MacArthur Foundation and the Rockefeller Foundation, began to express growing interest in addressing issues related to sexuality, first as an extension of their support for work on HIV and AIDS, and then later – especially at the Ford Foundation – as a programme area in its own right. In 1992, the Ford, MacArthur and Rockefeller Foundations together provided support for the creation of an international Working Group on Sexual Behaviour Research, loosely linked to the AIDS and Reproductive Health Network. This Working Group, which was active over much of the next decade, aimed to strengthen a focus on social science research, emphasising the social and cultural construction of sexuality as its overarching theoretical framework, and highlighting the social structures and the social and political processes shaping sexuality. It sought to support the research and theorising that was beginning to develop in the Global South, organising a series of small seminars and conferences over the course of the 1990s, and publishing a number of edited volumes bringing together work on these themes (Parker and Gagnon 1995; Parker and Aggleton 1999; Parker et al. 2000).

The making of a new journal

Together, these factors were influential in creating legitimacy for a new form of academic enterprise: namely the cross- and interdisciplinary exploration of issues relating to sexuality, culture and health. It was into this space that a new journal, entitled *Culture, Health & Sexuality* (CHS), stepped. Subtitled 'an international journal for research, intervention and care' and first published in 1999 by Routledge in the form of four slim issues a year, CHS offered a setting for the publication of research papers, reviews of methodology, and conceptual contributions. With respect to its aims and scope, the journal set out to provide:

- an international forum for the analysis of culture and health, health beliefs and systems, social structures and divisions, and the implications for these for sexual health, and individual, collective and community well-being;
- an environment in which the policy and practice implications of research in the fields of culture and health, and culture and reproductive and sexual health, can be considered;
- a setting for critical scholarly debate about how best to analyse the cultural dimensions of health issues in general, and reproductive and sexual health issues in particular.

By the year 2014, CHS had grown rapidly to become the number one journal internationally publishing in its field, publishing no less than 14 issues in 2013 (4 of them special issues), and with an impact factor placing it among the best in its class. Published in association with the International Association for the Study of Sexuality, Culture and Society (IASSCS), the journal engages with a diverse range of issues and topics, providing a window into the contemporary and evolving field of sexuality research.

An overarching emphasis on cultural systems and social contexts characterises the majority of the articles published in the journal, with a significant topical focus on issues such as the interaction between sex and gender, the complex forms of sexual diversity found across different cultures, the social organisation of sex work and transactional sex, and the ways in which globalisation and related historical transformations have been remaking the sexual landscape in the early twenty-first century. What might be described as the darker side of sex has also been explored in many articles, with a focus on issues such as sexual stigma and discrimination, the social production of sexual oppression, and the challenges of sexual violence. Issues such as the use of new technologies, bodily cutting and modification, parenting and parenthood, the sexual experiences of young people, innovative methods and methodologies in research on sex and sexuality, and new conceptualisations and approaches in sexuality research have all found place in CHS, as has work on topics as diverse as gender dynamics of HIV testing, sexual discourse among minority ethnic groups, links between body esteem and safe sex practices, and the parenting rights of same-sex couples.

This book

Many of these themes are taken up in this present volume, which brings together some of the most read and most cited contributions to the journal over the last 16 years. Our aim in editing it has been to offer a concise introduction both to the field of research that currently comprises culture, health and sexuality, and the work of key authors who, between them, have charted the development of this significant area of work.

Thematically, the book covers a wide range of important topics that have helped to further understanding and define ongoing research agendas and priorities within the field. The role of *culture and context* in shaping sexuality is one such theme that underpins many of the works published in this volume. A focus on the intersections between *sex and gender* as they relate to health is also a central theme, with chapters in this area helping to develop understanding of the various ways in which societal expectations concerning men and women – alongside other variables such as class, age and ethnicity – can impact upon health and well-being.

Sexual diversity and practice are also examined, with chapters on this theme highlighting the complex interrelationships between sexual identities, sexual practices and sexual communities, and the challenges faced expressing diversity and resisting dominant, and often oppressive, normative systems.

A focus on the transactional nature of sex forms a further important element of the book with chapters here challenging more conventional, and often judgemental, assumptions made about *sex work*, by demonstrating the diverse nature of the actors involved within it and the contexts in which it occurs.

Sexual violence is the thematic focus for another section of the book, with chapters in this area emphasising not only the vulnerabilities of particular population groups, but also stressing the need to consider the wider social, cultural, economic and political context in which rape and sexual violence persists. Finally, in an increasingly globalised world, understanding how *mobility and migration* interrelate with culture, health and sexuality is of paramount importance. The focus that is placed upon these issues in another section of this volume highlights cutting-edge research from across the globe.

In addition to the chapters included in this volume, we have assembled an additional set of readings which can be accessed via a specially created website, www.routledge.com/cw/aggleton. These provide opportunities to explore more deeply some of the issues highlighted here. They also encourage readers to access the journal's own website to read around a topic or to delve more deeply into relevant concerns.

Taken together, the chapters included in the print version of this volume, along with the additional papers that can be accessed electronically, offer an exciting vision of the cutting edge in contemporary research on culture, health and sexuality. They highlight the work of some of the most important authors currently shaping this field. They also point in the direction of some of the key themes and lines of investigation that we might expect to see in the future: the importance of rethinking the role of culture in shaping the nexus between sexuality and health, the central role of structures, and of structural violence, in relation to sexuality and health, and the growing importance of sexual rights and understandings of practical justice in this rapidly evolving field of research.

Beyond this, however, the chapters reprinted here provide a compelling portrait of an exceptionally vibrant field of investigation and analysis – one that will surely continue to evolve in the future, and to engage with important issues in the contemporary world.

References

Berkowitz, R. 2003. *Stayin' Alive: The Invention of Safe Sex*. New York: Basic Books.
Berkowitz, R. and Callen, M. with Sonnabend, J. 1983. *How to Have Sex in an Epidemic: One Approach*. New York: News From The Front Publications.

Chateauvert, M. 2014. *Sex Workers Unite: A History of the Movement from Stonewall to Slutwalk*. Boston, MA: Beacon Press.

Dowsett, G. and Aggleton, P. 1999. *Sex and Youth: Contextual Factors Affecting Risk for HIV/AIDS. A Comparative Analysis of Multi-site Studies in Developing Countries*. Geneva: UNAIDS Best Practice Collection. Available at: http://data.unaids.org/publications/irc-pub01/jc096-sex_youth_en.pdf [Accessed 15 September 2014].

Mann, J. and Carballo, M. 1989. Social, cultural and political aspects: Overview. *AIDS* 3(Suppl. 1): S221–S223.

Parker, R. and Gagnon, J. (eds) 1995. *Conceiving Sexuality: Approaches to Sex Research in a Postmodern World*. New York and London: Routledge.

Parker, R. and Aggleton, P. (eds) 1999. *Society, Culture, and Sexuality: A Reader*. London: UCL Press.

Parker, R., Barbosa, R.M. and Aggleton, P. (eds) 2000. *Framing the Sexual Subject: The Politics of Gender, Sexuality and Power*. Berkeley, Los Angeles and London: University of California Press.

Riley, D. and O'Hare, P. 2000. Harm reduction: History, definition, and practice. In: J.A. Inciardi and L.D. Harrison (eds) *Harm Reduction: National and International Perspectives*. Thousand Oaks, CA, and London: SAGE, 1–26.

Treichler, P.A. 1987. AIDS, homophobia and biomedical discourse: An epidemic of signification. *Cultural Studies* 1(3): 263–305.

WHO. 1975. *Education and Treatment in Human Sexuality: The Training of Health Professionals. World Health Organization Technical Report Series No. 572*. Geneva: WHO. Available at: http://whqlibdoc.who.int/trs/WHO_TRS_572.pdf [Accessed 21 December 2014].

Section 1

Culture and context

A growing emphasis on the importance of both culture and context characterizes much recent thinking about sexuality and sexual relations. Cultural systems shape the meaning of sexual experience and the ways in which people interpret and understand sexual practices. Alongside this, it is possible to identify a range of other, broader contextual factors that also contribute to what has been described as the social and historical construction of sexuality, and that have also provided a focus for analysis and investigation. The three chapters in this section all explore the ways in which both culture and context shape and influence sexuality, and the reasons why they are therefore increasingly central in sexuality research. In the first chapter, Richard Parker analyses the role of culture, social systems and political economy in shifting paradigms in sexuality research over the past three decades. He identifies three major phases in the development of this work. In the first phase, work focusing on the social construction of sexual experience developed an important critique of the biomedical and sexological approaches that had dominated the field over much of the twentieth century. In the second phase, increasingly detailed studies of sexual life were developed which highlighted the cross-cultural diversity of sexual cultures, sexual identities and sexual communities. In the most recent phase, there has been a growing recognition of the complex relationship between culture and power, and increasing attention to the political and economic dimensions of sexuality. The chapter ends by highlighting a number of important silences and invisibilities that continue to characterize much sexuality research and the challenges that must still be confronted in seeking to expand our understanding of these issues.

In the second chapter, Juanne Clarke examines the portrayal of sexuality and sexual health in US magazines for teenage and middle-aged women from 2000 to 2007. She develops an exploratory content analysis of the portrayal of sexuality, sexual health and disease in select magazines designed for two groups of women: teenagers and women in the 40 to 50-year-old age category in the USA. She argues that this portrayal was both similar for the two groups of women and yet also distinctly different. Magazines for both these audiences emphasized women's responsibility for controlling sexual expression. In the case of young women, the focus was on avoiding sex in order to prevent pregnancy, protect themselves from sexually transmitted infections, and guard against untrustworthy male partners, and abstinence was identified as the only way to fully achieve these goals. For the older group of women, emphasis was placed on their responsibility for maintaining their marriages and monitoring of the sexuality of their female children. Neither group of magazines explored women's sexual desires or sexual satisfaction, focusing, on the contrary, on controlling and regulating women's sexuality.

The last chapter in this section, by Mark Hunter, draws on extended ethnographic research together with archival sources in order to examine the perceived importance of multiple-sexual partners in KwaZulu-Natal, a South African province where as many as one in three people are thought to be HIV positive. Hunter argues that a full understanding of contemporary multiple-partner relations requires examining them in historical perspective, and exploring the gendered cultural politics through which they have been produced over time. Calling into question stereotypes relating to promiscuity and African masculinity, he examines the ways in which changing conditions associated with capitalist development, migrant labour and Christianity have shaped changing expressions of masculinity and manliness. Unable to draw upon the resources available to them in earlier historical periods, Hunter argues, has meant that men now seek multiple partners as a way of expressing masculinity.

Chapter 2

Sexuality, culture and society
Shifting paradigms in sexuality research

Richard Parker

Introduction

Over the course of the past three decades, we have seen a veritable explosion in the field of sexuality research. From a relatively limited field, dominated primarily by biomedical and sexological research, the study of sexuality has in recent years expanded most rapidly across a wide range of social sciences. The signs of a field coming of age are everywhere: new scholarly and scientific journals focusing on sexuality have been launched; new interdisciplinary sexuality research centres have been formed; innovative academic degree programmes have been created; established foundations and research funding agencies have made sexuality a programmatic priority; and the volume of publications reporting sexuality research findings has increased rapidly in recent years. While many of these developments are concentrated in the leading intellectual centres of resource-rich societies, the trend is clearly global, with important new developments taking place as much in the South as in the North.

As with any rapidly evolving field, in order to think about the further development of sexuality research, it is important to pause periodically in order to take stock of where the field has been and to reflect on where it might seek to go in the future. Examining the questions and approaches that have oriented investigation in the past and in the present is an essential step in seeking to articulate the kinds of issues and theoretical frameworks that might open up new ground in the future. With this goal in mind, in this chapter I want to try to examine some of the most important ways in which we have thought about the social and cultural dimensions of sexuality in recent years and some of the ways in which investigation on sexuality has evolved, giving particular attention to the epistemological assumptions and challenges that have guided this work, and the paradigms that have organized it. In short, I want to reflect on the development of research on the social and cultural dimensions of sexuality, highlighting what seem to be the kinds of questions that we have asked – and, by extension, some of the questions that we have perhaps *failed* to ask. Some suggestions will also be offered as to the key challenges currently confronting the field of sexuality research – the kinds of questions and research priorities which are especially important to pursue in order to ensure the continued development of this field in the future.

With these goals in mind, the chapter will look first at three main sets of issues that over the course of roughly the past 25 to 30 years – the past three decades – seem to have been central to much of the work that has been carried out in studying the social and cultural dimensions of sexuality. For lack of better labels, and at the expense of some probable oversimplification, these are flagged as: (1) Thinking sexuality: diversity, difference and the epistemology of sexuality research; (2) Sexual cultures, identities and communities; and (3) Structure and agency: toward a political economy of the body. Finally, I will also try to highlight at least some of the things that may have been left out of current analyses and investigations and some of the questions that we have failed to ask or even articulate. The goal will be to flesh out a fourth set of issues around what might be described as Sexuality and Silence – both the silence that results from the questions that we, as investigators, fail to ask and the discursive silence that is perhaps produced by what may be our own (over) attention in recent years to issues of discourse and culture.

Thinking sexuality: diversity, difference and the epistemology of sexuality research

It was only in the 1970s and the early 1980s that concepts such as culture and society began to emerge as a powerful conceptual tool for thinking about sexuality – in large measure in opposition to the concept of nature. This was itself, of course, the result of a long-term series of changes in the ways in which sexuality has been conceptualized and interrogated. As Michel Foucault and others have pointed out, since at least the Middle Ages, the social articulation of sexuality had been organized primarily by religion, and it was fundamentally the religious monopoly over the sins of the flesh that late nineteenth and early twentieth century biomedical science began to undercut (Foucault 1978; Weeks 1985, 1991). By the beginning of the twentieth century, this emerging set of discursive practices had begun to offer an alternative (to religious), 'scientific' vision of sexuality and its consequences, based less on accepted moral precepts than on empirical investigation and observation (Robinson 1976; Weeks 1985, 1991).

To the extent that human sexuality was re-conceptualized as the province not of religious morality but rather of human nature, the study of sexuality was constituted as the scientific domain of biology and medicine, of psychiatry and the emerging discipline of sexology (Weeks 1985). For much of the twentieth century, in spite of a number of important changes that have taken place over time, research and analysis in the sexological tradition generally shared a number of important commonalities (Gagnon and Parker 1995). Nearly all of the work emerging from this tradition (and indeed much of the undercurrent at sexology conferences today) has conceived of sex as a kind of natural force that exists in opposition to civilization, culture or society.

While researchers have differed on whether or not the sex drive was a positive force warped by a negative civilization (as Havelock Ellis and Alfred Kinsey tended to see it) or a negative force in need of social control (as Freud and most of his followers tended to view it), they all generally agreed on the power of sexuality to define who we are as human beings (Robinson 1976). In both of these directions, however, in spite of the important differences that might be cited to distinguish between them, there has nonetheless been an equally strong propensity to reduce the question of sex to some kind of underlying reality: to a biological or psychological imperative which ultimately determines the meaning of even the most seemingly disparate beliefs and practices. It is this underlying 'essentialism' of the sexological project that has continued, on up to the present, to provide the dominant framework for the investigation and understanding of human sexuality across both time and space.

By the mid- to late 1960s, however, it began to become apparent to many that key elements within the 'sexological paradigm' were beginning to dissolve. To the extent that a paradigm can be understood as an interrelated set of widely accepted explanations, based on agreed-upon methods and empirical observations, the certainties of a positivist or scientific explanation of sexual life had begun to be shaken. Whether in structuralist thought,

Marxist theory or certain streams of psychoanalysis, the 1970s and 1980s were characterized by a new willingness to call into question the 'naturalness' of all human experience. Since much of the power of sex seemed somehow linked to biological being and the experience of the body, sexuality was perhaps more resistant to such interrogation than many other areas of human life. But even here, important doubts began to be raised from a number of different theoretical vantage points. The primary challenge to such supposedly scientific explanations came from social theorists and social science researchers working on issues related to gender and sexuality, as well as from activists, particularly from the feminist and the emerging gay and lesbian movements, who sought to question key elements of the sexological paradigm that they viewed as antithetical to their most important interests (Gagnon and Parker 1995).

It was within this broader context that a new focus on sexuality – and, in particular, on sexual diversity – as a social, cultural and historical construction began to emerge in the 1970s and early 1980s (Plummer 1984). In opposition to the conceptualization of sexual life and experience as rooted in biology and nature, social researchers began to rethink sexual experience, like all human experience, less as the result of some immutable human nature, than as the outcome of a complex set of social, cultural and historical processes. This conceptualization, in turn, began to refocus research attention on the symbolic dimensions of sexual experience and on the intersubjective cultural forms that shape and structure the experience of sexual life in different social settings (Parker 1991). It also shifted attention, implicitly, from the search for natural laws and empirical uniformity to a new emphasis on cross-cultural comparisons and contrasts and a new focus on sexual diversity and difference (see, for example, Ortner and Whitehead 1981; Caplan 1987; Parker and Gagnon 1995; Szasz and Lerner 1996; Manderson and Jolly 1997; Parker et al. 2000).

Pioneering social research carried out on sexual diversity and non-normative sexualities in a wide range of different settings during the late 1970s and the early 1980s made a major contribution to these emerging debates (see, for example, Carrier 1976; Herdt 1981; Fry 1982; Blackwood 1986; Lancaster 1988). Influenced not only by theoretical academic frameworks, but also by the emerging feminist and gay and lesbian movements, and focusing on issues related to both women's sexuality and male homosexuality, this work helped to shape the emerging field of sexuality studies in the 1980s by using specific case studies to call attention to sexual diversity and difference (Ortner and Whitehead 1981; Vance 1984; Blackwood 1986).

The focus on cultural difference that was central to much of the emerging sexuality research during this period was constructed in at least two somewhat distinct ways. On the one hand, many anthropological researchers working on same-sex interactions sought to differentiate between the social construction of same-sex relations in non-Western cultures and so-called developing countries, as opposed to the social construction of homosexuality and gay communities and cultures in the countries of North America or Western Europe. They tended to articulate a comparison (or contrast) between two very different models for the constitution of sexual identities based on the relationship between sexual practice and individual subjectivity (Carrier 1976; Herdt 1981; Blackwood 1986; Jackson 1989; Nanda 1990; Parker 1991; Lancaster 1992; Murray 1992b).

A somewhat different focus could be found in detailed ethnographic work carried out by Latin American and, somewhat later, Asian and African researchers during the 1980s and over the course of the 1990s on sexual subcultures and non-normative sexualities. In this work, the locus of comparison and contrast was both between North and South, but also centre and periphery, hegemonic and what we might describe as subaltern patterns in the organization of gender and sexuality. In this line of research, ethnographies and other descriptive studies have focused on female sex workers and their venues, male same-sex sexual networks and settings (movie theatres, parks, public toilets, etc.), male hustlers and transgender sex workers, and similar sexual subcultures (or alternative cultures), with the goal of documenting sexual diversity and difference within these societies rather than in contrast to Northern settings (see, for example, Gaspar 1985; Perlongher 1987; Gayatri 1995; Gevisser and Cameron 1995; Tan 1996; Thandani 1996; Denizart 1997).

Sexual cultures, identities and communities

The understanding of sexuality as being socially constructed that had begun to emerge in the late 1970s and early 1980s thus refocused research attention on the social and cultural systems which shape not only our sexual experience, but the ways in which we interpret and understand that experience. This view of sexuality and sexual activity increasingly focused research attention on the intersubjective nature of sexual meanings – their shared, collective quality, not as the property of atomized or isolated individuals, but of social persons integrated within the context of distinct and diverse sexual wholes. Within this framework, sexual conduct has been seen as largely intentional, yet its 'intentionality' is always shaped within the specific contexts of socially and culturally structured interactions. In this sense, understanding individual behaviour is less important than understanding the context of sexual interactions – interactions which are necessarily social and which involve complex negotiations between different individuals. Attention has thus increasingly turned to what have been described as the sexual 'scripts' that exist in different social settings, and that organize the structure and possibilities of sexual interaction in a range of specific ways (Gagnon and Simon 1973; Simon and Gagnon 1984; Parker 1991; Paiva 2000; Carrillo 2002). This focus, in turn, has led to a new concern with the wider cultural scenarios, the discursive practices, and the complex systems of knowledge and power which quite literally produce the meaning and experience of sexuality in different historical, social and cultural settings (see Simon and Gagnon 1984; see, also, Rubin 1984 and Weeks 1985).

In much recent social research on sexuality and sexual conduct, this emphasis on the social organization of sexual interactions, on the contexts within which sexual practices occur and on the complex relations between meaning and power in the constitution of sexual experience, has led to a new focus on the investigation of diverse 'sexual cultures' (Parker 1991). Research attention has thus increasingly shifted from sexual behaviour, in and of itself, to the cultural settings within which it takes place – and to the cultural rules that organize it. Special emphasis has been given to analysing the cultural categories and the systems of classification that structure and define sexual experience in different social and cultural contexts (Parker 1991).

As research attention began to focus on such issues, it quickly became apparent that many of the key categories and classifications that have been used to describe sexual life in Western biomedicine (and, more recently, in public health epidemiology) are in fact far from universal or given in all cultural settings. On the contrary, categories as diverse as 'homosexuality', 'prostitution' and even 'masculinity' and 'femininity' may be very differently structured in diverse social and cultural settings – while any number of other significant categories may well be present that fail to conform or fit neatly into the classificatory systems of Western science. By focusing more carefully on local categories and classifications, social researchers have thus sought to move from what, in anthropology or linguistics, might be described as an 'outsider' perspective to what is described as an 'insider' perspective – from the 'experience-distant' concepts of science to the 'experience-near' concepts that the members of specific cultures use to understand and interpret their own reality (Geertz 1983; Parker 1991).

Nowhere has the importance of understanding the specific, or 'experience-near', concepts organizing sexual life been more clearly evident than in examining the complex relationship between sexual behaviour and sexual identity. Early in the HIV/AIDS epidemic, for example, it became apparent that epidemiological categories related to homosexuality and heterosexuality were at best a poor gloss on the complexity and diversity of lived sexual experience, and that neither homosexual nor heterosexual behaviour was necessarily associated with a distinct sense of self or sexual identity – that even 'heterosexuality' as a category would need to be problematized in many social and cultural settings (Parker 1987; Carrier 1989; Daniel and Parker 1993). As a result of this understanding, significant research attention has focused on the different ways in which sexual interactions are structured and on the diverse sexual identities that are organized around such interactions. In many settings, for example, notions of activity and passivity in sexual interactions, translated into gendered symbols of masculinity and femininity, proved to be more important in defining sexual identity than one's sexual object choice or the sex/gender of one's partner (Parker 1987; Carrier 1989; Tan 1995; Kahn 1996). Indeed, while biomedical models of sexual experience have often posited a necessary relationship between sexual desire, sexual behaviour and sexual identity, research in diverse cultural contexts quickly called this relationship into question, demonstrating an extensive range of possible variations that seem to be present across different social and cultural settings (Lancaster 1988; Jackson 1989; Kennedy and Davis 1993; Carrier 1995; Jackson 1997, 2000; Kulick 1998; Prieur 1998; Blackwood and Wieringa 1999; Parker 1999; Chao 2000).

While much of the cross-cultural research carried out on sexual identity has focused on relations between men who have sex with other men and, increasingly, women who have sex with women (see, for example, Blackwood and Wieringa 1999), the same kind of critical reflection has also been applied to a number of other epidemiological categories, particularly in relation to perceived HIV/AIDS 'risk groups'. Studies of sex work, for example, have documented the fact that relations of sexual and economic exchange are far more complex and varied than originally assumed (Truong 1990; de Zalduondo 1991; Kempadoo and Doezema 1998; Aggleton 1999; Kempadoo 1999). In many contexts, the exchange of sexual services for money, gifts or favours is a common part of sexual interaction that implies no special sexual (or, for that matter, social) identity, while in others such exchanges may be specifically organized around a distinct sense of shared identity on the part of sex workers (Aggleton 1999; Fábregas-Martínez and Benedetti 2000; Hunter 2002). The social sanctions and stigma associated with female or male prostitution in some settings do not necessarily exist in others, and the relationship between behaviour and identity is as problematic, and as situationally variable, in relation to sex work as it is in relation to same-sex interactions (Daniel and Parker 1993; Kempadoo and Doezema 1998; Kulick 1998; Prieur 1998; Brennan 2004). Indeed, in much recent work on sexual cultures and the social construction of sexual interactions, even notions of gender, and of gender identity, have increasingly been called into question. What it is to be male or female, masculine or feminine, in different social and cultural contexts may vary greatly, and gender identity is clearly not reducible to any underlying biological dichotomy. All biological males and females must undergo a process of sexual socialization in which culturally specific notions of masculinity and femininity are shaped across the life course. It is through this process of sexual socialization that individuals learn the sexual desires, feelings, roles and practices typical of their cohorts or statuses within society – as well as the sexual alternatives that their culture opens up to them (Parker *et al.* 2000).

Perhaps as a result, research in diverse settings has increasingly focused on the processes of sexual socialization and on the sexual experience of young people, not only in and of itself, but also as an especially important window to the dynamics of sexual life – to the ways in which intersubjective sexual meanings are internalized and reproduced in social and sexual interaction (Irvine 1994; Holland *et al.* 1998; Cáceres 1999; Paiva 2000; Amuchástegui 2001; Tolman 2002; Aggleton *et al.* 2006). Key public health concerns with issues, such as HIV-related risk behaviours on the part of young people and of unwanted pregnancy during adolescence, have increasingly been translated in sophisticated, multisite and multiple-methodology studies of the sexual, reproductive and life histories of youth from diverse social classes and ethnic groups (Heilborn *et al.* 2006).

One of the most important new areas of research to emerge in the mid-1990s was the study of masculinity (Connell 1995; Kimmel 1996; Viveros 2001). While the HIV epidemic, together with attention to women's reproductive health, had previously focused attention on sexual minorities and on heterosexual women, work on masculinity more generally (and on heterosexual men in particular) had, for the most part, received little attention. A new focus on gender and sexual identities, and on questions of gender relations and gender equity, brought new attention to the social construction of masculinity – and to the diversity of men's sexual cultures in different settings, with especially important emphasis being given to the need to understand the influence of both social class and racial and ethnic identity as they intersect with and impact upon masculine identities and subjectivities (Cornwall and Lindisfarne 1994; Gutmann 1996; Valdés and Olavarria 1998; Castro 2001; Morrell 2001; Louie 2002; Viveros 2002). Stereotypical conceptions of masculinity were called into question, and the role of men in reproductive processes and decision-making became an important area of investigation. This in turn made possible an important re-conceptualization of the complexity of conjugal relationships, as well as a growing understanding of the multiple forms of social differentiation that structure the diversity of masculinities in different social contexts (Connell 2001; Whitehead and Barrett 2001; Hirsch 2003; Gear 2005; Hunter 2005; Ouzgane and Morrell 2005).

This focus on the social construction of sexual identities has also been associated with an increasing emphasis on the organization of distinct sexual communities (Weeks and Holland 1996). Indeed, just as recent research initiatives have demonstrated that there is no necessary or intrinsic relationship between sexual behaviours and sexual identities, many studies have also demonstrated the complex (and sometimes contradictory) links between sexual identity and the formation of sexual communities (Herdt 1992; Plummer 1992; Kennedy and Davis 1993; Dowsett 1996; Levine *et al.* 1997; Weeks 2000). The different ways in which sexual communities take shape and evolve have thus become especially important questions for research aimed at understanding the broader social and cultural context of sexual conduct (Murray 1992a; Rubin 1997; Parker 1999; Peacock *et al.* 2001).

As in the case of work on sexual identities, research on the sexual subcultures and communities associated with men who have sex with men has been especially important. Early studies of behaviour changes in response to HIV/AIDS within the gay communities of a number of developed countries have pointed to the importance of community development and support structures as correlates for the reduction of sexual risk behaviour (Kippax *et al.* 1993; Dowsett 1996). Research carried out in a range of other social and cultural contexts, and particularly in a number of developing societies where the emergence of a gay community has been more limited, on the contrary, has pointed to the lack of such structures as equally important in seeking to understand limited behavioural change (Daniel and Parker 1993), as well as to the importance of emerging community structures as part of a broader process of social and sexual change (Parker 1999; Tan 2001; Boellstorff 2005).

This awareness of fundamental differences in the organization of sexual communities, in turn, has led to greater research attention for the diverse sexual subcultures that exist in many societies. Particularly in relation to men who have sex with men, the different social and sexual networks and value systems associated with same-sex interactions between lower or working class men as opposed to men from the middle and upper classes, the specific contexts associated with transgender experience, with male prostitution and a range of other variations, have all become a focus for study and have demonstrated the complex ways in which sexual practices are organized within social systems (Kulick 1998; Prieur 1998; Parker 1999; Jackson 2000; Peacock *et al.* 2001; Carrillo 2002; Manalansan 2003; Luibheid and Cantu 2005; Melendez and Pinto 2007).

Many of the same approaches and insights gained through the study of diverse sexual communities associated with men who have sex with men have also been applied as well to other groups such as sex workers, youth cultures and the sexual subcultures of different class and ethnic groups. Attention has focused on the complex ways that such diverse communities structure the possibilities of sexual interaction between individual social actors, defining a range of potential sexual partners and practices. Who one is permitted to have sex with, in what ways, under what circumstances and with what specific outcomes are never simply random questions. Such possibilities are defined through the implicit and explicit rules and regulations imposed by the sexual cultures of specific communities. Research has thus turned increasingly to the study of social and sexual networks in an attempt to investigate the systems of meaning and the social structural principles that organize the possibilities of sexual interaction in different communities (Laumann and Gagnon 1995; Laumann *et al.* 2004).

Structure and agency: toward a political economy of the body

While the work carried out over the course of the past 10 to 15 years on sexual cultures, identities and communities has opened new insights into the study of sexuality – and has offered an important alternative to mainstream epidemiological and public health approaches to questions such as HIV and AIDS, women's and men's reproductive and sexual health and related concerns – from roughly the mid-1990s to the present, growing concern has also focused on the ways in which sexual cultures are integrated within and cross-cut by complex systems of power and domination. This increasing engagement with issues of power, and with the relationship between culture and power, in recent years has increasingly forced research on sexuality to address a range of broader structural issues that, in interaction with culturally constituted systems of meaning, also play a key role in organizing the sexual field and defining the possibilities that may be open to sexual subjects. This, in turn, has led to a new emphasis on seeking to move beyond a number of the theoretical limitations of exclusively cultural approaches to sexuality studies, in particular by framing social constructionism with political economy – with a fuller awareness of the fact that transformations in socially constituted sexual and gender relations always reflect broader political, economic and cultural changes (see Lancaster and di Leonardo 1997; Parker *et al.* 2000; Parker and Aggleton 2007).

Much recent research has thus sought to reach beyond post-modernism, although still embracing post-modernist problematizations of traditionally defined categories of sex, gender, race and class – but has also abandoned earlier mechanistic models of political economy, in which an economic base is deterministic of a cultural super-structure, in favour of a more complex, interactive model. The result has been an attempt to build a more grounded and politically relevant social constructionist theory – or what some have described as a new 'political economy of the body' and its sexual pleasures (Lancaster 1995; Lancaster and di Leonardo 1997; Parker 1999, 2001). Research attention has thus come increasingly to focus on the historical and political-economic analysis of structural factors such as gender power differentials and sexual discrimination and oppression – and, importantly, on the synergistic effects of these factors with other forms of social inequality such as poverty and economic exploitation, racism and ethnic discrimination and social exclusion more generally.

Within this framework, research has increasingly focused on what have been described as the forms of 'structural violence' that determine the social vulnerability of both groups and individuals (Farmer *et al.* 1996; Parker 2001; Farmer 2004). Researchers have sought to more fully understand the ways in which these forms of structural violence are situated in historically constituted political and economic systems – systems in which diverse political and economic processes and policies related to issues such as economic development, housing, labour, migration or immigration, health, education and welfare impact upon communities and cultures, shaping health and well-being, as well as the possibilities for agency, self-determination and sexual freedom.

In seeking to respond to this growing perception of the importance of structural factors and structural violence in shaping sexual experience, attention has increasingly focused on the ways in which societies and communities inform sexual interaction between social actors. Such possibilities are defined through the implicit and explicit rules and regulations imposed by the sexual cultures of specific communities as well as the economic and political power relations which underpin these sexual cultures – and they can never be fully understood without examining the importance of issues such as 'class', 'race' or 'ethnicity' and the other multiple forms through which different societies organize systems of social inequality and structure the possibilities for social interaction along or across lines of social difference.

This awareness of the ways in which social orders structure the possibilities (and obligations) of sexual contact has drawn special attention to socially and culturally determined differentials in power (Parker 2001). Just as detailed cross-cultural and comparative investigation of the social construction of same-sex interactions provided perhaps the key test case for demonstrating the importance of cultural analysis in relation to sexuality and HIV/ AIDS, work casting the body as both a symbolic and a material product of social relations – a construct that is necessarily conditioned by a whole range of structural forces – has provided an especially important way of reframing recent research on sexuality, sexual cultures and sexual communities. In some of the most dynamic work currently being carried out, these concerns have led researchers to focus new attention on the diverse social movements related to sexuality, sexual health and sexual rights – including the feminist and the lesbian and gay movements, but also movements for sex worker rights, for transgender identity and autonomy, the sexual rights of young people and a range of related issues (see, for example, Adam *et al.* 1998; Petchesky and Judd 1998; Martinot and James 2001; Petchesky 2003; Terto Jr *et al.* 2004).

Sexuality and silence

Over the course of the past three decades, then, we have seen a set of major developments in social research on sexuality and sexual cultures. There has been a far-reaching critique of essentialist assumptions concerning the nature of sexual life and the articulation of an increasingly sophisticated alternative framework that focuses on the social and cultural dimensions of sexual experience, within a perspective that is sensitive to historical processes and political and economic forces. This is no small accomplishment, and any review of the development of this field of research in recent decades cannot help but highlight the significant advances that have taken place in our understanding of the social and cultural dimensions of sexuality.

Before ending, however, it is also worth reflecting briefly on what issues may have been left outside our view in the light of the kinds of issues that have been prioritized thus far. In other words, what questions have we failed to ask? What answers have we perhaps failed to reach because of the kinds of questions that we have asked? What are the kinds of issues that we might want to focus on in the future with the goal of moving this field forward? While my answers to these queries will be tentative at best, there are a number of points that I would like to offer in the hope of opening up possible lines for discussion and debate in the future.

In particular, it seems to me that the strong emphasis that we have placed on issues of culture – and, as a surrogate for culture, language and discourse – may unintentionally have diverted our attention away from the importance of certain kinds of 'silence'. Indeed, it may unintentionally have produced some kinds of silence that would not have been the case had we adopted other theoretical perspectives and methodological approaches. In particular, I am struck by the fact that in much recent sexuality research, sex itself seems to be increasingly absent – the actual sexual practices that at some level are the point of departure for the development of sexuality research as a field somehow seem to have disappeared (perhaps in a kind of inverse relationship to the development of theoretical frames and methodological tools).

There are times when it might be asked whether the growing legitimacy of sexuality research as a field – with its own institutional centres, the attention of funding agencies and the like – might not have taken place at the expense of a certain kind of 'sanitization' of our subject matter. Sexuality research may have become legitimate, but the price of increased legitimacy may have been the loss of a certain kind of transgressive power that characterized some of the most important early work in this field – and with that, perhaps, some of its potential as a source of resistance, as a source of meaningful social, political and cultural critique in relation to what really underlies the power of hegemonic mainstream sexual moralities.

In thinking about this issue, I have found myself remembering a chance conversation now more than 25 years ago with the British anthropologist (one of the first researchers to carry out work on the social construction of sexuality in Brazil), Peter Fry, about the languages of sexuality, when he made the offhand comment that in his experience most of what actually happens in sexual exchanges happens in silence. I also found myself thinking back to reading a remarkable master's thesis written in the late 1980s by the Brazilian social psychologist and ethnographer, Veriano Terto, *No escurinho do cinema* (In the darkness of the cinema), in which he described the orgiastic interactions of men on weekday afternoons in the pornographic movie theatres of Rio de Janeiro – an elaborate dance not only of meanings and identities, but also of bodies and pleasures, that took place (as, in at least some settings, it continues to take place today) in total silence, with a very different set of signifiers than what we have come to focus on in much of our most sophisticated contemporary sexuality research (Terto Jr 1989).

In short, borrowing from Paul Boyce, Peter Aggleton and their co-authors in an article on HIV research (Boyce *et al.* 2006), perhaps the time has come to put the sex back in sex research and to pay renewed attention to the complex choreography of bodies, caresses and sensations that our own work may ironically have left aside in our rush to legitimacy and professional recognition.

Pushing this question further, as important as our attention to culture, and to voice, may have been in the development of recent sexuality research, this focus may well have drawn our attention away from at least some issues that ought rightfully to be at the centre of our concerns – away from sex itself, as well as from what can be described as some of the kinds of 'discursive silence' (Lützen 1995) that might well be crucial in thinking about social and cultural change, and about the grassroots politics of social and sexual transformation. The fact that something may have yet to be articulated does not mean that it is not taking place – sometimes right before our eyes.

It is important to link this recognition back to some of the key questions of political economy discussed previously. Power, in this field as in others, has not only the capacity to throw some issues into sharp relief (inequalities, for example) or to trigger change (through resistance, for example), but it also has the potential to silence and, by silencing, to 'invisibilize' as well. This is particularly important when it comes to understanding new forms of sexuality, emerging modes of sexual expression and ways of sexual-relating (e.g. the power of new technologies such as the Internet, or the invisibilization of clear-cut sexual identities and categories that occur in night spaces, or in the darkness of the cinema, and so on). Indeed, invisibility may well be the other side of silence, and we would be well advised not to ignore their interactions and intersections.

Silence and invisibility can of course take many forms. At the same time that we celebrate the continued development of the field of sexuality research – our dis/organized pleasures, the growing richness of our understanding of sexual cultures and our ongoing struggle for sexual rights – it is worth remembering that these very real accomplishments still exist side-by-side with ongoing forms of oppression and exclusion that continue to be characterized more by their silences and their invisibility than by the freedoms that we ultimately hope our work will contribute to.

What might a notion of dis/organized pleasure mean, for example, for impoverished women struggling to escape domestic violence in their daily lives? What constitutes a notion of sexual rights for female or transgender sex workers in the most marginalized and excluded settings? Or for the poor youth of the peri-urban communities that ring modern metropolitan urban centres in countries and cultures around the world? How can we begin to address these forms of exclusion through our research, in ways that will be meaningful for those in the front lines of such on-the-ground struggles? These are just some of the questions that we will only be able to begin to answer if we are willing to listen to the silences, and to open our eyes to the invisibilities, that are still so much a part of sexual life for so many people around the world.

References

Adam, B., Duyvendak, J. and Krouwel, A. (eds) 1998. *The Global Emergence of Gay and Lesbian Politics: National Imprints of a Worldwide Movement*. Philadelphia: Temple University Press.

Aggleton, P. (ed.) 1999. *Men Who Sell Sex: International Perspectives on Male Prostitution and HIV/ AIDS.* Philadelphia: Temple University Press.

Aggleton, P., Ball, A. and Mane, P. (eds) 2006. *Sex, Drugs and Young People: International Perspectives.* London and New York: Routledge.

Amuchástegui, A. 2001. *Virgindad e Iniciación Sexual en México: Experiencias y Significados.* México, DF: EDAMEX S.A.

Blackwood, E. (ed.) 1986. *Anthropology and Homosexual Behavior.* New York: Haworth.

Blackwood, E. and Wieringa, S. (eds) 1999. *Female Desires: Same-Sex Relations and Transgender Practices Across Cultures.* New York: Columbia University Press.

Boellstorff, T. 2005. *The Gay Archipelago: Sexuality and Nation in Indonesia.* Princeton: Princeton University Press.

Boyce, P., Huang Soo Lee, M., Jenkins, C., Mohamed, S., Overs, C., Paiva, V. *et al.* 2006. Putting sexuality (back) into HIV/AIDS: Issues, theory and practice. *Global Public Health* 2: 1–34.

Brennan, D. 2004. *What's Love Got to Do with it? Transnational Desires and Sex Tourism in the Dominican Republic.* Durham: Duke University Press.

Cáceres, C. 1999. *Nuevos Retos: Investigaciones Recientes sobre Salud Sexual y Reproductive de los Jovenes en el Peru.* Lima: REDESS Jovenes.

Caplan, P. (ed.) 1987. *The Cultural Construction of Homosexuality.* London: Tavistock Publications.

Carrier, J. 1976. Family attitudes and Mexican male homosexuality. *Urban Life* 5: 359–375.

Carrier, J. 1989. Sexual behavior and the spread of AIDS in Mexico. *Medical Anthropology* 10: 129–142.

Carrier, J. 1995. *De Los Outros: Intimacy and Homosexuality among Mexican Men.* New York: Columbia University Press.

Carrillo, H. 2002. *The Night is Young: Sexuality in Mexico in the Time of AIDS.* Chicago, IL: University of Chicago Press.

Castro, R. 2001. 'When a man is with a woman, it feels like electricity': Subjectivity, sexuality and contraception among men in Central Mexico. *Culture, Health & Sexuality* 3: 149–165.

Chao, A. 2000. Global metaphors and local strategies in the construction of Taiwan's lesbian identities. *Culture, Health & Sexuality* 2: 377–390.

Connell, R.W. 1995. *Masculinities.* Berkeley and Los Angeles: University of California Press.

Connell, R.W. 2001. *The Men and the Boys.* Berkeley, Los Angeles and London: University of California.

Cornwall, A. and Lindisfarne, N. (eds) 1994. *Dislocating Masculinity: Comparative Ethnographies.* London and New York: Routledge.

Daniel, H. and Parker, R. 1993. *Sexuality, Politics and AIDS in Brazil.* London: The Falmer Press.

Denizart, H. 1997. *Engenharia Erótica: Travestis no Rio de Janeiro / Erotic Engineering: Transvestites in Rio de Janeiro.* Bilingual edition. Rio de Janeiro: Jorge Zahar Editor.

de Zalduondo, B. 1991. Prostitution viewed cross-culturally: Toward re-contextualizing sex work in AIDS research. *The Journal of Sex Research* 22: 223–248.

Dowsett, G. 1996. *Practicing Desire: Homosexual Sex in the Era of AIDS.* Stanford: Stanford University Press.

Fábregas-Martínez, A.I. and Benedetti, M.R. (eds) 2000. *Na Batalha: Identidade, Sexualidade e Poder no Universo da Prostituição.* Porto Alegre: Dacasa/Palmarica.

Farmer, P. 2004. An anthropology of structural violence. *Current Anthropology* 45: 304–324.

Farmer, P., Connors, M. and Simmons, J. (eds) 1996. *Women, Poverty and AIDS: Sex, Drugs and Structural Violence.* Monroe, ME: Common Courage Press.

Foucault, M. 1978. *The History of Sexuality, Volume 1: An Introduction.* New York: Random House.

Fry, P. 1982. *Para Inglês Ver: Identidade e Política na Cultura Brasileira.* Rio de Janeiro: Zahar Editores.

Gagnon, J. and Simon, W. 1973. *Sexual Conduct: The Social Sources of Human Sexuality.* Chicago, IL: Aldine.

Gagnon, J. and Parker, R. 1995. Conceiving sexuality. In: R. Parker and J. Gagnon (eds) *Conceiving Sexuality: Approaches to Sex Research in a Postmodern World.* New York and London: Routledge, 3–16.

Gaspar, M. 1985. *Garotas de Programa: Prostituição em Copacabana e Identidade Cultural*. Rio de Janeiro: Zahar.

Gayatri, B. 1995. Indonesian lesbians writing their own script: Issues of feminism and sexuality. In: M. Reinfelder (ed.) *From Amazon to Zami: Towards a Global Lesbian Feminism*. London: Cassell, 86–98.

Gear, S. 2005. Rules of engagement: Structuring sex and damage in men's prisons and beyond. *Culture, Health & Sexuality* 7: 195–208.

Geertz, C. 1983. *Local Knowledge*. New York: Basic Books.

Gevisser, M. and Cameron, E. (eds) 1995. *Defiant Desire: Gay and Lesbian Lives in South Africa*. London and New York: Routledge.

Gutmann, M. 1996. *The Meanings of Macho: Being a Man in Mexico City*. Berkeley and Los Angeles, CA: University of California Press.

Heilborn, M.L., Aquino, E., Bozon, M. and Knauth, D.R. (eds) 2006. *O Aprendizado da Sexualidade: Reprodução e Trajetórias Sociais de Jovens Brasileiros*. Rio de Janeiro: Editora Fiocruz and Editora Garamond.

Herdt, G. 1981. *Guardians of the Flutes: Idioms of Masculinity*. New York: McGraw-Hill.

Herdt, G. (ed.) 1992. *Gay Culture in America: Essays from the Field*. Boston, MA: Beacon Press.

Hirsch, J. 2003. *A Courtship After Marriage: Sexuality and Love in Mexican Transnational Families*. Berkeley and Los Angeles, CA, and London: University of California Press.

Holland, J., Ramazanoglu, C., Sharp, S. and Thompson, R. 1998. *The Male in the Head*. London: Tufnell Press.

Hunter, M. 2002. The materiality of everyday sex: Thinking beyond 'prostitution'. *African Studies* 61: 99–120.

Hunter, M. 2005. Cultural politics and masculinities: Multiple-partners in historical perspective in KwaZulu-Natal. *Culture, Health & Sexuality* 7: 209–223.

Irvine, J. (ed.) 1994. *Sexual Cultures and the Construction of Adolescent Identities*. Philadelphia: Temple University Press.

Jackson, P. 1989. *Dear Uncle Go: Male Homosexuality in Thailand*. Bangkok: Bua Luang Publishing Company.

Jackson, P. 1997. Kathoey Gay Man: The historical emergence of gay male identity in Thailand. In: L. Manderson and M. Jolly (eds) *Sites of Desire/Economies of Pleasure: Sexualities in Asia and the Pacific*. Chicago, IL: University of Chicago Press, 166–190.

Jackson, P. 2000. An explosion of Thai identities: Global queering and re-imagining queer theory. *Culture, Health & Sexuality* 2: 405–424.

Kahn, S. 1996. Under the blanket: Bisexualities and AIDS in India. In: P. Aggleton (ed.) *Bisexualities and AIDS: International Perspectives*. London: Taylor & Francis, 161–177.

Kempadoo, K. (ed.) 1999. *Sun, Sex and Gold: Tourism and Sex Work in the Caribbean*. Lanham, MD: Rowman and Littlefield.

Kempadoo, K. and Doezema, J. 1998. *Global Sex Workers: Rights, Resistance, and Redefinition*. New York and London: Routledge.

Kennedy, E.L. and Davis, M. 1993. *Boots of Leather, Slippers of Gold: The History of a Lesbian Community*. New York: Penguin.

Kimmel, M. 1996. *Manhood in America: A Cultural History*. New York: Free Press.

Kippax, S., Connell, R.W., Dowsett, G. and Crawford, J. 1993. *Sustaining Safe Sex: Gay Communities Respond to AIDS*. London: Falmer Press.

Kulick, D. 1998. *Travestí: Sex, Gender and Culture among Brazilian Transgendered Prostitutes*. Chicago, IL: University of Chicago Press.

Lancaster, R. 1988. Subject honor and object shame: The construction of male homosexuality and stigma in Nicaragua. *Ethnology* 27: 111–125.

Lancaster, R. 1992. *Life is Hard: Machismo, Danger, and Intimacy of Power in Nicaragua*. Berkeley and Los Angeles, CA: University of California Press.

Lancaster, R. 1995. 'That we should all turn queer?' Homosexual stigma in the making of manhood and the breaking of a revolution in Nicaragua. In: R. Parker and J. Gagnon (eds) *Conceiving Sexuality: Approaches to Sex Research in a Postmodern World.* New York and London: Routledge, 135–156.

Lancaster, R. and di Leonardo, M. (eds) 1997. *The Gender/Sexuality Reader: Culture, History, Political Economy.* New York and London: Routledge.

Laumann, E. and Gagnon, J. 1995. A sociological perspective on sexual action. In: R. Parker and J. Gagnon (eds) *Conceiving Sexuality: Approaches to Sex Research in a Postmodern World.* New York and London: Routledge, 183–213.

Laumann, E., Ellingson, S., Mahay, J., Paik, A. and Youm, Y. (eds) 2004. *The Sexual Organization of the City.* Chicago, IL: The University of Chicago Press.

Levine, M., Nardi, P. and Gagnon, J. (eds) 1997. *In Changing Times: Gay Men and Lesbians Encounter HIV/AIDS.* Chicago, IL: The University of Chicago Press.

Louie, K. 2002. *Theorising Chinese Masculinity: Society and Gender in China.* Cambridge: Cambridge University Press.

Luibheid, E. and Cantu, L. 2005. *Queer Migrations: Sexuality, US Citizenship, and Border Crossings.* Minneapolis: University of Minnesota Press.

Lützen, K. 1995. *La mise en discours* and silences in research on the history of sexuality. In: R. Parker and J. Gagnon (eds) *Conceiving Sexuality: Approaches to Sex Research in a Postmodern World.* New York and London: Routledge, 19–32.

Manalansan, M. 2003. *Global Divas: Filipino Gay Men in the Diaspora.* Durham: Duke University Press.

Manderson, L. and Jolly, M. (eds) 1997. *Sites of Desire/Economies of Pleasure: Sexualities in Asia and the Pacific.* Chicago, IL: The University of Chicago Press.

Martinot, S. and James, J. (eds) 2001. *The Problems of Resistance: Studies in Alternate Political Cultures.* Amherst, NY: Prometheus Books.

Melendez, R. and Pinto, R. 2007. 'It's really a hard life': Love, gender and HIV risk among male-to-female transgender persons. *Culture, Health & Sexuality* 9: 233–245.

Morrell, R. 2001. *Changing Men in Southern Africa.* London: Zed Books.

Murray, S. 1992a. *Oceanic Homosexualities.* New York: Garland.

Murray, S. 1992b. Components of gay community in San Francisco. In: G. Herdt (ed.) *Gay Culture in America: Essays from the Field.* Boston, MA: Beacon Press, 107–146.

Nanda, S. 1990. *Neither Man Nor Woman: The Hijras of India.* Belmont, CA: Wadsworth Publishing.

Ortner, S. and Whitehead, H. (eds) 1981. *Sexual Meanings: The Cultural Construction of Gender and Sexuality.* Cambridge: Cambridge University Press.

Ouzgane, L. and Morrell, R. (eds) 2005. *African Masculinities: Men in Africa from the Late 19th Century to the Present.* New York: Palgrave Macmillan.

Paiva, V. 2000. *Fazendo Arte com a Camisinha: Sexualidades Jovens em Tempos de Aids.* São Paulo: Summus Editorial.

Parker, R. 1987. Acquired immunodeficiency syndrome in urban Brazil. *Medical Anthropology Quarterly,* new series 1: 155–175.

Parker, R. 1991. *Bodies, Pleasures and Passions: Sexual Culture in Contemporary Brazil.* Boston, MA: Beacon Press.

Parker, R. 1999. *Beneath the Equator: Cultures of Desire, Male Homosexuality, and Emerging Gay Communities in Brazil.* New York and London: Routledge.

Parker, R. 2001. Sexuality, culture and power in HIV/AIDS research. *Annual Review of Anthropology* 30: 163–179.

Parker, R. and Gagnon, J. (eds) 1995. *Conceiving Sexuality: Approaches to Sex Research in a Postmodern World.* New York and London: Routledge.

Parker, R. and Aggleton, P. (eds) 2007. *Culture, Society and Sexuality: A Reader.* 2nd edition. London and New York: Routledge.

Parker, R., Barbosa, R.M. and Aggleton, P. (eds) 2000. *Framing the Sexual Subject: The Politics of Gender, Sexuality, and Power.* Berkeley, Los Angeles and London: University of California Press.

Peacock, B., Eyre, S., Quinn, S.C. and Kegeles, S. 2001. Delineating differences: Sub-communities in the San Francisco gay community. *Culture, Health & Sexuality* 3: 183–201.

Perlongher, N. 1987. *O Negócio do Michê: A Prostituição Viril*. São Paulo: Editora Brasiliense.

Petchesky, R. 2003. *Global Prescriptions: Gendering Health and Human Rights*. London: Zed Books.

Petchesky, R. and Judd, K. (eds) 1998. *Negotiating Reproductive Rights: Women's Perspectives Across Countries and Cultures*. London: Zed Books.

Plummer, K. 1984. Sexual diversity: A sociological perspective. In: K. Howells (ed.) *Sexual Diversity*. Oxford: Basil Blackwell, 219–253.

Plummer, K. (ed.) 1992. *Modern Homosexualities*. London and New York: Routledge.

Prieur, A. 1998. *Mema's House, Mexico City: On Transvestites, Queens, and Machos*. Chicago, IL: The University of Chicago Press.

Robinson, P. 1976. *The Modernization of Sex: Havelock Ellis, Alfred Kinsey, William Masters and Virginia Johnson*. Ithaca, NY: Cornell University Press.

Rubin, G. 1984. 'Thinking sex': Notes for a radical theory of the politics of sexuality. In: C. Vance (ed.) *Pleasure and Danger: Exploring Female Sexuality*. London: Routledge and Kegan Paul, 267–319.

Rubin, G. 1997. Elegy for the Valley of Kings: AIDS and the leather community in San Francisco, 1981–1996. In: M. Levine, P. Nardi and J. Gagnon (eds) *In Changing Times: Gay Men and Lesbians Encounter HIV/AIDS*. Chicago, IL: The University of Chicago Press, 101–144.

Simon, W. and Gagnon, J. 1984. Sexual scripts. *Society* 22: 53–60.

Szasz, I. and Lerner, S. (eds) 1996. *Para Compreender la Subjetividad*. México, DF: El Colégio de México.

Tan, M. 1995. From bakla to gay: Shifting gender identities and sexual behaviors in the Philippines. In: R. Parker and J. Gagnon (eds) *Conceiving Sexuality: Approaches to Sex Research in a Postmodern World*. New York and London: Routledge, 85–96.

Tan, M. 1996. Silahis: Looking for the missing Filipino bisexual male. In: P. Aggleton (ed.) *Bisexualities and AIDS: International Perspectives*. London: Taylor & Francis, 207–225.

Tan, M. 2001. Survival through pluralism: Emerging gay communities in the Philippines. *Journal of Homosexuality* 40: 117–142.

Terto Jr, V. 1989. *No escurinho do cinema: sociabilidade orgiástica nas tardes cariocas*. Master's Dissertation in Psychology. Rio de Janeiro: PUC.

Terto Jr, V., Victora, C.G. and Knauth, D.R. (eds) 2004. *Direitos sexuais e repredutivos como direitos humanos, Corpus* (Special Issue) (1).

Thandani, G. 1996. *Sakhiyani: Lesbian Desire in Ancient and Modern India*. London: Cassell.

Tolman, D. 2002. *Dilemmas of Desire: Teenage Girls Talk about Sexuality*. Cambridge, MA: Harvard University Press.

Truong, T.D. 1990. *Sex, Money and Morality: Prostitution and Tourism in South East Asia*. London: Zed Books.

Valdés, T. and Olavarria, J. (eds) 1998. *Masculinidades y Equidad de Género en América Latina*. Santiago, Chile: FLACSO-Chile.

Vance, C. (ed.) 1984. *Pleasure and Danger: Exploring Female Sexuality*. Boston, MA: Routledge and Kegan Paul.

Viveros, M. 2001. Contemporary Latin American perspectives on masculinity. *Men and Masculinities* 3: 237–260.

Viveros, M. 2002. Dionysian Blacks: Sexuality, body, and racial order in Colombia. *Latin American Perspectives* 29: 60–77.

Weeks, J. 1985. *Sexuality and its Discontents*. London: Routledge and Kegan Paul.

Weeks, J. 1991. *Against Nature: Essays on History, Sexuality and Identity*. London: Rivers Oram Press.

Weeks, J. 2000. *Making Sexual History*. Cambridge: Polity Press.

Weeks, J. and Holland, J. (eds) 1996. *Sexual Cultures: Communities, Values and Intimacy*. New York: St. Martins Press.

Whitehead, S. and Barrett, F. (eds) 2001. *The Masculinities Reader*. Oxford: Polity Press.

Chapter 3

Women's work, worry and fear

The portrayal of sexuality and sexual health in US magazines for teenage and middle-aged women, 2000–2007

Juanne Clarke

Introduction

The purpose of this chapter is to report on a comparative investigation of the social construction of sexuality, sexual health and disease in the highest circulating print mass media magazines directed towards two groups of women in the USA. The first group of magazines, designed for teenage women, includes *Seventeen*, *CosmoGirl!* and *Teen Vogue*. The second group of magazines, directed to women aged between 40 and 50 years, includes *Good Housekeeping*, *Redbook* and *O, The Oprah Magazine*.

The study of sexuality is particularly important today because of the major changes that have occurred in the past half-century or so with respect to the widespread availability and utilization of birth control techniques such as the contraceptive pill and the consequent separation of sexual intercourse from procreation, marriage and family. At the same time as this sex-promoting social and pharmaceutical shift has occurred, so too have increasingly dire threats to life and health posed by various sexually transmitted infections (STIs), including HIV/AIDS, become apparent. As background to these shifts, there have been significant changes in the worlds of women and men in the labour market, in relationships and in marriage (Baker 2005), along with a continuation of gender inequalities. The political and economic alterations evident in the rise of neo-liberalism along with conservative social policies, particularly in the USA, must also be seen as background to this investigation of sexuality (Casper and Carpenter 2008).

One of the possible avenues for our understanding of sexuality and its changing meanings is its portrayal in the mass media. The media are indispensable to life in modern mass societies. Television, newspapers, radio, films and magazines are taken-for-granted aspects of daily living. Lives are lived, relationships forged, disagreements stated, views constructed and deconstructed, policies explained and justified and worries and solutions identified through media stories. Media both create and reflect social realities. Indeed, one theorist has argued that our lives in modern societies today are ultimately mediated (Altheide 2002).

There has been a tradition of studying the media portrayal of the sexualities of young, mostly teenaged women (see for instance Frith and Kitzinger 1997; Jackson and Cran 2003; Jackson 2005a, 2005b). These studies have focused on the presentation of sexuality in a variety of mass media, including, most significantly, magazines, television and movies (Tincknell *et al.* 2003; Batchelor *et al.* 2004; Tally 2006; Jensen and Jensen 2007), girls' comics and romantic fiction (Walkerdine 1990; Radway 1991; Jackson 1993; Gill and Herdieckerhoff 2006), video rental jackets (Oliver *et al.* 2003) and websites (Lambiase

2003). Research has demonstrated both varying and stable interpretations of sexuality over the past 30 or so years (Fine 1988; Allen 2003; Flood 2003; Ussher 2005).

Studies of the portrayal of sexuality in magazines devoted to a teenage audience have documented ongoing ambivalence toward sexuality and a variable adherence to two hegemonic discourses, heterosexuality and the double standard (Muehlenhard and Peterson 2005; Ussher 2005). Heterosexuality is generally represented as normative. Same-sex sexuality has tended to be invisible or staged for titillation such as the Madonna/Britney kiss at the MTV awards in 2003 (Ussher 2005: 27). Furthermore there is a relative silence about masturbation and self-pleasure (Carpenter 1998). What still counts as sex is penile-vaginal penetration (Medley-Rath 2007).

The double standard of sexuality is coupled with heterosexism. The double standard asserts the idea that sex is a natural right and a strong, even irresistible drive for men, and non-existent or repressed among teenage women who are nevertheless charged with the responsibility of satisfying the sexual needs of men, protecting themselves (Carpenter 1998; Jackson 2005a, 2005b; Medley-Rath 2007) and determining how far to go (Batchelor *et al.* 2004). Young women are sometimes described as the victims of male sexual desire (Jackson 2005a, 2005b). They are not expected to enjoy sex and, if they do, they can be labelled with disparaging epithets. Teenage women must avoid being thought of as easy (Kitzinger 1995; Ussher 1997) or risk sexual violence (Ussher 1997). Virginity is portrayed as a prize among women to be offered to a man, usually upon marriage or, at least, in the context of a committed relationship. For young men, in contrast, virginity is a problem to be overcome as soon as possible and preferably outside of a committed relationship (Carpenter 2002).

It is important to point out that over time the variety of sexual scripts present in magazines may have expanded. Investigating 244 stories in *Seventeen* magazine from 1974 to 1994, Carpenter (1998) found a growth in the inclusion of the possibility of female desire, and homosexuality, masturbation and even mention of recreational sex. Sometimes there are paradoxical messages within national magazines. Ussher (2005), for example, noted that young women are portrayed as sexually free and also warned against being too pushy. Moreover, in general, the studied magazines seem to show a small but increasing similarity over time between men and women regarding the meanings of virginity loss (Carpenter 2002). However, whenever a conflict was portrayed it was always resolved in favour of the hegemonic double standard and heterosexuality (Carpenter 1998).

Jackson (2005b), in a study of letters written asking for advice to a teenage magazine from Australasia, noted how responses to teenage questions about sexual desire, through discourses of romance, sexual safety and adolescence, often seemed to dampen desire through focusing on fears of pregnancy and disease and promoting a love relationship. In a second study using the same data, Jackson (2005a) found that young women were constructed as ever possible candidates for disease.

Little attention has been paid to cultural, racialized or class-based differences in magazine portrayal. This echoes McRobbie's (2000) findings regarding the UK magazine, *Jackie*, which was described as presenting 'a classless, raceless sameness, a kind of false unity which assumes a common experience of womanhood or girlhood' (69). In one weak exception to this generalization, Carpenter (2001) undertook a cross-national comparison of the highest circulating magazine for teenagers in Germany, *Bravo*, with the highest circulating American magazine of the same genre, *Seventeen*, and found some similarities as well as some striking differences. The most important difference was that the German magazine offered a consistently more positive portrayal of teenage sexuality.

There have been no scholarly studies of the representation of sexuality in magazines for middle-aged women. McRobbie (1996), studying the UK magazine *More*, designed for young women in their late teens and early twenties, documented a highly positive portrayal of all types of sexualities. This is similar to the positively pro-sex character of two US magazines designed for women in this same, slightly older than the teen years, age range: *Glamour* and *Cosmo* (Clarke 2008). Despite the lack of investigation into the media portrayal of sexuality among middle-aged women, some investigations of the actual experiences of sexuality have suggested that heterosexism and the double standard largely continue even in the context of the gender 'tug of war and ambivalence' about sexuality (Wouters 1998: 244) and as a reflection of capitalism and patriarchy (Winship 1987). Women appear as responsible for the emotional well-being of their marriages, including the sexual components (Rubin 1990; Duncombe and Marsden 1998), in the context of ongoing gender inequalities in power and access to resources. In the absence of any available literature on sexuality in magazines designed for middle-aged women, the purpose of this chapter is to present a comparative analysis of magazines designed for two different age groups: teenage women and women between 40 and 50 in the years 2000–2007.

Magazine stories were selected as data both to build on the research on teenagers previously discussed and because magazines form an important part of the lives of many women (Winship 1987) and apparently have done so since 1693 (White 1970). Moreover, magazines appear to be a fundamental source for and reflection of the ideal practice of the feminine. They are broadly circulated and may be passed from person to person. Magazines are accessible, often cheap, readily available and read all over the Western world. They may be viewed in private and read more than once. It is likely that most young women have seen at least one teenage magazine (Batchelor *et al.* 2004). The high circulation rates for the magazines for the older age group suggest that this is likely true of this demographic as well.

Although widely circulated, there is no evidence that magazines are read as instruction manuals. Instead, they, as all media, are approached in contradictory ways by their audiences and with a combination of cynicism, resistance and acceptance (Jackson 2005b). However, young women do say that such magazines are as important for them as parents are for information about sex (Medley-Rath 2007). Currie (1999) found that teenage girls reported that they valued magazines for providing them with role models. In Jackson's (2005b) study, young women reported that teenage magazines were an important source of information about doing 'girl' and doing 'sexuality'. Another investigation found a direct correlation between magazine exposure and attitudes to sexuality (Kim and Ward 2004).

Methods

Sample

This chapter reports on a qualitative content analysis of the highest circulating mainstream mass print magazines during the years 2000 to 2007, designed for two age groups of women in the USA. The magazines for teenage women include *Seventeen*, *CosmoGirl!* and *Teen Vogue*. The magazines for middle-aged women include *Good Housekeeping*, *Redbook* and *O, The Oprah Magazine*. All of the magazines indicate that they are directed towards a general adult audience. None of the magazines is specifically directed towards a specific subcultural or 'racial' group. Table 3.1 summarizes the available information about circulation rates and average age and income of audience.

Table 3.1 Circulation rates, median age and household income of magazine audiences

Magazine	Circulation	Median audience age (years)	Household income ($)
CosmoGirl!****	2,908,861	18.3	60,000–100,000
Seventeen***	2,013,357	16.2	70,260
Teen Vogue**	972,555	16.0	65,584
Good Housekeeping*	4,609,209	50.7	51,163
Redbook*	2,370,707	45.8	55,788
O, The Oprah Magazine*	2,336,426	43.2	62,990

Notes:
* Hearst magazines: https://www.hearst.com/magazines/hearst-integrated-media
** Conde nast media kit: http://condenastmediakit.com
*** http://seventeenmediakit.com/r5/cob_page.asp?category_code=circ
**** www.quantcast.com/cosmogirl.com

This study was based on all available full text articles (without graphics) found indexed under the key word 'sexuality' and the subtopics of sexual health, Chlamydia, gonorrhoea, herpes, human papillomavirus (HPV), AIDS, syphilis, pelvic inflammatory disease, bacterial vaginosis, hepatitis and pregnancy in *The Reader's Guide to Periodical Literature* (H. W. Wilson Company n.d.) and found in the specified magazines. In accepting this source and classification of key terms we must accept the decisions regarding what counts as relevant and acknowledge that the editors of the *Reader's Guide* will have been influenced by changing definitions regarding sex, for instance, in an immeasurable manner over time. However, relying on the definitional decisions of the *Reader's Guide* does offer some consistency and would allow for replication of this research and a comparison over time (Clarke 1991, 1992).

The years in question were selected in order to provide enough data over a long enough period of time to avoid the bias of the selection of one year only when a particular event occurred, such as the announcement of a new sexually transmitted disease such as HIV/AIDS, for example, or a new pharmaceutical treatment such as the vaccine for the human papillomavirus (HPV). They were also chosen to amass a large enough sample of articles on sexuality for meaningful content, but not for a trend, analysis. There were 51 articles in the magazines for teenagers and 24 articles in the magazines for the older age group available and included in this cross-sectional analysis.

Analysis

Initially all articles were read to ensure their topical applicability. Then all articles were read repeatedly and inductively (Berg 1989; Neuman 2000). The coding categories emerged as the data was read alongside sensitizing concepts such as heterosexism and the double standard (Bryman 2004). New themes were noted when observed. Numerous quotations were highlighted and some are used to illustrate the dominant ideas reflected in these magazines.

Results

Sexuality in teenage magazines

Sex, fear and pregnancy

In US teenage magazines, sexual relations are presented as fraught with fear, and a generalized fear is presented as a reasonable response to engaging in sex: 'The bottom line is, any physical intimacy (not just sex) has serious health and emotional risks. So keep that in mind the next time you hook up with someone' (Geary 2005, Your body questions answered, *Seventeen*). One specific concern is the prospect of pregnancy. This is described as an ever-ready possibility whenever girls engage in any type of sexual relations. The magazines hint that there are dangers lurking in all sorts of sexual interaction both at the time of the sexual relations and even much later. For instance, 'lots of girls think that pregnancy-free zones exist, but they don't' (Marks 2002, Ask Dr. Marks, *CosmoGirl!*). In the following quotation, note the stereotypical positioning of the reader as an 'innocent young schoolgirl' who can get pregnant long after the sexual event, when menstruating and even while sitting in class:

> Q: Can you get pregnant if you have sex during your period?
> A: Yes. A girl can ovulate (release an egg) just after her period. And since sperm can live for up to a week, she can have sex during her period – and then get pregnant five days later while sitting in class.
>
> (Maher 2005, How not to get pregnant, *Seventeen*)

Sperm itself, divorced from sexual penetration but spread across panties, is described as potentially causing pregnancy: 'But a wad of semen may not get absorbed, so if a girl's vagina comes in contact with it, she could get pregnant' (Maher 2005, How not to get pregnant, *Seventeen*).

Young women are ultimately held responsible if a woman does get pregnant. Unlike young men, they cannot avoid a pregnancy by running away:

> He has the option to bolt; you don't. The simple fact is that not taking care of yourself isn't smart – or mature – so if you don't want to deal with the birth control part, you definitely aren't psychologically ready to get into the sex part.
>
> (Anonymous 2002, Sex and the suburb, *CosmoGirl!*)

Even more fearsome than pregnancy itself are the possible horrifying consequences. In the following story, a young girl not only has to manage the pregnancy on her own but also bleeds to death alone in her college dormitory:

> On January 29, 2002, Karen Hubbard bled to death after secretly delivering her baby in a bathroom stall at her college dorm. Up until that night, no one even knew she was pregnant.
>
> (Grigoriadis 2002, Death, *CosmoGirl!*)

Sex, fear and STDs, STIs and HIV

Young women are also told to fear seemingly ever-present STDs and STIs including HIV. That STDs are virulent, gruesome and endemic is emphasized: 'You might feel like you're the only person going through this, but you're not alone. Three million teens get diagnosed with an STD each year' (Leone 2002, All about STDs, *CosmoGirl!*). The signs, symptoms and natural histories of various types of STIs and STDs are described in great and repulsive detail including Chlamydia, gonorrhoea, syphilis, HPV, HIV, hepatitis B and herpes (Byrd 2006, I'm like you but I have HIV, *Seventeen*). Exacerbating worry is the following description enumerating the many different subtypes of the human papillomavirus: 'There are about 30 strains of the virus that infect the genitals' (Marks 2002, Ask Dr. Marks, *CosmoGirl!*). HIV/AIDS, too, is featured as a particular worry: 'But the truth is anyone can get HIV. In fact, teen girls will make up one-eighth of all new cases diagnosed this year' (Almasi 2003, STDs: Exposed, *CosmoGirl!*) and 'HIV/AIDS is spreading like fire among girls and young women' (Almasi 2003, STDs: Exposed, *CosmoGirl!*).

Sex and fear of betrayal

Young girls are advised not to trust young men because the majority of them are undependable: 'Beware! 52% of guys who have had an STD don't tell their partners' (Anonymous 2006, I got an STD, *Seventeen*). Young men are described as wanting their own sexual pleasure at any expense. Young women are described as having less power than young men, wanting to be liked and, thus, 'giving in': 'I figured he'd use a condom, but he didn't. I knew it wasn't safe, but I was more worried that if I told Tom to stop, he'd think I was lame' (Anonymous 2006, I got an STD, *Seventeen*). In another story a young woman's vulnerability is described as follows: 'He said it felt better without condoms, so we didn't use birth control' (Crain 2001, What's up doc?, *CosmoGirl!*).

In the following two stories, the young women's sexual partners withhold information about their STIs: 'Three weeks later, I found out that I have HIV' (Crain 2001, What's up doc?, *CosmoGirl!*); 'I was positive. The medicine had eliminated it, but I was still scared – I'd had it for months. If you don't treat Chlamydia, it can lead to infertility. By not telling me, Tom put me even more at risk' (Kemp 2004, Your most private sex questions, *CosmoGirl!*).

Medicalization

Sex is repeatedly contextualized by concerns about disease and routine but frightening doctor visits, medical treatments and vaccines. Regular visits to a gynaecologist are recommended 'once-a-year, starting at 13–15' (Greco 2005, Checkup!, *CosmoGirl!*). This general point of view is that 'If you're sexually active, you must ask a doctor to test you for sexually transmitted diseases at least once a year, even if you use condoms and don't show any signs of infection' (Karras 2007, I had unprotected sex … now what?, *Seventeen*).

Both getting and refusing medical care may be problematic and fraught with various qualms: 'Not getting medical treatment means the virus will be that much harder to control later – it could actually be too late' (Byrd 2006, I'm like you but I have HIV, *Seventeen*). Young women are presented as afraid that the doctor will know whether or not they are virgins: 'Will my gynaecologist know I've had sex?' (Joiner and Leonard 2005, Am I gay?, *Seventeen*). That young women will be embarrassed by their necessary doctor visits is reinforced: 'What's up doc? Your doctor has seen it all, so don't be embarrassed to ask her anything' (Grumman 2005, Do you have this STD?, *Seventeen*).

Young women's fear and anxiety about sex is even given a medical label in this next illustration in which one teen asks whether she may be experiencing 'erotophobia', to which Dr Judy responds: 'I doubt that there's anything "wrong" with you. It's normal for teens to feel anxious about (or even be afraid of) having sex ... Besides the scary consequences of STDs and unintended pregnancy, sex involves some heavy emotions you may not be ready to deal with yet' (Crain 2001, What's up doc?, *CosmoGirl!*).

Abstinence is the answer

Fear of all sorts of dangers that might be related to sex leads to a repeated emphasis on abstinence. This is illustrated by the numerous admonitions to abstain not only from sexual intercourse but also from sex play. Some illustrations follow:

> 'Remember the only way to get 100% safe is to not have sex' (Karras 2007, I had unprotected sex ... now what?, *Seventeen*); 'Even without vaginal intercourse, there are still risks to consider' (Karras 2007, I had unprotected sex ... now what?, *Seventeen*); 'Abstinence from sexual activity is the only truly 100-percent effective option' (Anonymous 2004, Your sex dilemmas – resolved, *Seventeen*); 'Abstinence is the only way to truly protect yourself' (Anonymous 2004, Your sex dilemmas – resolved, *Seventeen*); 'And since condoms don't always cover HPV infected areas, abstinence is the only sure way to protect yourself' (Crain 2002, HPV alert, *CosmoGirl!*); 'And please remember that since condoms can break or leak without your knowing it, the only truly safe sex is no sex' (Crain 2002, What's up doc?, *CosmoGirl!*); 'Look, the only "safe" sex is no sex, since condoms can break, slip off, or not cover the infected area' (Leone 2002, All about STDs, *CosmoGirl!*).

Sex in magazines for women aged 40–50

Sex as woman's work and responsibility in marriage

Sex is usually described as a burden, a type of work for women, who are assumed to be married and mothers, in magazines for 40 to 50-year-olds. In the following example, sex is positioned as one of the types of work that modern women must do. In general: 'multiple orgasms have been replaced by multitasking, and amid the dishes, diapers and company reports, all too many of us look up one day to realize our sexuality has been stuffed into the back of a sock drawer' (Brody 2003, Here's to your health!, O, *The Oprah Magazine*).

Despite women's double day of work, and whether they themselves have sexual desire, they are portrayed as being accountable for their husband's happiness, sexual fulfilment and the well-being of their marriages: 'But when sex evasion turns into a daily habit, marriage can become an arctic zone' (Mahoney 2007, Romance, *Good Housekeeping*) and 'sometimes you have to make love for the benefit of the other person, even though you may not need it yourself at the moment' (Mahoney 2007, Romance, *Good Housekeeping*).

Women are described as being in an exchange or bargaining role with their husbands. They are portrayed as if they are expected to manage the complex calculations necessary to maintain a balanced marital equation. The next quotation suggests that in agreeing to marry, women implicitly consent to be available for sex: 'Remember your wedding day? When you said "I do", you said "I do" to sex too' (Mahoney 2007, Romance, *Good Housekeeping*). The assumption here is that he gives something and she gives something in return. He takes away and she, in turn, takes something away.

The next quotation quantifies the bargain further and likens it to a bank account:

> 'It helps many couples to think of sex as a bank account,' says Lana Holstein MD, author of *Your Long Erotic Weekend*. 'If you just got back from a vacation where you had lots of time alone, then saying "I'm too wiped out tonight" isn't a problem. But if you haven't had much sex in the last 6 months, then it took your husband some courage to ask. If you say no that can be damaging.'
> (Mahoney 2007, Romance, *Good Housekeeping*)

Women are held implicitly responsible if their husbands masturbate or 'use' pornography (both of which are portrayed as problematic): 'When a wife turns down sex, what does she want her husband to do instead? Should he go masturbate? My clients usually say, "No, I don't want him to do that!" Nor do they want him to spend an hour on a pornography Web Site' (Mahoney 2007, Romance, *Good Housekeeping*). The bargain becomes a power struggle that the woman is asked to end in the next illustration: 'Don't allow yourself to see sex as a power struggle – intercourse or nothing – because nothing will always win,' points out McCarthy (Mahoney 2007, Romance, *Good Housekeeping*).

Fearmongering is evident, too, in discussing the possible negative consequences of refusing a husband's request for sex: 'When couples drift into the celibate zone – feeling as if it would take a $150 meal or act of Congress to spark some interest – there's trouble ahead' (Mahoney 2007, Romance, *Good Housekeeping*). Women's responsibility includes not only the sexual encounter but also for feeling desire for their husbands. Even if it takes a visit to the opera the woman is portrayed as having a duty to be happily ready for sex: 'If your husband doesn't like the opera, go with your sister,' says Ruth Westheimer, 'You'll come home alive, happy – and ready for an intimate encounter' (Mahoney 2007, Romance, *Good Housekeeping*). The emotional work of being responsible to be ready for a sexual encounter is highlighted in the next quotation, too. Under the heading 'What to say to him' women are advised to promise regular sexual activity: 'From now on, you can count on me to be in the mood every Wednesday morning' (Mahoney 2007, Romance, *Good Housekeeping*).

Following from the theme of work is the idea that sex can be viewed as a workout and of benefit to women's health. Again intrinsic pleasure and pleasuring are ignored: 'Think of it [sex] as working out. You may not be excited to get on the treadmill, but most of us enjoy the exercise glow once we're "in the zone" ' (McGraw 2002, Dr. Phil, 'Get past the awkwardness of talking about s-e-x!', O, *The Oprah Magazine*); 'Sexuality may not be the first thing that you think of when tending to your health. But what a great natural source of energy. It's more powerful and lasting than any smoothie or protein bar, not to mention calorie-free' (McGraw 2002, Dr. Phil, 'Get past the awkwardness of talking about s-e-x!', O, *The Oprah Magazine*); 'Whether you have sex or simply a healthy appetite for it, when that drive is activated, no matter what your age, you feel resilient, vibrant, ready for the rush of life' (Brody 2003, Here's to your health! Who says good sex requires a push-up bra and candlelight?, O, *The Oprah Magazine*).

The double standard of sexuality is also evident in these magazines. Men are viewed as desiring a variety of types of sex. Women are seen as giving or withholding it in turns. Women are entreated to provide, not just sex per se, but an array of different 'types' of sex and to act as if they want to. The following is a quote from a man who is trying to explain what sex means to men. It is as ordinary as pizza and men are positioned as liking all sorts of toppings: 'Sex for us is like pizza, okay? You put anchovies on it, you put pineapple on it – all of it's good' (Elins 2004, How sex is like pizza … and other startling features of the male mind, O, *The Oprah Magazine*). Women are told that oral sex is fundamental to their husband's well-being and self-esteem: 'Again, guys say there's no such thing as a good blow job – just the fact that it's a blow job is good. But they want you to show love to the phallus because it's a reflection of them' (Elins 2004, How sex is like pizza … and other startling features of the male mind, O, *The Oprah Magazine*).

Sex is also described as a litmus test of a marriage: 'A couple's sexual relationship often mirrors the rest of their relationship' (McGraw 2002, Dr. Phil, 'Get past the awkwardness of talking about s-e-x!', O, *The Oprah Magazine*). Declining sex is equated with rejection of a husband. Being unwilling to engage in sex at one point in time is generalized beyond the moment to reflect a woman's whole attitude to her partner:

> Nobody likes to be rejected and no rejection strikes closer to home than when your partner, the person in whom you have invested the most, says by word or deed: 'I am not attracted to you, do not desire you, and do not want you.'
>
> (McGraw 2002, Dr. Phil, 'Get past the awkwardness of talking about s-e-x!', O, *The Oprah Magazine*)

Worry about sex and one's children

The other major theme in these magazines for middle-aged women is that women should worry about the sexual behaviours of their teenage children, particularly girls. One worry for mothers is the teenage graduation trip to a holiday destination:

> Teens on 'party trips' face many potential dangers, from alcohol poisoning to date rape and STDs. These kinds of spring-break and graduation vacations often involve teens flashing bare breasts, passing out drunk and living by the motto 'what happens in Cancun, stays in Cancun'.
>
> (Jones 2006, Will your teen be safe on a party trip?, *Good Housekeeping*)

Mothers are portrayed as worrying about their daughters engaging in an increasingly popular pastime, oral sex: 'In addressing mother–daughter groups around the country, I've learned that many middle school girls view oral sex as a bargain. When they do it, the girls say they are in control and can't get pregnant' (Snyderman 2002, Your health, *Good Housekeeping*).

Sometimes, oral sex is believed to be a type of abstinence: 'A survey of Southern college students in the mid-1990s found that fully 37% of them considered oral sex to be abstinence' (Snyderman 2002, Your health, *Good Housekeeping*); 'A lot of teens have this idea that it's no big deal. Kids who think this may be missing crucial messages about sexually transmitted diseases and self-esteem' (Whitaker 2006, Teen dating – a mom's guide, *Good Housekeeping*).

Anomalous findings

The data analysis so far has emphasized the dominant discourses. It must also be said that there were instances of anomalous findings in both groups of magazines. For instance, three articles touched on homosexuality in an accepting and compassionate way in the teenage magazines. Two examples follow: 'There are times when it's hard, like when people say anti-gay stuff, but having family and friends who are there for me always helps me get through it' (Marks 2002, Ask Dr. Marks, *CosmoGirl!*) and 'I was a junior in high school when my older brother told our family that he's gay. Mom and Dad were fine with it – they taught me that being gay is something you're born with' (Marks 2002, Ask Dr. Marks, *CosmoGirl!*).

In a few of the stories for teenagers there was also an uncritical acceptance of pharmaceuticals as a ready and easy solution for an unwanted pregnancy or STI. The following offers an example: 'We hung out a few times, and a week later in the heat of the moment – we had sex. We didn't use a condom, and it crossed my mind that I might get an STD, but I didn't care. I figured if I caught something, I'd just take a pill and it would go away' (Byrd 2006, I'm like you but I have HIV, *Seventeen*).

In the stories for middle-aged women, there were two articles that mentioned that mothers should be worrying about their innocent sons in the face of sexually aggressive girls. For instance, 'Boys need to be told that it's OK to say no. And girls need to be taught how to be respectful of a boy's feelings' (Whitaker 2006, Teen dating – a mom's guide, *Good Housekeeping*). And one story held out the possibility that sexual problems are a couple's responsibility. However, since the magazine readers are women, the implicit message is that women are to take responsibility for telling their partners to change: 'Sexual incompatibility is not an individual's problem. It's a couple's problem, and nothing short of both of you being actively involved will do the trick' (McGraw 2002, Tell it like it is, O, *The Oprah Magazine*); 'As a society of couples, we have behaved and miscommunicated our way into a problem of epidemic proportions … I'm talking about millions of relationships in which sexual appetites don't match' (McGraw 2002, Tell it like it is, O, *The Oprah Magazine*).

There was also some evidence of the medicalization of sexuality for middle-aged women. In this case, the focus is not on STIs but on the biomedically defined benefits: ' "Sex, and the cuddling that comes with it, releases all kinds of chemicals that women need," says Dr Holstein, "including mood-boosting hormones like dopamine, norepinephrine and oxytocin" ' (McGraw 2002, Dr. Phil, 'Get past the awkwardness of talking about s-e-x!', O, *The Oprah Magazine*). It was found that 'couples who had sex regularly had higher levels of disease-fighting antibodies than those who didn't' (McGraw 2002, Dr. Phil, 'Get past the awkwardness of talking about s-e-x!', O, *The Oprah Magazine*).

Discussion

There is an underlying anti-sex message for both teenage and middle-aged women in the magazines addressed to these two different age groups. In neither kind of magazine is sex described as being for the pleasure of the woman reader. In magazines directed to both groups, sex is described as the work and worry of women. Teenage and older women are held responsible for sex and its consequences. Young women must work to avoid sex because of disease, pregnancy, doctor visits and betrayal of boyfriends. Middle-aged women must work to ensure that their marriages continue. In both cases, women are deployed as managers of sexual expression in the interest of the continuation of heterosexual marriage.

Young, presumed unmarried, women are discouraged from engaging in sex and advised to practise abstinence (until marriage). Married women are encouraged to engage in sex with their husbands whether they want to or not for the benefit of their husbands. Ultimately, in both groups of magazines, this portrayal reflects a double standard because sex is to be avoided until marriage and then engaged in for the sake of the happiness of husbands and the longevity of marriage.

The negative portrayal of the possibility of sex for women's own pleasure may be a reactionary response to the heightened concern in the USA about such issues as teenage sexuality, adolescent pregnancy, abortion and gay rights (Casper and Carpenter 2008). Such social arrangements destabilize the heterosexual marriage and in the case of adolescent pregnancy may lead to dependence on the state. This certainly corresponds to the cotemporaneous, strong anti-sex and pro-heterosexual marriage messages, policies and programmes planned and instituted by the Bush administration in the interests of neo-liberal economic policies and supported by his electoral support by social conservatives, sometimes called 'the moral majority' or the Christian Right. This may also reflect a post-feminist backlash (McRobbie 2004) against the gains of women in equality and autonomy (Baker 2005) wherein sex for the pleasure of independent women is rejected. As Fine (1988) argued, discourses of desire (in women) are missing.

It is worth speculating about how the link between neo-liberal and socially conservative policies might work. Magazines are commercial products. Among other things, content responds to editorial policy, audience wishes and advertising demands (Curran *et al.* 1996). In the social climate of the USA during the years focused on in this study, it is likely that stories supporting the maintenance of heterosexual marriage and patriarchy would likely be looked on more favourably by profit-seeking media conglomerates because such a portrayal reinforces existing power relations.

These findings also support the argument that sexuality is becoming more rationalized and medicalized (Jackson and Scott 1997; Tiefer 2000; Marshall 2002). Sex as the desire of women has been distorted, by and large into sex as another part of women's work to be rationally organized and managed. Both age groups are subject to the fundamental trends of modernity and post-modernity, including the spread of medicalization and rationalization.

Gill and Herdieckerhoff (2006) argue that neo-liberal rationality has spread to all areas of life. The idea that sexuality is medicalized and risky is but one aspect of the overall medicalization of US life (Conrad 2005) in a risk society (Beck 1992). Rather than being contextualized by concerns about emotional well-being and women's personal pleasure and desire, the stories for young women focused on the links between sex and gruesomely described diseases and regular doctor visits. Biomedicine is deployed in the descriptions of the health benefits of sexual expression in the magazines for middle-aged women.

There are, however, various small signs of resistance to the dominant discourses. These include some positive references to homosexuality and to the effectiveness of medications in the face of STIs in the magazines for teenage girls. In the magazines for middle-aged women, there was some recognition that sexual issues are sometimes a couple's problem and that mothers need to be concerned about their sons because of sexually aggressive girls.

Limitations and future directions for research

There are a number of study limitations that need to be mentioned, all of which suggest new directions for future research. First, this study has relied on an analysis of one medium only, over a limited time period, and has used individual stories indexed under particular keywords. It would be valuable to trace possible changes over time in a variety of media and with different keywords associated with sexuality. Second, while the magazines selected were high circulating, we cannot make any claims about their actual level of pragmatic influence on, or reflection of, their audience. This remains a topic worthy of investigation. Third, this analysis relied on text only. Observations of accompanying photographs might allow for more nuanced findings regarding the potential diversity of the audience being addressed. Fourth, this method of topical analysis is also limited in that it takes the studied stories out of the context of the whole magazine. A contextual analysis may provide more data about possible contradictions between these findings and other visual, advertising or written materials within these magazines or between different types of stories such as advice columns as compared to personal stories.

Conclusion

In conclusion, this study has demonstrated how magazines devoted to both teenage and middle-aged women describe women as responsible for sexual expression that is portrayed as being ultimately intended for the maintenance of heterosexual, patriarchal marriage in the context of a double standard. In both groups of magazines, the possibility of women's sexual desires is largely invisible. In the magazines for teenage girls, desire is obfuscated by a focus on various fears and an admonition to abstain. In magazines for older women, sexual desire is hidden by a spotlight on the satisfaction of the needs of husbands and the requirement to monitor the sexual expression of children, particularly girls.

References

Allen, L. 2003. Girls want sex, boys want love: Resisting dominant discourses of (hetero) sexuality. *Sexualities* 6: 215–36.

Altheide, D.L. 2002. *Creating Fear: News and the Construction of Crisis*. New York: Aldine de Gruyter.

Baker, M. 2005. *Families Changing Trends in Canada*. Toronto: McGraw Hill.

Batchelor, S.A., Kitzinger, J. and Burtney, E. 2004. Representing young people's sexuality in the 'youth' media. *Health Education Research* 19: 669–76.

Beck, U. 1992. *Risk Society: Towards a New Modernity*. London: SAGE.

Berg, B.L. 1989. *Qualitative Research Methods for the Social Sciences*. Boston, MA: Allyn & Bacon.

Bryman, A. 2004. *Social Research Methods*. 2nd ed. Oxford: Oxford University Press.

Carpenter, L. 1998. From girls into women: Scripts for sexuality and romance in *Seventeen* magazine, 1974–1994. *Journal of Sex Research* 35: 158–68.

Carpenter, L. 2001. The first time / *Das erstes mal*: Approaches to virginity loss in US and German teen magazines. *Youth and Society* 33: 31–61.

Carpenter, L. 2002. Gender and the meaning and experience of virginity loss in the contemporary United States. *Gender & Society* 16: 345–65.

Casper, M.J. and Carpenter, L.M. 2008. Sex, drugs and politics: The HPV vaccine for cervical cancer. *Sociology of Health and Illness* 30: 886–99.

Clarke, J. 1991. Media portrayal of disease from the medical, political economy and life-style perspectives. *Qualitative Health Research* 1: 287–308.

Clarke, J. 1992. Cancer, heart disease and AIDS: What does the media tell us about these diseases? *Health Communication* 4: 105.

Clarke, J. 2008. *Sexuality in Cosmo Magazine: 2000–2007*. Unpublished manuscript, Wilfrid Laurier University.

Conrad, P. 2005. The shifting engines of medicalization. *Journal of Health and Social Behavior* 46: 3–14.

Curran, J., Morley, D. and Walkerdine, V. (eds) 1996. *Cultural Studies and Communications*. London: Arnold.

Currie, D. 1999. *Girl Talk: Adolescent Magazines and Their Readers*. Toronto: University of Toronto Press.

Duncombe, J. and Marsden, D. 1998. 'Stepford wives' and 'hollow men'? Doing emotion work, doing gender and 'authenticity' in intimate heterosexual relationships. In: G. Bendelow and S.J. Williams (eds) *Emotions in Social Life: Critical Themes and Contemporary Issues*. New York: Routledge, 211–27.

Fine, M. 1988. Sexuality, schooling and adolescent females: The missing discourse of desire. *Harvard Educational Review* 58: 29–53.

Flood, M. 2003. Lust, trust and latex: Why young heterosexual men do not use condoms. *Culture, Health & Society* 5: 353–69.

Frith, H. and Kitzinger, C. 1997. Talk about sexual miscommunication. *Women's Studies International Forum* 20: 517–29.

Gill, R. and Herdieckerhoff, E. 2006. Rewriting the romance: New femininities in chick lit. *Feminist Media Studies* 6: 487–504.

H. W. Wilson Company n.d. *The Reader's Guide to Periodical Literature*. Available at: https://library.wlu.ca/research-materials/databases/rgft [Accessed 9 March 2015].

Jackson, S. 1993. Love and romance as objects of feminist knowledge. In: M. Kennedy, C. Lubelska and V. Walsh (eds) *Making Connections: Women's Studies, Women's Movements, Women's Lives*. London: Taylor & Francis, 38–49.

Jackson, S. 2005a. 'Dear Girlfriend …': Constructions of sexual health problems and sexual identities in letters to a teenage magazine. *Sexualities* 8: 258–305.

Jackson, S. 2005b. 'I'm 15 and desperate for sex': 'Doing' and 'undoing' desire in letters to a teenage magazine. *Feminism & Psychology* 15: 295–313.

Jackson, S. and Scott, S. 1997. *Gut Reactions to Matters of the Heart: Reflections on Rationality, Irrationality and Sexuality*. Oxford: Blackwell.

Jackson, S. and Cran, F. 2003. Disrupting the sexual double standard: Young women's talk about heterosexuality. *British Journal of Social Psychology* 42: 113–27.

Jensen, R.E. and Jensen, J.D. 2007. Entertainment media and sexual health: A content analysis of sexual talk, behaviour and risks in a popular television series. *Sex Roles* 56: 275–84.

Kim, J.L. and Ward, L.M. 2004. Pleasure reading: Associations between young women's sexual attitudes and their reading of contemporary women's magazines. *Psychology of Women Quarterly* 28: 48–58.

Kitzinger, J. 1995. 'I'm sexually attractive but I'm powerful': Young women negotiating sexual reputation. *Women's Studies International Forum* 18: 187–96.

Lambiase, J. 2003. Sex: Online and in Internet advertising. In: T. Reichert and J. Lambiase (eds) *Sex in Advertising: Perspectives on the Erotic Appeal*. Mahwah, NJ: Erlbaum, 247–72.

Marshall, B.L. 2002. 'Hard science': Gendered constructions of sexual dysfunction in the 'Viagra Age'. *Sexualities* 5: 131–58.

McRobbie, A. 1996. More! New sexualities in girls and women's magazines. In: J. Curran, D. Morley and V. Walkerdine (eds) *Cultural Studies and Communications*. New York: St Martin's Press, 172–94.

McRobbie, A. 2000. *Feminism and Youth Culture*. 2nd ed. New York: Routledge.

McRobbie, A. 2004. Post-feminism and popular culture. *Feminist Media Studies* 4: 257.

Medley-Rath, S.R. 2007. 'Am I still a virgin?': What counts as sex in 20 years of *Seventeen*. *Sexuality and Culture* 11: 24–38.

Muehlenhard, C.L. and Peterson, Z.D. 2005. Wanting and not wanting sex: The missing discourse of ambivalence. *Feminism & Psychology* 15: 15–20.

Neuman, W.L. 2000. *Social Research Methods: Qualitative and Quantitative Approaches*. 4th ed. Toronto: Allyn and Bacon.

Oliver, M.B., Banjo, O. and Kim, J. 2003. Judging a movie by its cover: A content analysis of sexual portrayals on video rental jackets. *Sexuality & Culture* 38(7): 38–56.

Radway, J.A. 1991. Interpretive communities and variable literacies: The functions of romance reading. In: C. Mukerji and M. Schudson (eds) *Rethinking Popular Culture: Contemporary Perspectives in Cultural Studies*. Berkeley: University of California Press, 465–86.

Rubin, L. 1990. *Erotic Wars*. New York: Farrar, Straus and Giroux.

Tally, M. 2006. 'She doesn't let age define her': Sexuality and motherhood in recent 'middle-aged chick flicks'. *Sexuality & Culture* 10: 33–55.

Tiefer, L. 2000. Sexology and the pharmaceutical industry: The threat of co-optation. *Journal of Sex Research* 37: 273–83.

Tincknell, E., Chambers, D., Van Loon, J. and Hudson, N. 2003. Begging for it: 'New femininities', social agency and moral discourse in contemporary teenage and men's magazines. *Feminist Media Studies* 3: 47.

Ussher, J. 1997. *Fantasies of Femininity: Reframing the Boundaries of Sex*. Harmondsworth: Penguin Books.

Ussher, J.M. 2005. The meaning of sexual desire: Experiences of heterosexual and lesbian girls. *Feminism & Psychology* 15: 27–32.

Walkerdine, V. 1990. *Schoolgirl Fictions*. London: Verso.

White, C. 1970. *Women's Magazines 1693–1968*. London: Michael Joseph.

Winship, J. 1987. *Inside Women's Magazines*. London: Pandora.

Wouters, C. 1998. Changes in the 'lust balance' of sex and love since the sexual revolution: The example of the Netherlands. In: G. Bendelow and S.J. Williams (eds) *Emotions in Social Life: Critical Themes and Contemporary Issues*. New York: Routledge, 228–49.

Chapter 4

Cultural politics and masculinities

Multiple partners in historical perspective in KwaZulu-Natal

Mark Hunter

Introduction

Seventy per cent of the total number of HIV-positive people worldwide – 28.5 million people – live in sub-Saharan Africa. Unlike North America and Europe, where HIV/AIDS predominates among men who have sex with men, and injecting drug users, in Africa most transmissions take place through heterosexual sex. Although there is now considerable agreement that gender is central to any understanding of male–female transmission, the social values surrounding manhood have been less examined (Mane and Aggleton 2001). Yet studies have shown the benefits of such an approach. In South Africa, for instance, scholars have noted how dominant masculinities can shape men's sometimes violent control over women, demand for 'flesh to flesh' sex, and celebration of multiple partners (Campbell 1997; Wood and Jewkes 2001; Hunter 2002).

From a somewhat different perspective, an important recent theme in HIV/AIDS research is that of 'sexual networking'. Epidemiologists have argued that multiple-partnered relationships may play an important part in driving the HIV pandemic; the same number of overall partners but organized within concurrent rather than serial relationships leads to a considerably more rapid advance of sexually transmitted diseases (Morris and Kretzschmar 1997; though also see Legarde *et al.* 2001). Positioning multiple-partnered relations as one element of what they call a 'distinct and internally coherent African system of sexuality', the influential demographers Pat and John Caldwell and their collaborators have stressed the prevalence of such relationship patterns within African society and their embeddedness within its underlying social structure (Caldwell *et al.* 1989: 187). Drawing (somewhat uncritically) on early ethnographies, they view such relations in the context of African wives' sexual unavailability for long periods because of both high fertility rates and long periods of post-partum abstinence. Yet, in contrast to this somewhat static approach, I attempt to show how sexual networks have emerged and changed over time. Moreover, I adopt a masculinities framework to demonstrate how men's 'tradition' of having multiple partners both result from and shape male power.[1]

This chapter is situated geographically in KwaZulu-Natal (KZN), a province where one in three people are thought to be HIV-positive (Department of Health 2002). Showing how masculinities emerge out of changing material conditions, it is influenced by the work of the Italian Marxist Antonio Gramsci, who devoted his short life (he died in an Italian fascist prison cell in 1937) to interpreting and challenging the dominant political and cultural forces that shape a society's 'common sense'. Connell's (1987, 1995) seminal writings on masculinities draw strongly on this Gramscian tradition, stressing how women and men, the gay and the straight, contest and produce a plurality of masculinities. Applied to Zulu society, this conception of culture rejects the search for some kind of static logic to Zulu sexuality that public health workers can easily 'map' and then 'modify' perhaps through 'education'. Instead, it posits an understanding of Zulu-ness as being constructed through contestations in everyday life where material and cultural change are inseparable and co-determining and where 'education' is but one of a number of shapers of 'culture'.[2]

To contextualize and historicize masculinities is especially important because the frightening reality of HIV/AIDS causes much research to gravitate towards the present day.[3] Additionally, popular discourse tends to characterize African people as inherently 'diseased' and 'promiscuous', making it imperative to problematize representations of static African masculinities (on racialized colonial representation of 'promiscuous' Africa see Vaughan 1991 and McClintock 1995). At a time when gender is now correctly a taken-for-granted concept in the study of AIDS, there is value in stepping back and considering how male power has been assembled over time. What gendered battles took place to produce today's taken-for-granted traditions? How are men's social and ideological strengths maintained and what contradictions do they face?

Following a brief methodological note, this chapter charts the rise and fall of *isoka*, broadly a man with multiple sexual partners, a powerful though fluid concept in isiZulu. The importance of the notion of *isoka* has been noted in KwaZulu-Natal (see, for example, Varga 1997), but the concept has not been historicized. This chapter argues that colonial rule and capitalist penetration significantly altered paths to manhood and reworked the meanings and practices surrounding multiple partners. Evidence suggests that in nineteenth-century KwaZulu-Natal, multiple partners were not men's sole prerogative and that unmarried women could also enjoy limited sexual relations with more than one boyfriend. In contrast, by the 1940s and 1950s, most oral testimonies suggest that *umthetho* (the law) allowed only men to have multiple sexual partners. An *isoka* was sharply juxtaposed to an *isifebe*, a loose woman engaging in plural relations. Men, however, did not enjoy unlimited freedom. An unmarried man who played with multiple girls whom he would not or could not marry was castigated as being *isoka lamanyala* (literally a dirty *isoka*). Men among men were expected to marry, establish an independent household, and oversee the enlargement of this domestic unit through childbirth.

This chapter draws particular attention to the period from the 1980s when many informants recount tremendous difficulty securing affordable housing and stable, if any, employment. Consequently, most young men today are unable to marry because of the high cost of *ilobolo* (bridewealth) and find it difficult to establish an independent *umuzi* (homestead or home) and become *umnumzana* (homestead head). The expansion of women's work opportunities in the last 50 years has also disrupted men's position as the sole provider, although many women face harsh poverty particularly as unemployment has increased since the 1990s. In this context, once celebrated as a youthful pastime, securing multiple partners has taken on an exaggerated significance for men and, indeed, for some women desperate to secure money or gifts. The chapter ends by noting the rising doubts that men now harbour around the *isoka* masculinity in the era of AIDS.

Context and method

The following analysis combines ethnographic, archival and secondary sources collected for the author's doctoral dissertation based in Mandeni, a municipality 120 kilometres north of

Durban on the North Coast of KwaZulu-Natal. The principal data that this chapter draws from is approximately 300 interviews with informants aged between 16 and 80 (all of the names of people appearing in this chapter are pseudonyms). Interviews were semi-structured and geared towards understanding informants' life histories, with a special emphasis on relationships. Some informants were questioned as many as five times. These interviews, alongside 15 meetings with same-sex groups of three to four young people, were mined for clues as to how sexuality has transformed from the 1940s. Virtually all interviews were conducted and transcribed in isiZulu. Useful supplementary sources include the Zulu newspapers *Ilanga* and *Isolezwe* and the radio station *Ukhozi* FM.

These sources were interpreted in conjunction with numerous informal conversations and observations. Beginning with a 4-month stay in 2000, the author lived in Mandeni for 18 months in total, staying in Isithebe Informal Settlement with the Dlamini family. The contradictions inherent in the author's position as a White male born in the UK, studying in the USA, of course need to be acknowledged. Just a stone's throw away from this informal settlement where the author stayed in the Dlamini family's large *umuzi* is Isithebe Industrial Park; driving from the informal settlement on the dirt, often mud, roads, past the many *imijondolo* (rented one-room accommodation) and into the adjacent factory complex quickly repositioned the author as a probable factory manager with power over hundreds of lives. This is just one example of the power dynamics involved in conducting research in a country where so starkly the 'racial becomes the spatial' (Pred 2000: 98).

Nineteenth-century masculinities: the homestead economy and women with multiple partners

Zulu society emerged from a period of military warfare at the turn of the twentieth century, and bravery and fighting skills were important attributes associated with manliness. The central economic focus for isiZulu speakers, however, was *umuzi* (the homestead), and, in turn, the physical and symbolical centre of this institution was *isibaya* (cattle kraal). Big men accumulated many cattle, took several wives, and thus built a successful homestead; the more wives a man had the more labour he was able to control and the richer and more esteemed an *umnumzana* (household head) he became (see Carton 2000 on masculinities at the turn of the century among isiZulu speakers). The commencement of courting was thus a significant step towards marriage and manhood and this is suggested by the fact that one meaning of the word *isoka* was unmarried man. More fully, Colenso's (1861) dictionary gives the nineteenth-century meaning of the noun *isoka* as: 'Unmarried man; handsome young man; sweetheart; accepted lover; a young man liked by the girls.' With its emphasis in this era on denoting the courting stage, it is perhaps not surprising that the noun *isoka* bears close similarity to the verb *ukusoka* (circumcision) – a prior rite of passage from boyhood abolished by Shaka (who founded the Zulu kingdom in the early nineteenth century). As is evident from the definition, an *isoka* was also seen as a man popular with girls.

Controlling fertility was paramount in pre-colonial society since an *umuzi* could grow only through childbirth or the acquisition of additional wives (see Guy 1987). Nevertheless, sexual practices that avoided childbirth were relatively freely permitted. Evidence from court cases, oral testimonies collected by the colonial official and historian James Stuart at the turn of the twentieth century, and early ethnographies all suggest that non-penetrative forms of sex (*ukusoma*, or thigh sex) were widely practised among unmarried persons.[4]

Somewhat surprisingly in light of future attitudes, records also indicate a certain level of acceptance around women having more than one *soma* (intercrural sex) partner, although it is true that those overstepping the mark could be chastised as being *izifebe* (pl. of *isifebe*, a loose woman). Hunter [Wilson] (1936: 182), writing about Mpondolond albeit in the 1930s, describes the attitude of unmarried women having multiple boyfriends as 'the more skulls the better'. Extramarital affairs also appear to have been quite well accepted in southern Africa well before the onset of migrant labour (see Delius and Glaser 2003). Indeed, before the introduction of Christian notions of 'the body as the Temple of God', the essence of *ukugana* (a verb translated sometimes too quickly into 'to marry') was childbirth and building an *umuzi* and not sexual fidelity for its own sake. Such relatively open attitudes around certain forms of sexuality at certain times should not, however, be drawn upon to suggest that African society was in any way promiscuous. Virginity-testing ceremonies institutionalized the enormous value placed on premarital virginity for young women, and chaste demeanour was essential if a woman was to be seen as marriageable. In certain respects, African society could be extremely sexually conservative.

Multiple partners in rural areas in the 1940s and 1950s: men being *isoka*, women behaving badly

If nineteenth-century Zulu society was structured around largely self-sufficient homesteads, by the 1950s most rural areas were dependent on migrant labour. Drawn first to the diamond and gold mines in the late nineteenth century, men increasingly found work in the twentieth century in the mushrooming industries of large towns such as Johannesburg and Durban. A greater number of women too began to build livelihoods in urban areas, often as domestic workers or engaging in informal activities such as the brewing of beer. Wage labour gave men new powers but it also imparted on them fresh expectations; in assuming the position of breadwinner, men took on primary responsibility for supporting the *umuzi* (Silberschmidt 2001).

Interviews with elderly informants in rural areas suggest that, against this transforming terrain, accepted thinking on multiple-sexual partners in the 1940s/1950s had transmuted significantly from the nineteenth century. Notably, men and women's rights to have multiple partners had diverged sharply. Transformations are most evident in premarital sexuality where, in contrast to the nineteenth century, all informants are adamant that *umthetho* (the law) only allowed women to have a single lover; multiple partners were the prerogative of *isoka* alone. That a growing asymmetry emerged between men and women's rights to have multiple partners is suggested by an apparent change in the meaning of *isoka*. Doke *et al.*'s (1990) dictionary compiled in the 1940s and 1950s differentiates between an original meaning of *isoka*, 'a man old enough to commence courting', and later meanings that encompass a 'young man popular among girls'. Vilakazi (1962: 47) describes in powerful terms the Don Juan or Casanova status of *isoka* in the mid-century, a strong theme in testimonies: 'Courting behaviour among traditional young men is a very important part of their education; for a young man must achieve the distinction of being an *isoka*, i.e., a Don Juan or a Casanova.'

According to informants, being an *isoka* and having several girlfriends was countered to the ignominy of life as an *isishimane*, a man too scared to talk with girls and without a single girlfriend. With its symbolic crutch as polygamy, the *isoka* concept was widely circulated, and at times challenged, in everyday discourse, as demonstrated by its prominent position in *izibongo* (oral praise poetry) (Koopman 1987; Gunner and Gwala 1994; Turner 1999). If the archetypal *isoka* figure in the 1950s was a single young man famous for his prowess in courting several women, the *isoka* masculinity had a much wider ambit, one example being its bolstering of the husband's position that they alone should enjoy extramarital liaisons, especially important at a time when polygamy had become extremely rare.

This *isoka* masculinity was dominant but not universal. Christianity sanctioned a single, monogamous, moral code that was endorsed, if not always strictly followed, by male *amakholwa* (Christians/believers). Schooling and Christianity certainly seems to have influenced a more critical attitude among women to their husbands' extramarital affairs (see Lo`ngmore 1959; Wilson and Mafeje 1963). The existence of same-sex relations also suggested a further challenge to heterosexual norms, the Zulu words for a homosexual man being *isitabane* or *ingqingili* (see also Epprecht 1998 on same-sex relations in Zimbabwe). Moreover, being *isoka*, even in the 1950s, could lead to embarrassing illnesses. Especially for urban men, penetrative sex (as opposed to *ukusoma*) had become a mark of manliness, and yet the embarrassing symptoms of STIs such as syphilis reminded men of the hazards of a masculinity that celebrated multiple-sexual conquests.[5] The harsh reality of migrant labour also meant that, although women's sexuality was jealously guarded in some circumstances, a number of women did have extramarital affairs with a certain level of implicit approval: many of my older female informants smiled wryly when relating how a secondary lover was dubbed *isidikiselo*, the top of a pot, while the first man, the *ibhodwe*, was the main pot; metaphors closely linked to a woman's need for sexual relations, and sometimes support, when her husband was working in the towns.

Moreover, the *isoka* masculinity faced restrictions precisely because other paths to manhood were ultimately more valued. While an *isoka* could *ukusoma* (engage in thigh sex) with several partners, in order to become a respected *umnumzana* he had to have a wife and build an *umuzi*. The phrase *isoka lamanyala* (*amanyala* means dirt or a disgraceful act), used to rebuke men with too many girlfriends, signified an unseemly masculinity, a masculinity gone too far. Though some men did recall a certain status associated with being *isoka lamanyala*, for most it was a reproach. Men with more than one girlfriend, including married men partaking in extramarital relations, could be called to account for their intention to marry their girlfriends particularly by parents with a heavy stake in their daughter's future *ilobolo*. Indeed, most informants were adamant that an *isoka*'s ability to attract women was heavily dependent on his control over cattle and other resources necessary to marry; hence in the 1940s and 1950s, despite the bravado around the language of *isoka*, men who had not yet secured work found it difficult to be *qoma*'d (chosen) by even a single woman.

What forces mid-century consolidated this *isoka* masculinity and, compared to the nineteenth century, frowned on women who had multiple partners? A persistent theme in writings on colonial Africa is how African men and the colonial state looked towards customary law to solidify patriarchal traditions (on the detrimental effects of customary law `` 1982; Marks 1989). The apparent new tradition that limited women, particularly the unmarried, to only one boyfriend seemed to have emerged out of this subtle blend of Zulu and Christian values. Demonstrating this, while most informants said that a woman's restriction to only one boyfriend was part of a timeless Zulu *umthetho* (law), tellingly some sourced the rule as coming from God. Yet these struggles over tradition did not take place in a social or geographical vacuum. They were underpinned by shifts in bargaining power as a consequence of migrant labour and the erosion of agricultural capacity in rural society. Instead of being dependent on their fathers for bridewealth, young migrant workers, now able to save *ilobolo* themselves, were in a strong position to demand that their girlfriends adopt a chaste demeanour and refrain from having secondary partners.

Though some women, of course, did develop intimate relations with more than one man, those doing so, especially the unmarried, were chastised as being *izifebe* (loose women). So severe was this insult that it could result in a claim of defamation.[6] Indeed, in the eyes of many men, the *ihlazo* (disgrace) of having a child before marriage or being seen as *isifebe* positioned women as lacking *inhlonipho* (respect) and therefore undesirable to marry – condemned to a low status in society or forced to escape derision by moving to towns. Young girls' chaste living was further supervised by *amaqhikiza* (girls who had already selected a boyfriend) and elder women who periodically tested girls' virginity. While parents set firm limits, notably against pregnancy, they were rarely involved in the day-to-day socialization of young men or women's sexuality (on changing forms of sexual socialization see Delius and Glaser 2002).

As is common in the telling of oral histories, many respondents tended to remember the 1940s/1950s with nostalgia – as a period of stability, opulence and convention. The *umnumzana* figure that I have drawn attention to sometimes figured in these accounts as a marker of a static and romanticized manhood. Certainly, one can easily underestimate the extent that aspiring for manhood in the mid-century placed men in an extremely ambiguous position; building a rural home and family forced men to work in towns, and yet the consequences of this separation often undermined the very institution men sought to construct. A final important point of ambiguity results from the need to see sexuality as closely connected to broader gendered patterns. Parents, in particular, could position their daughters as being *izifebe* – or loose women – in order to deny them the opportunity to worship or school, both practices associated with possible desertion to the towns and the loss of labour and *ilobolo*. Sexuality, as Weeks (1985: 16) points out, is 'a transmission belt for wider social anxieties' – contestations over sexuality are about much more than simply sex. Put another way, the cultural politics of multiple partners overlapped with parallel contestations over the roles and duties of women in society.

In conclusion, the evidence suggests that having multiple partners was the subject of ongoing change and contestation in the 1950s. Tradition, rather than being simply passed down or lost, faced intense contestation at its every move. Although both men and women were engaging in multiple-partnered relations, compared to the nineteenth century, women, particularly unmarried women, faced much more public censure for doing so; the notion of *isoka* saw to it that this right was coded as male-only, pivoting on the tradition of polygamy. The following section explores contestations over multiple partners in the contemporary period.

Multiple partners in the era of democracy and unemployment

A persistent theme in oral accounts is the long and arduous investments men made in order to become *umnumzana* (a homestead head). In the colonial and apartheid era this was never an easy project. Indeed, as the twentieth century progressed, men became progressively dependent on wage labour to provide *ilobolo* (bridewealth). At work, in particular, African men faced the humiliation of being positioned as boys. Today, however, arguably two further forces threaten South African men's path to *umnumzana* status: the difficulty that men face in marrying and setting up an independent household and the greater participation of women in the labour market and thus their independence from men. Population census data suggests that marital rates began to drop from the 1960s. This was probably as a response to increased cohabiting in towns, more educated women gaining new work opportunities, and migrant labour biting deeper into the ability of men and women to form long-term relationships. From the 1970s, however, technological developments, slow economic growth, population rises and, since 1994, tariff reductions prompted a dramatic increase in unemployment and a greater casualization of work. Unemployment estimates today range from 30 to 42 per cent depending on the methodology used (Altman 2003). Though some African people have taken advantage of the post-apartheid deracialization of schooling and employment, for the great majority the prospects of steady work are very slim. Since the payment of *ilobolo* is so heavily dependent on a man's employment, weddings in many South African communities are infrequent events today. In KwaZulu-Natal, the common *ilobolo* figure of ten cows (plus one beast, the *ingqutu*, for the mother) was set as a maximum payment by the colonial administration in 1869 and later incorporated in the Natal Code of Native Law (Welsh 1971). Today in KwaZulu-Natal, 11 cows is ironically seen as one of the most timeless of all African traditions (although not in other provinces where, unlike in Natal, customary law was not codified). For sure, marriage has always been a process rather than an event and the institution is demonstrating flexibility – most families today utilize generous cattle-cash exchange rates. Nonetheless, wedlock continues to remain outside the scope of most young men's financial capacity. According to the most recent population census, less than 30 per cent of African men and women over 15 years of age in South Africa were in marital relations in 2001. Interlinked changes in women's status and roles also serve to undermine men's position as *umnumzana*. Many men are no longer the sole provider and some are even dependent on women for survival. This is the context in which marriage becomes not only undesirable but unnecessary from the perspective of women.

The seismic changes to the institution of African marriage in the twentieth century have long been noted in published work. Especially in urban areas, high levels of illegitimate children, extramarital relations and prostitution were seen as evidence for societal breakdown over half a century ago (see Krige 1936; Hellmann 1948; Longmore 1959). Yet, although urban areas undoubtedly did rework sexuality, it must be recognized that urban growth also fashioned the emergence of an alternative urban masculinity. Throughout the colonial and apartheid eras, elements in the state and society debated the extent to which African urban dwellers should be stabilized. In the 1950s and 1960s, although influx controls were severely tightened, formal township housing programmes expanded at their fastest rate for those with urban residential rights. According to Posel (1995: 237), 'This stabilization strategy included, at its very core, efforts to "build" stable African family units.' The advertisement in Figure 4.1 appearing in the Zulu-language newspaper *Ilanga lase Natal* in the 1950s draws on the imagery of a modern urban *umnumzana*, a man who aspired to Western standards of education and fashion. The important point to stress is that urbanization, often seen as a process that led to immorality, could also lead to new notions of manhood, ones in which notions of marriage and building a home still played a central part.

For East Africa, Silberschmidt (2001) has argued that high unemployment and low incomes created a context in which men's self-esteem could be bolstered through multiple-partnered relations and violence against women. South African society is perhaps even more divided than East Africa in terms of wealth and poverty both between and within races. At the bottom of the social hierarchy many unemployed or poorly paid women are forced to engage in transactional sex with men, often multiple men (see Hunter 2002). But another significant trend is men's frequent unemployment. The inability today of many

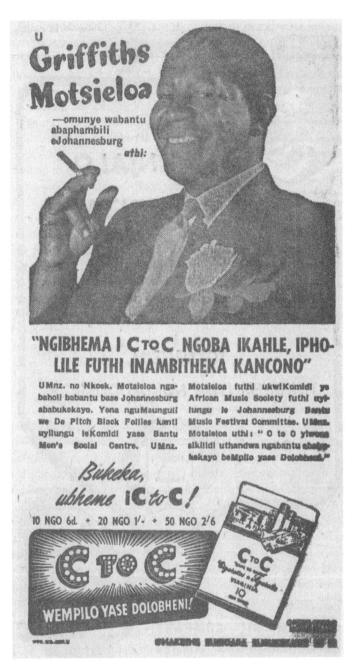

Figure 4.1 Griffiths Motsieloa, a well-known musician in the 1940s, advertises C to C cigarettes, markers of urban life. The newspaper *Ilanga*, from which this advert is sourced, was widely read in rural and urban areas by educated men and it helped to foster a modern image of *umnumzana* (household head) – a man confidently in control of his destiny and firmly at the helm of a domestic household

Source: *Ilanga lase Natal*, 18 March 1950, Killie Campbell Africana Library.

men to achieve *umnumzana* status through work, marriage and fulfilling a 'provider' role is the context in which expressions of manliness that celebrate numerous sexual conquests must be understood. Seventeen-year-old township resident Sipho describes the way some men position their quest for women: 'If he has six, I want seven, then he wants to have eight.' The numbers are very often much higher than the one or two girlfriends mentioned by the elder generation, and penetrative sex is invariably taken for granted; many youth, especially in urban areas, are unaware that the practice of *ukusoma* (thigh sex) ever existed. Despite the diverse history of the *isoka* masculinity noted here, men generally present *isoka* as a part of a seamless Zulu custom. Zandi, a 22-year-old township woman, describes how men conflate polygamy with multiple partners, to justify the latter: 'They say that it is their culture to have more than one girl. They say my grandfather had six wives, I want to be like him.' To denote an unacceptable side of the *isoka* masculinity, young men and women, like their grandparents, still speak of *isoka lamanyala* (dirty *isoka*), although today the concept has been partially unlinked from marriage. It is no longer common to hear of men being lambasted by the term *isoka lamanyala* for having many girlfriends and showing no intention of marrying any of them. A more likely usage of *isoka lamanyala* might be to describe a man who cheats on his girlfriend with her best friend, or a man who spreads HIV.

Certainly, AIDS is bearing heavily down on the *isoka* masculinity. HIV/AIDS-related illnesses transform some of the most virile and popular bodies into barely living skeletons, shunned by friends and neighbours. Outwardly confident about being *isoka*, at times men betray their inner doubt. The contradictions of being *isoka* in the era of HIV/AIDS are perhaps most tragically played out at the many funerals in the area; previous 'players' are buried by their friends who were once envious of their ability to attract women. Consequently, men and masculinities are under huge scrutiny and critique, even if women are still commonly blamed for promiscuity and AIDS. Men's own self-doubt is further propelled by women's often aggressive critique of irresponsible men infecting women with HIV. One 29-year-old woman told me that many women no longer use the tradition-laden concept of *isoka lamanyala* to criticize men: 'The young they just call [bad men] *izinja* (dogs).'

There is some evidence in South Africa that male doubt is being institutionalized in groups such as 'men for change' noted by Walker (2003) in Alexandra Township. These groups can counter the risk-taking and bravado implicit in dominant masculinities. Certainly, in the last three years of working in Mandeni, interviews have documented rising doubt among young men over the celebration of multiple partners. Nonetheless, sexuality is deeply enmeshed in a broader cultural politics, and its transformation takes place through contradictory tugs rather than unidirectional movements. Women seeking education and other opportunities have long been scorned as *izifebe* (loose women), and today the disciplining of rebellious women as loose still serves to bolster male power. One only has to spend a short time in many homes in South Africa's townships or rural areas to observe that women shoulder huge burdens of domestic responsibility. The insult of *isifebe* hovers over women who challenge traditional gendered roles in the home and elsewhere. With this in mind, it is easier to see how men can adhere to differential claims over multiple partners embodied in concepts such as *isoka/isifebe* that, while threatening to their lives if enacted in multiple-partnered relationships, reiterate gendered power in broader spheres of everyday life. These binary categories also, of course, help to reiterate the normativity of heterosexual masculinities.

But it is too simplistic to suggest that masculinities are simply defended by men and challenged by women. Women's efforts to secure livelihoods in harsh socio-economic circumstances can also serve to reproduce dominant masculinities. Many women are themselves quick to see the benefits of securing multiple partners, living in an environment where the prospects of work and marriage are slim and where they are often aware of their own boyfriends' unfaithfulness. As one young man recently put it: 'Now [the post-apartheid period] women say that it is 50/50 – if we have other girlfriends, they have other boyfriends', a sentiment of course with a long history. The pleasure of sex is openly celebrated, but these liaisons can also be brazenly about money, especially those relationships with sugar daddies. Although some unemployed men or schoolboys complain that they find it difficult to secure a single girlfriend, sugar daddies are usually said to work at well-paying firms in Mandeni. The type of acquired dispositions (Bourdieu 1990) that women would invest in in the 1940s, such as being seen to be chaste, *khutele* (hard working) and respectful, are much less important today, as it is a sexy demeanour that can secure men and money in contemporary South Africa.

Facing these circumstances, intervention messages are highly contradictory, often unable to reconcile themselves with the material realities of life for the majority in post-apartheid South Africa. At least publicly, churches tend to forcefully promote abstinence before marriage, though the message seems hollow when betrothal is such a rarity. In KwaZulu-Natal, the pandemic has led to attempts to revive the practice of virginity testing (see Scorgie 2002). In Mandeni's township, a local church now annually organizes a virginity-testing ceremony, an intervention not without irony given the historical role of churches in railing against 'heathen' traditions.

One theme running through the narratives of youth interventions in South Africa is the need to treat young people, particularly women, with respect. Young people's rights are championed, and the category of youth is symbolically reworked to place young people on a more even keel with adults. The postcard advert from Youth AIDS (Figure 4.2) is suggestive of this theme, appropriating the word *baba* (father) in its text: 'If you are going to have sex, use a condom *baba*.' Many young male readers will indeed be fathers, yet the postcard blends trendy youth images with a word usually reserved for older men, though now part of township lingo. It bestows on youth the duties of responsibility associated with manhood, in exchange for elevated male respect – respect being redefined away from traditional practices pivoting on gender and generational hierarchies. Such strategies of creating alternative values around manhood are also attempted by the most high profile AIDS institution in South Africa, Love Life, a large non-governmental organization (NGO) established to reduce teenage pregnancies and HIV infections through media campaigns, telephone advice lines and youth centres. The Love Life poster (Figure 4.3) encourages men to achieve respect through a healthy body, positioning sport as a desirable expression of manhood.

It is easy to see how these and other groovy intervention messages promoting choice, independence and self-respect can appeal to those who envisage bright prospects in the new South Africa. Certainly there is a growing African middle class in South Africa, and most South African Whites have relatively good prospects of work. However, for the majority of poorer, predominantly African, South Africans (the principal subject of this chapter), the resonations between choice, positive living and the lived experiences of poor schooling and unemployment are more muted. Notwithstanding these comments, it has perhaps become too easy to dismiss campaigns such as Love Life out of hand as simply being aimed at a relatively small elite. A more balanced assessment must also recognize how deeply hampered any interventions to rework masculinities, and more broadly sexuality, are by the extreme poverty in many areas of the country. Creating a new lifestyle brand, as Love Life has attempted, certainly does open up spaces for contestation by all South Africans,

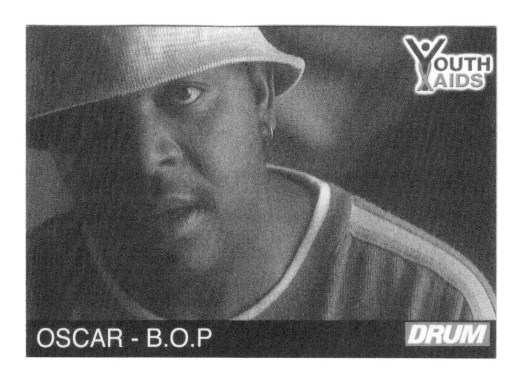

OSCAR - B.O.P

DRUM

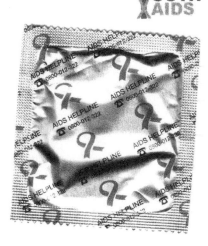

"If you are going to have sex,
use a condom baba."

www.youthaids.co.za

Figure 4.2 A postcard given away in July 2003 with popular magazine *Drum*. Oscar is a successful South African music personality. With a condom attached, the postcard speaks to young men through the word *baba* (father). *Baba*, a term historically used by older men, has been appropriated by young township men today as an informal, yet respectful, greeting. Youth AIDS thus doubly appropriates it in an attempt to bestow responsibility on youth to engage in safe sex

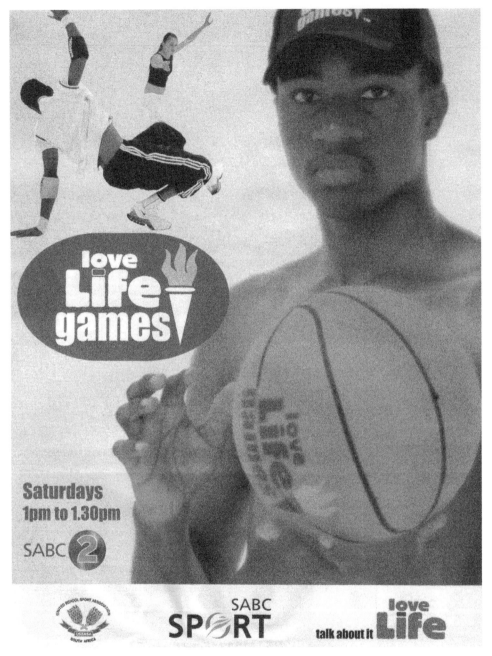

Figure 4.3 Love Life, South Africa's largest intervention campaign, portrays itself as a new lifestyle brand, competing with consumer icons such as Nike and Coke. In an era when *umnumzana* (head of household) status is denied to many men, sports are promoted as a fashionable alternative expression of manliness

Source: *S'camtoPRINT*, Issue 53, 17 August 2003.

rich and poor, and this must be seen as a positive development; at the moment, however, it seems that it is middle-class, urban-based, youth who have the strongest base from which to employ such symbols to challenge dominant expressions of sexuality.

Viewing masculinities and notions of respect through a historical lens also makes it possible to see why one of the key slogans of Love Life, 'Talk about it' – promoting parent/child dialogue on sex – is so controversial in South Africa. Sexual socialization historically took place through age-sets; talking about sex across generations could be seen as highly impertinent and counter to notions of *inhlonipho* (respect). Thus, opposition to new notions of mutual respect and universal rights may have more to do with attempts to preserve gendered and generational hierarchies than any kind of blanket African taboo on talking about sex, as some suggest. Supporters and critics of campaigns such as Love Life all arguably tend to focus too narrowly on sexuality rather than exploring its embeddedness within a multiplicity of gendered struggles and practices in everyday life.

Disaggregating male power and forefronting cultural politics

The notion of cultural politics captures the way that men and women, the young and the old, the gay and the straight, contest everyday cultural beliefs, ones that have real material consequences. The practice of multiple partners has never been static in South African history and is contested on the ebb and flow of changing material livelihoods. Gender is more than simply the one-dimensional expression of male power but, as historical analysis of the *isoka* masculinity demonstrates, is embodied in male vulnerabilities and weaknesses. It is the coming together of male power in some ideological and material domains with men's weakness in others, including their ability to achieve full manhood through building an *umuzi* (home), that can create the violence and risky masculinities so often tragically noted in the era of HIV/AIDS. Historically rooted analysis – rarely featuring in HIV/AIDS debates – has an important role to play in replacing stereotypes of static African masculinities or culture with accounts that recognize complex, contested, processes of cultural change.

Notes

1 See also Heald (1995) for this critique of the Caldwells' work.
2 See Morrell (1996) and also Hamilton (1998) for important historical writings on 'Zulu-ness'.
3 Particularly important exceptions combining contemporary ethnography with historical analysis are Schoepf (1988) and Setel (1999).
4 Ndukwana, in a long and complex testimony to James Stuart at the turn of the century, makes several references to unmarried women being allowed to have a number of *soma* partners, as long as she *soma*'d with only one per month so that pregnancy could be accounted for. Testimony of Ndukwana in Stuart Archive, Vol. 4, 300; 353 (Webb and Wright 1986). Accounts of courting contained in evidence for criminal court cases from this period also suggest that unmarried women had a significant degree of sexual freedom; see RSC II/1/42 Rex v Gumakwake (85/1887) and RSC II/1/44 Rex v Ulusawana (45/1888).
5 Describing the effect of STIs on masculinity, a doctor's assistant practising in the area in the 1960s remembers the embarrassment attached to syphilis and suggests that, like AIDS, it could provide a check on male masculinity, although its curability of course contrasts strongly with AIDS today.
6 Most of the small number of defamation cases that I have seen from this period are when a woman has been callled *isifebe* – a great offence for a Christian as well as a non-Christian woman. See Majozi v Khuzwayo (1/ESH uncatalogued civil case, 65/63) for a rural setting and Buthelezi v Ntuli

(1/ESH uncatalogued civil case, 66/66) for a more urban setting.

References

Altman, M. 2003. The state of employment and unemployment in South Africa. In: J. Daniel, A. Habib and R. Southall (eds) *State of the Nation: South Africa 2003–2004*. Cape Town: HSRC, 158–183.

Bourdieu, P. 1990. *The Logic of Practice*. Stanford: Stanford University Press.

Caldwell, J., Caldwell, P. and Quiggin, P. 1989. The social context of AIDS in sub-Saharan Africa. *Population Development Review* 15: 185–234.

Campbell, C. 1997. Migrancy, masculine identities and AIDS: The psychosocial context of HIV transmission on the South African gold mines. *Social Science and Medicine* 45: 273–281.

Carton, B. 2000. *Blood from Your Children: The Colonial Origins of Generational Conflict in South Africa*. Pietermaritzburg: University of Natal Press.

Colenso, J.W. 1861. *Zulu-English Dictionary*. Pietermaritzburg: Davis.

Connell, R. 1987. *Gender and Power*. Cambridge: Polity.

Connell, R. 1995. *Masculinities*. Berkeley, CA: University of California Press.

Delius, P. and Glaser, C. 2002. Sexual socialisation in South Africa: A historical perspective. *African Studies* 61: 27–54.

Delius, P. and Glaser, C. 2003. *The myth of polygamy: A history of extra-marital and multi-partnership sex in South Africa*. Paper presented to the Sex and Secrecy Conference, University of Witwatersrand, 22–25 June.

Department of Health. 2002. *National HIV and Syphilis Sero-prevalence Survey in South Africa 2001*. Pretoria: Department of Health, South African Government.

Doke, C., Malcolm, D., Sikakana, J. and Vilikazi, B. 1990. *English-Zulu Zulu-English Dictionary*. Johannesburg: Witwatersrand University Press.

Epprecht, M. 1998. Good God Almighty, what's this!: Homosexual crime in early colonial Zimbabwe. In: S. Murray and W. Roscoe (eds) *Boy-Wives and Female Husbands: Studies of African Homosexualities*. New York: St Martin's Press, 197–221.

Gaitskell, D. 1982. Wailing for purity: Prayer unions, African mothers and adolescent daughters 1912–1940. In: S. Marks and R. Rathbone (eds) *Industrialization and Social Change in South Africa*. Essex: Longman, 338–357.

Gunner, E. and Gwala, M. 1994. *Musho: Zulu Popular Praises*. Johannesburg: Witwatersrand University Press.

Guy, J. 1987. Analysing pre-capitalist societies in southern Africa. *Journal of Southern African Studies* 14(1): 18–37.

Hamilton, C. 1998. *Terrific Majesty: The Powers of Shaka Zulu and the Limits of Historical Invention*. Cambridge, MA: Harvard University Press.

Heald, S. 1995. The power of sex: Some reflections on the Caldwells' 'African Sexuality' thesis. *Africa* 65: 489–505.

Hellmann, E. 1948. *Rooiyard: A Sociological Survey of an Urban Slum Yard*. Manchester: Manchester University Press.

Horrell, M. 1968. *The Rights of African Women: Some Suggested Reforms*. Johannesburg: Institute of Race Relations.

Hunter, M. 1936. *Reaction to Conquest: Effects of Contact with Europeans on the Pondo of South Africa*. London: Oxford University Press.

Hunter, M. [Wilson] 2002. The materiality of everyday sex: Thinking beyond 'prostitution'. *African Studies* 61: 99–120.

Ilanga lase Natal. 1950. 18 March, p. 1.

Isolezwe. 2003. 28 July, p. 9; 2 August, p. 2.

Koopman, A. 1987. The praises of young Zulu men. *Theoria* 70: 41–54.

Krige, E. 1936. Changing conditions in marital relations and parental duties among urbanized natives. *Africa* 1: 1–23.

Legarde, E., Auvert, B., Caräel, M., Laourou, M., Ferry, B., Akam, E., Sukwa, T., Morison, L., Maury, B., Chege, J., N'Doye, I., Buvé, A. and the study group on heterogeneity of HIV epidemics in African cities. 2001. Concurrent sexual partnerships and HIV prevalence in five urban communities of sub-Saharan Africa. *AIDS* 15: 877–884.

Longmore, L. 1959. *The Dispossessed: A Study of the Sex-life of Bantu Women in Urban Areas around Johannesburg*. London: J. Cape.

Mane, P. and Aggleton, P. 2001. Gender and HIV/AIDS: What do men have to do with it? *Current Sociology* 496: 23–37.

Marks, S. 1989. Patriotism, patriarchy and purity: Natal and the politics of Zulu ethnic consciousness. In: L. Vail (ed.) *The Creation of Tribalism in Southern Africa*. Berkeley, CA: University of California Press, 215–240.

McClintock, A. 1995. *Imperial Leather: Race, Gender and Sexuality in the Colonial Conquest*. London: Routledge.

Morrell, R. (ed.) 1996. *Political Economy and Identities in KwaZulu-Natal: Historical and Social Perspectives*. Durban: Indicator Press.

Morris, M. and Kretzschmar, M. 1997. Concurrent partnerships and the spread of HIV. *AIDS* 11: 641–48.

Posel, D. 1995. State, power and gender: Conflict over the registration of African customary marriage in South Africa c. 1910–1970. *Journal of Historical Sociology* 8: 223–256.

Pred, A. 2000. *Even in Sweden: Racisms, Racialized Spaces and the Popular Geographical Imagination*. Berkeley, CA: University of California Press.

S'camtoPRINT. 2003. Issue 53, 17 August.

Schoepf, B. 1988. Women, AIDS and economic crisis in Central Africa. *Canadian Journal of African Studies* 22: 625–644.

Scorgie, F. 2002. Virginity testing and the politics of sexual responsibility: Implications for AIDS intervention. *African Studies* 61: 55–75.

Setel, P. 1999. *Plague of Paradoxes*. Chicago, IL: University of Chicago Press.

Silberschmidt, M. 2001. Disempowerment of men in rural and urban East Africa: Implications for male identity and sexual behaviour. *World Development* 29: 657–671.

Simons, J. 1968. *African Women: Their Legal Status in South Africa*. London: C. Hurst & Co.

Turner, N.S. 1999. Representations of masculinity in the contemporary oral praise poetry of Zulu men. *South African Journal of African Language* 19: 196–203.

Varga, C. 1997. Sexual decision making and negotiation in the midst of AIDS: Youth in KwaZulu-Natal, South Africa. *Health Transition Review* 7(Suppl 3): 45–67.

Vaughan, M. 1991. *Curing Their Ills: Colonial Power and African Illness*. Oxford: Basil Blackwell.

Vilakazi, A. 1962. *Zulu Transformations: A Study of the Dynamics of Social Change*. Pietermaritzburg: University of Natal Press.

Walker, L. 2003. *Men behaving differently: South African men since 1994*. Paper presented to the Sex and Secrecy Conference, University of Witwatersrand, 22–25 June.

Webb, C. and Wright, J. 1986. *The James Stuart Archive of Recorded Evidence Relating to the History of the Zulu and Neighbouring Peoples, Volume 4*. Pietermaritzburg: University of Natal Press.

Weeks, J. 1985. *Sexuality and its Discontents: Meaning, Myths and Modern Sexualities*. London: Routledge.

Welsh, D. 1971. *The Roots of Segregation: Native Policy in Colonial Natal, 1845–1910*. Cape Town: Oxford University Press.

Wilson, M. and Mafeje, A. 1963. *Langa: A Study of Social Groups in an African Township*. Cape Town: Oxford University Press.

Wood, K. and Jewkes, R. 2001. 'Dangerous love': Reflections on violence among Xhosa township youth. In: R. Morrell (ed.) *Changing Men in Southern Africa*. Pietermaritzburg: University of Natal Press, 317–36.

Natal Archives, Durban

Civil cases, Eshowe District (1/ESH): Majozi v Khuzwayo (uncatalogued civil case, 65/63); Buthelezi v Ntuli (uncatalogued civil case, 66/66).
Criminal cases, Natal: RSC II/1/42 Rex v Gumakwake (85/1887); RSC II/1/44 Rex v Ulusawana (45/1888).

Section 2

Sex and gender

It is commonplace nowadays to assert that while the term 'sex' refers to biological differences in the form of chromosomes, hormonal profiles, and internal and external sex organs, gender describes the characteristics that a society or culture delineates as masculine or feminine. Yet all too often discussion ends there. Yet, both historically and cross-culturally, there exist enormous variations in societal expectations concerning women and men, with major differences in terms of class, age, ethnicity and sexuality among other factors. All too often, in both the academic and policy and programme literatures, gender is associated with women, who are portrayed as relatively powerless in their negotiations and relationships with men. Men, if they appear at all, often figure somewhat stereotypically as women's oppressors, unconcerned both about their own health and the well-being of others. The chapters in this section question some of these assumptions, offering a more sophisticated understanding of the intersections between sex, gender and other variables as they impact on, and relate to, health.

In the first chapter, Rosina Cianelli, Lilian Ferrer and Beverly J. McElmurry explore how sociocultural factors and misinformation about HIV transmission contribute to an increasing number of Chilean women becoming infected. In spite of this trend, few culturally specific HIV prevention interventions have been developed for women and girls in that country, particularly for those from socially marginalised communities and backgrounds. The goal of the study reported on was to elicit the perspectives of low-income Chilean women regarding HIV and relevant sociocultural factors, as a forerunner to the development of culturally appropriate forms of intervention. As part of a mixed-methods study, data were collected from low-income Chilean women by means of a survey and in-depth interviews. Results provide evidence of widespread misinformation and misconceptions related to HIV and AIDS. Cultural beliefs and practices rooted in machismo and marianismo, including the roles and responsibilities of men and women linked to these, constitute major barriers to HIV prevention development. Future prevention efforts should aim to support women's empowerment, partner communication and the education of women vulnerable to HIV.

In their chapter, Lisa Bowleg, Michelle Teti, Jenne S. Massie, Aditi Patel, David J. Malebranche and Jeanne M. Tschann point to the fact that while much existing research documents the links between ideologies of masculinity and sexual risk among multi-ethnic young men and White male college students in the USA, similar research with Black heterosexual men was scarce at the time the chapter was written. Their exploratory study aimed to address this gap. Interviews took place with Black low- to middle-income heterosexual men aged 19 to 51 years in Philadelphia. Analyses highlight the presence of two explicit ideologies of masculinity: namely, that Black men should have sex with multiple women, often concurrently, and that Black men should not be gay or bisexual. Findings also point to the existence of two more implicit ideologies of masculinity: the first supportive of the notion that Black heterosexual men cannot decline sex, even risky sex, and the second suggestive of the fact that women should be responsible for condom use. The study's important implications for HIV prevention with Black heterosexual men in the USA are outlined.

Finally, Tsitsi B. Masvawure's chapter adds complexity to the notion that women are largely powerless in their sexual relationships with men. It also challenges two common perceptions regarding transactional sex relationships, particularly in Africa: first, that such relationships are primarily resorted to as survival strategies by economically disadvantaged young women, and second, that sex and money are always exchanged within these relationships. Instead, the author shows how, in reality, young women and the men they date may use these relationships primarily to compete for social status in their peer groups, as well as to fashion themselves as high-status, successful modern subjects. Often, for female students, and indeed the men they date, transactional sex often involves more than a straightforward exchange of sex and money. Ethnographic data was collected at the University of Zimbabwe using participant observation and in-depth interviews, with findings highlighting the importance of taking into account the contexts in which transactional sex occurs. Transactional sex takes different shapes and holds different meanings depending on when and where it takes place.

Chapter 5

HIV prevention and low-income Chilean women

Machismo, marianismo and HIV misconceptions

Rosina Cianelli, Lilian Ferrer and Beverly J. McElmurry

Introduction

Approximately 35 million people were living with HIV infection and 2.3 million of new cases were reported worldwide at the end of 2012. Although the HIV-related death rate has decreased by 30 per cent since 2005, HIV continues to be one of the leading causes of death (Kaiser Family Foundation 2013; UNAIDS 2013a). In the Latin American region, 1.6 million people live with HIV, accounting for 4 per cent of people infected worldwide (UNAIDS 2013a). In Chile, 50,000 people were living with HIV in 2011, and this number increased to 69,860 in 2012 (UNAIDS 2013b). Recent data demonstrate that women are one of the most vulnerable groups in terms of its acquisition. Globally, half of all people living with HIV today are women (UNAIDS 2013a). In Chile, the number of new HIV infections among women continues to rise. Between 1986 and 1990, the ratio of men to women living with HIV was 7:1; however, as of 2011 the ratio had dropped to 3.6:1 (MINSAL 2013).

Gender inequalities, socio-economic disadvantage, violence, substance abuse, inadequate prevention messages and inappropriate programmatic responses to the epidemic have been identified as factors that increase women's vulnerability to HIV infection worldwide (Schneider and Stoller 1995; Buzy and Gayle 1996; Patz et al. 1999; Gilbert and Walker 2002; Peragallo et al. 2005; Miner et al. 2011; Cianelli et al. 2012). In general, women who are vulnerable to HIV do not perceive themselves to be at risk. They believe that HIV is something that happens to homosexually active men or to other women, not something that happens to women in an ongoing 'stable' relationship. Women may not acknowledge that their partners have other sexual partners. Therefore, they do not view their partners as a possible way of acquiring HIV (Guimaraes 1994; Pesce 1994; Cianelli 2003; Cianelli et al. 2012).

In many cases, HIV-positive women confront issues that negatively impact their quality of life such as poverty and violence. Many of them are of low educational level with no paid employment, making them more vulnerable to HIV. New cases are most often reported among young women (20–49 years old) who are living in poverty, have only an elementary education and are unemployed housewives (MINSAL 2013). In most cases, women have become infected through sexual contact with their husbands or other partners. Infection rates continue to rise, and the development of effective programmes for low-income Chilean women has become a serious public health need.

Central to the reproduction of gender inequalities in Latin America are concepts of *machismo* and *marianismo*. Machismo is related to the social domination and privilege that men have over women in economic, legal, judicial, political, cultural and psychological spheres. Ideas about machismo can be explicit or otherwise; however, they contribute to discrimination against women. Boys typically grow up learning that they are strong and can obtain their goals by being aggressive. They also learn that in the future they must be the 'protector' of their wife and family (Strait 1999; Gilchrist and Sullivan 2006). As noted by Gissi (1978), in a *machista* society the macho man is strong, active, independent, polygamous, unfaithful and sexually experienced. It is expected that such men will have multiple partners before and after marriage and this increases the risk of acquiring HIV (Marin *et al.* 1993; Sabogal and Catania 1996; Ferrer *et al.* 2005). In contrast men often expect an affectionate, submissive and faithful woman who plays a passive and dependent role in the sexual sphere and who is able to work inside and outside of the home as necessary (Rosenbluth and Hidalgo 1978; Arciniega *et al.* 2008).

The complement to machismo is marianismo (Pinel 1994), with the submission of women to men being a significant component (Pesce 1994). This produces a double standard whereby women are placed either in the category of good mothers and wives, or in the category of bad women who are sexually available and knowledgeable (Raffaelli and Suarez-Al-Adam 1998). In a context of marianismo, girls learn that they must be good wives and mothers and be respectful of and dependent on men (Peragallo 1996; Peragallo *et al.* 2005). Under the influence of marianismo, the most important values for women are chastity, motherhood, submissiveness, self-sacrifice and caretaking (Strait 1999). In the psychological sphere, submission is expressed by constrained ideas, opinions, choices and feelings. In the physical aspect of submission, the body of the woman is considered an object for the pleasure of men. Women must subordinate their pleasure to the decisions and feelings of men. This hierarchical structure supports discrimination, sexual harassment and the economic manipulation of women (Pinel 1994; Valencia-Garcia *et al.* 2008).

Other factors that place women at risk are lack of HIV knowledge and misconceptions and myths that women have about the virus, particularly about how it can be transmitted, acquired or avoided. It is important to learn more about women's sources of HIV-related information because these can be the source of lack of HIV knowledge and misconceptions. The general awareness that women have about HIV transmission is often not enough for them to perceive themselves as being at risk because of their partners' behaviour (Praca and Gualda 2000).

Methods

Design and setting

A mixed-methods design was used to elicit a reasonably comprehensive picture of the HIV-prevention needs of low-income women in an urban area in Chile. Data were collected via a survey of 50 women and 20 in-depth interviews conducted at a community clinic located in La Pintana County in the south-east of Santiago. The area is considered one of the most socio-economically disadvantaged communities in the city, with 31 per cent of the 190,000 inhabitants living in poverty (Gobierno-Región-Metropolitana 2003; Metropolitana and Chile 2003). In addition, the area has a high incidence of alcohol and drug abuse, adolescent pregnancy and sexually transmitted infections (CONACE 1998, 2002; CONASIDA 2000; Ministerio-Educación-Chile 2005).

Purposive sampling was used to select the research respondents (Bernard 1995; Patton 2002). Quantitative data was collected from a survey of 50 women. Qualitative data from in-depth follow-up interviews with 20 women was sufficient to reach saturation (National

Institutes of Health and Office of Behavioral and Social Sciences Research 2001). Inclusion criteria for the study specified that respondents should be Chilean women (1) aged 18 to 49 years old, (2) sexually active with a male partner during the last three months, (3) living in La Pintana County of Santiago, Chile, and (4) receiving care at a community clinic.

The Office for the Protection of Research Subjects at the University of Illinois at Chicago and the Ethics Committee at the Pontificia Universidad Catòlica de Chile approved the study. Recruitment of participants at the community clinic consisted of having the researcher personally ask women in the waiting area whether they would like to participate. Snowball recruitment was also used. Women who agreed to participate were invited to a private room within the clinic where inclusion criteria were assessed.

The survey consisted of 20 demographic items and 22 true–false statements to assess HIV-related knowledge. Participants took approximately 50 minutes to complete the survey with the assistance of the researcher. Twenty of these women then participated in a two-hour face-to-face semi-structured follow-up interview, which explored women's views on machismo, marianismo and HIV/AIDS.

Descriptive statistics were performed to analyse the quantitative data obtained from the questionnaires. A database was developed to facilitate the processes of data storage, coding, retrieval and analysis using SPSS. Content analysis was used to analyse the qualitative data to identify and define the major themes that emerged from the interviews. The verbatim transcriptions of the interviews were imported into the N5 (Nud*ist 5) program. Memos with observations and notes concerning the interview were incorporated into the program by the researcher. Content analysis was used to identify, code and categorise text data (Patton 1990).

Results

The mean age of the sample was 31 years (Standard Deviation [SD] = 9.7), with a mean of six years of formal education. A quarter of the women were currently living with a spouse or partner, and 42 per cent were legally married. The mean number of years living with a spouse or partner was 3.1 (SD = 1.8). Two-thirds of the participants identified themselves as Roman Catholic. The mean income per person per month was US$54, with a range from US$19 to US$189. Nearly all (82 per cent) of the participants were economically dependent housewives.

HIV-related knowledge

Quantitative analysis of the responses to the survey questions indicated that most participants were knowledgeable about HIV and AIDS, in particular about the virus being sexually transmitted. The questions related to the statements on this topic were answered correctly by 60–98 per cent of participants. Statements related to condom use were given correct responses by 90 per cent of the participants, but 64 per cent did not recognise abstinence as a means of protection against HIV. The statement 'HIV/AIDS cannot be transmitted by using public toilets' was given an incorrect response by 40 per cent of participants. Twenty per cent of the women gave an incorrect response to the statement 'A pregnant woman who is infected with the AIDS virus can transmit the AIDS virus to her unborn child'.

Participants were asked to estimate the percentage of women infected with HIV in the community by answering the following question: 'In your community, how many women out of 100 do you think are infected by HIV?' The estimates ranged from 0 to 80; the median was 10 and the mean was 16.2 (SD = 16.5). Eight participants (16 per cent) estimated that no women locally were infected with HIV. Eighteen (36 per cent) of the respondents estimated that the HIV infection rate among women was between 1 and 10 per cent.

The results for questions associated with discrimination or stigma are presented in Table 5.1. The participants believed that homosexually active men (88 per cent) and sex workers (86 per cent) were the only people to have HIV. Fifty-four per cent of the women checked 'true' to the statement 'All women infected by the AIDS virus have many sexual partners', and over half (60 per cent) indicated 'true' to the statement 'Most people who are infected by HIV look sick'.

Knowledge scores on the surveys were not reflected by the qualitative analysis of in-depth interviews, which revealed that lack of understanding was a major barrier to HIV prevention. Misinformation from various media sources, fear and lack of knowledge about transmission and effective prevention measures were recurrent themes. Gaps in understanding were identified, connected with the fact that women are afraid of knowing more:

> I learned about this disease from the TV, but sometimes the information is contradictory, so I feel confused. Ignorance related to AIDS is big: people do not ask about this disease, they prefer to not know.
>
> (Maria, 24 years old, seamstress)

Critically, women did not understand the difference between being HIV infected and having AIDS:

> You can meet a man that looks clean and respectable, but you do not know if he has some infection after you go to bed with him, because he is not going to tell you.
>
> (Isabel, 32 years old, clerk worker)

Instead, they believed that AIDS is a dangerous and painful illness, like being condemned to death. They believed that there is no available cure for this disease and that treatment is only there to decrease the pain.

Overall, interviews revealed that women's understanding of HIV transmission and prevention is very limited. When asked about HIV prevention, some women mentioned condoms, but many of the responses reflected myths and misconceptions common among community members such as the importance of having a stable partner, proper hygiene, the

Table 5.1 Number and percentage of women responding 'True' to questions of relevance to HIV-related discrimination and stigma (n = 50)

Question	n	%
Only homosexual men can be infected by the 'AIDS virus' (f)	44	88
Sexual workers (prostitutes) are the only women who get HIV/AIDS (f)	43	86
All women infected by the 'AIDS virus' have had many sexual partners (f)	27	54
Most people who are infected by the 'AIDS virus' look sick (f)	30	60

Note: (f) = false

use of birth control pills and intrauterine devices. Pregnancy and breastfeeding were not mentioned as ways to transmit the infection to children.

Sociocultural factors: machismo and marianismo

All of the respondents mentioned the concept of machismo when referring to their partners and/or other men (e.g. fathers, brothers, fathers-in-law). Women described machismo in different ways. The majority of the participants said that *machista* men believed in their superiority:

> When a man is a *machista*, the couple's relationship is centred on him. This means that everything the woman does must be for him.
>
> (Maria, 24 years old, seamstress)

Almost all participants said that *machista* men expected women to do everything for them:

> My neighbour is a *machista* man who likes everything done in his house by 11 am. When he needs something, he just gives the order to his wife [my friend] and she runs to do what he wants.
>
> (Carmen, 42 years old, baby sitter)

Sixteen women mentioned that it was common for *machista* men not to allow their partner to work outside the household, study or have friends. Women must ask them for permission to participate in activities outside of the home.

A greater challenge is the risk of HIV infection for women as a result of their partner's behaviour. Forty per cent of the women believed that they were at risk of HIV because of their partner's behaviour: lack of condom use, infidelity, non-injecting drug use and/or daily alcohol consumption that may result in risky sexual behaviours. The women mentioned that most men in the community do not feel at risk of HIV because they believe that it is something that happens to other people but not to themselves. Male infidelity, related to the culturally accepted idea that men should have more than one sexual partner, was clearly identified as a potential risk factor for HIV. Infidelity was justified or tolerated by the majority of the women. To be unfaithful is part of the culture of machismo. Women usually forgive their husbands after they have an affair. As a consequence, women recognise that male infidelity tends to be repetitive. Moreover, some women even blame themselves for their partners' infidelities:

> Women accept and forgive men's infidelity. This is like a vicious circle between men's infidelity and women's forgiveness.
>
> (Patricia, 33 years old, baby sitter)

Women indicated that women are intimately involved in perpetuating machismo because they are the ones who teach their children to follow the traditional *machista* system:

> We [women] are responsible for having *machista* men, because we raise and educate our children differently, depending on whether they are girls or boys.
>
> (Sandra, 28 years old, waitress)

Women also recognised that spousal abuse affects their HIV risk. Domestic violence, primarily sexual violence, is prevalent in the local community:

> Domestic violence is very common in my community. When you suffer partner aggression, you feel like you are dying, but you are still alive. However, something inside of me is dead.
>
> (Patricia, 26 years old, seller)

Participants drew a connection between sexual violence and HIV. Over half of the women in this study reported abuse by their current partner. They pointed out that not accepting male infidelities could result in violence against a woman.

While women did not talk overtly about marianismo, its effects are clear. All of the women interviewed perceived their role as centred on the household and taking care of their children. Their partners were the ones who made all the decisions, including those that had to do with women's aspirations and goals in life. Some of the participants mentioned women's rights being violated by the men in the community. During the interviews, all women described themselves as 'good women' because they cared and were concerned about their children, partners and families in general. Participants mentioned that men did not recognise this dedication because caring is seen as part of the woman's role:

> I take care of my husband; however, he does not recognise this.
>
> (Rosa, 39 years old, warehouse worker)

Taking care of children was mentioned by all participants as the most important responsibility that women have:

> We [women] give all our time to our children sometimes … we cannot work because we have to stay home to take care of them.
>
> (Angelica, 20 years old, factory worker)

All of the women stated that men have more rights and privileges than women and this is something that women have to deal with and tolerate every day:

> Males are more liberal; they can do everything they want. But women cannot do what they would like to do.
>
> (Marta, 29 years old, housewife)

According to ten interviewees, women's infidelity is present in the community, but is of lesser proportion than that of men. In addition, women's infidelity remains secret for two main reasons: the fear that husbands may find out, and because women do not want their children to know about their situation:

> Unfaithful women try to cover their infidelity, especially thinking about their children.
>
> (Patricia, 26 years old, seller)

Condoms were mentioned as being used by women when they had sexual intercourse outside their marriage, but only to avoid unwanted pregnancies, not to protect themselves from sexually transmitted diseases such as HIV:

My female friends told me that sometimes they use condoms with other sexual partners to avoid getting pregnant, but not with their husbands.

(Claudia, 35 years old, housekeeper)

Discussion

Data from this study offer insight into Chilean women's knowledge of HIV and AIDS and what this disease means for them. Findings from in-depth interviews indicated misconceptions and confusion about AIDS. Common misconceptions include the lack of distinction between HIV and AIDS; the mechanisms by which the virus is spread; and how a person looks if he/she has HIV infection. This led to confusion about prevention strategies and how to challenge stereotypes of people who were HIV-positive. Women expected the person who had HIV to look sick. Thus, if they had sex with someone who looked healthy, they did not believe they would be at risk.

Women had common misconceptions about HIV transmission. Participants identified the use of public toilets and shared tableware as well as lack of good genital hygiene and deep kissing as possible means of HIV transmission. During interviews, none of the women mentioned breastfeeding as a source of newborn infection with HIV. This is an important consideration for developing prevention programmes because it is a common practice among Chilean women to use a 'substitute mother' to breastfeed their children, which may elevate the risk of HIV infection for the newborn child.

It was clear that mass media played an important role in diffusing information about HIV to women in this community. However, sometimes the information produces confusion and the messages are contradictory. Television soap operas, television medical reports and the radio were the main sources of information about HIV mentioned by the women.

Machismo and marianismo present significant barriers to HIV prevention. In Latino culture, macho men represent male domination, and women are under their power. As a result, women lack the ability to make personal decisions and have difficulty adopting effective preventive actions (Peragallo et al. 2005; Cianelli et al. 2012). The sociocultural factors expressed as machismo and marianismo include gender inequality, lack of communication between partners about sexuality, and violence in relationships.

Domestic violence and gender roles, particularly male dominance, are important factors placing women at risk of HIV. Gender roles have been identified as barriers to HIV risk reduction among women (Gupta and Weiss 1993; Heise and Elias 1995; Miner et al. 2008) and specifically among Latino women (Gomez and Marin 1993; Amaro 1995; Peragallo et al. 2005). Women do not perceive that they have the support and the strategies for changing a situation considered normal in their community. Similar findings have been reported by Davila and Brackley (1999) and Del Rosario Valdez (2001).

In general, women continue to tolerate abusive situations. A few women indicated that they are trying to change the situation with their partners. However, for the majority of the participants, resignation was a significant characteristic. The absence of choices for women in a community is the clearest expression of machismo and marianismo. As a result, women lack the ability to make personal decisions and have difficulty adopting effective HIV preventive actions. These findings are consistent with those of Peragallo et al. (2005) and Villegas et al. (2011).

The number of women infected with HIV is increasing globally, and Chile is no exception to this trend (MINSAL 2013). In the context in which this study took place, future actions must take into account the sociocultural factors specific to this group of women (Cianelli 2003; Ferrer *et al*. 2005; Peragallo *et al*. 2005; Cianelli *et al*. 2012). In low-income urban areas such as those investigated in this study, women experience male dominance that often translates into violence, lack of opportunity for personal development, economic dependence and inability to negotiate with partners. Within this context, empowerment must be an important component of future HIV-prevention efforts. Programmes are needed to increase women's self-esteem, self-confidence and self-efficacy, as well as to decrease their dependence and depression. In addition, training in communication strategies and negotiation skills with male partners is important.

References

Amaro, H. 1995. Love, sex and power: Considering women's realities in HIV prevention. *American Psychologist* 50: 437–447.

Arciniega, G.M., Anderson, T.C., Tovar-Blank, Z.G. and Tracey, T.J.G. 2008. Toward a fuller conception of machismo: Development of a traditional machismo and caballerismo scale. *Journal of Counseling Psychology* 55(1): 19–33.

Bernard, H. 1995. *Research Methods in Anthropology*. Walnut Creek, CA: Altamira Press.

Buzy, J. and Gayle, H. 1996. The epidemiology of HIV and AIDS in women. In: L. Long and M. Ankrah (eds) *Women's Experiences with HIV/AIDS: An International Perspective*. New York: Columbia University Press, 181–204.

Cianelli, R. 2003. *HIV/AIDS Issues among Chilean Women: Cultural Factors and Perception of Risk Acquisition*. Chicago, IL: University of Illinois.

Cianelli, R., Ferrer, L., Norr, K. F., Miner, S., Irarrazabal, L., Bernales, M., Peragallo, N., Levy, J., Norr, J. and McElmurry, B. 2012. Mano a Mano-Mujer: An effective HIV prevention intervention for Chilean women. *Health Care for Women International* 33(4): 321–341.

CONACE. 1998. *Estudio Nacional de Drogas en la Población General de Chile, 1998*. Available at: www. senda.gob.cl/wp-content/uploads/2013/10/EstudioDrogas2012.pdf [Accessed 15 January 2015].

CONACE. 2002. *Sexto Estudio Nacional de Drogas en la Población General de Chile*. Available at: www. senda.gob.cl/wp-content/uploads/2011/04/2004_sexto_estudio_nacional.pdf [Accessed 15 March 2006].

CONASIDA. 2000. *May 11, 2001 Bulletin ETS (STD Bulletin) # 2*. Santiago: CONASIDA.

Davila, Y.R. and Brackley, M.H. 1999. Mexican and Mexican American women in a battered women's shelter: Barriers to condom negotiation for HIV/AIDS prevention. *Issues in Mental Health Nursing* 20(4): 333–355.

Del Rosario Valdez, M. 2001. A metaphor for HIV-positive Mexican and Puerto Rican women. *Western Journal of Nursing Research* 23(5): 517–535.

Ferrer, L., Issel, M. and Cianelli, R. 2005. Stories from Santiago: HIV/AIDS and needed health systems change. *Advances in Health Care Management* 5: 31–72.

Gilbert, L. and Walker, L. 2002. Treading the path of least resistance: HIV/AIDS and social inequalities: A South African case study. *Social Science & Medicine* 54: 1093–1110.

Gilchrist, H. and Sullivan, G. 2006. The role of gender and sexual relations for young people in identity construction and youth suicide. *Culture, Health & Sexuality* 8(3): 195–209.

Gissi, J. 1978. *El machismo en los dos sexos*. In: P. Covarrubias and R. Franco (eds) *Chile Mujer y Sociedad*. Santiago, Chile: Fondo de las Naciones Unidas para la Infancia, 550–573.

Gobierno-Región-Metropolitana. 2003. *Diagnostico del Territorio de la Región Metropolitana de Santiago, Resumen Ejecutivo*. Santiago: Gobierno de Chile: División de Análisis y Control de Gestión, Departamento de Ordenamiento Territorial y Medio Ambiente, Proyecto OTAS, Universidad de Chile: Instituto de Asuntos Públicos.

Gomez, C.A. and Marin, B.V. 1993. *Can women demand condom use? Gender and power in safer sex.* Paper presented at the IXth International Conference on AIDS. Berlin, Germany.

Guimaraes, C. 1994. Male bisexuality, gender relations and AIDS in Brazil. In: P. Wijeyaratne, J. Roberts, J. Kitts and L. Arsenault (eds) *Gender, Health, and Sustainable Development: A Latin American Perspective.* Ottawa: International Development Research Center, 26–34.

Gupta, G.R. and Weiss, E. 1993. Women's lives and sex: Implications for AIDS prevention. *Culture, Medicine and Psychiatry* 17: 399–412.

Heise, L. and Elias, C. 1995. Transforming HIV prevention to meet women's needs: A focus on developing countries. *Social Science & Medicine* 40: 931–943.

Kaiser Family Foundation. Kaiser global report. 2013. Available at: http://kff.org/global-health-policy/fact-sheet/the-global-hivaids-epidemic [Accessed 5 January 2015].

Marin, B.V., Tschann, J.M., Gomez, C.A. and Kegeles, S.M. 1993. Acculturation and gender differences in sexual attitudes and behaviors: Hispanic versus non-Hispanic white unmarried adults. *American Journal of Public Health* 83(12): 1759–1761.

Metropolitana, G.R.R. and Chile, U.D. 2003. *Diagnostico del Territorio de la Región Metropolitana de Santiago, Resumen Ejecutivo.* Santiago: Gobierno de Chile: División de Análisis y Control de Gestión, Departamento de Ordenamiento Territorial y Medio Ambiente, Proyecto OTAS, Universidad de Chile: Instituto de Asuntos Públicos.

Miner, S., Ferrer, L., Cianelli, R., Bernales, M. and Cabieses, B. 2011. Intimate partner violence and HIV risk behaviors among socially disadvantaged Chilean women. *Violence Against Women* 17(4): 1–5.

Ministerio-Educación-Chile. 2005. *Estrategia de Promoción de la Permanencia de las Adolescentes Embarazadas y Madres en el Liceo, 2005.* Mineduc: Nivel de Enseñanza Media, Programa Liceo para Todos, Unidad de Apoyo a la Transversalidad.

MINSAL. 2013. *Informe nacional evolucion del VIH-SIDA, Chile, 1984–2011.* Available at: http://epi.minsal.cl/epi/html/bolets/reportes/VIH-SIDA/InformePais_1984-2011_vih_sida.pdf [Accessed 6 January 2015].

National Institutes of Health and Office of Behavioral and Social Sciences Research. 2001. *Qualitative Methods in Health Research: Opportunities and Consideration and Review.* Available at: http://obssr.od.nih.gov/pdf/qualitative.pdf [Accessed 24 February 2002].

Patton, M. 1990. *Qualitative Evaluation and Research Methods.* 2nd ed. Newbury Park, CA: SAGE.

Patton, M. 2002. *Qualitative Research and Evaluation Methods.* Newbury Park, CA: SAGE.

Patz, D., Mazin, R. and Zacarias, F. 1999. *Women and HIV/AIDS: Prevention and Care Strategies.* Washington, DC: PAHO.

Peragallo, N. 1996. Latino women and AIDS risk. *Public Health Nursing* 13(3): 217–222.

Peragallo, N., Deforge, B., O'Campo, P., Lee, S.M., Kim, Y.J., Cianelli, R. and Ferrer, L. 2005. A randomized clinical trial of an HIV-risk-reduction intervention among low-income Latina women. *Nursing Research* 54(2): 108–118.

Pesce, L. 1994. AIDS research from a gender perspective. In: P. Wijeyaratne, J. Roberts, J. Kitts and L. Arsenault (eds) *Gender, Health, and Sustainable Development: A Latin American Perspective.* Ottawa, Canada: International Development Research Center, 19–25.

Pinel, A. 1994. Besides carnival and soccer: Reflections about AIDS in Brazil. In: P. Wijeyaratne, J. Roberts, J. Kitts and L. Arsenault (eds) *Gender, Health, and Sustainable Development: A Latin American Perspective.* Ottawa, Canada: International Development Research Center, 61–71.

Praca, N. and Gualda, D. 2000. A cuidadora e o (ser) cuidado: uma relação de dependência no enfrentamento da AIDS. *Revista Paulista de Enfermagem* 19(1): 43–52.

Raffaelli, M. and Suarez-Al-Adam, M. 1998. Reconsidering the HIV/AIDS prevention needs of Latino women in the United States. In: N. Roth and L. Fuller (eds) *Women and AIDS: Negotiating Safer Practices, Care and Representations.* New York: Haworth Press, 7–26.

Rosenbluth, C. and Hidalgo, C. 1978. *La mujer desde una perspectiva.* In: P. Covarrubias and R. Franco (eds) *Chile Mujer y Sociedad Santiago.* Chile: Fondo de las Naciones Unidas para la Infancia, 435–457.

Sabogal, F. and Catania, A. 1996. HIV risk factors, condom use and HIV antibody testing among heterosexual Hispanics: The national AIDS behavioral surveys. *Hispanic Journal of Behavioral Sciences* 18(3): 367–391.

Schneider, B. and Stoller, N. 1995. Introduction: Feminist strategies of empowerment. In: B. Schneider and N. Stoller (eds) *Women Resisting AIDS: Feminist Strategies of Empowerment.* 1st ed. Philadelphia, PA: Temple University Press, 339.

Strait, S. 1999. Drug use among Hispanic youth: Examining common and unique contributing factors. *Hispanic Journal of Behavioral Sciences* 2(1): 89–103.

UNAIDS. Global report. 2013a. Available at: www.unaids.org/sites/default/files/en/media/unaids/contentassets/documents/unaidspublication/2004/GAR2004_es.pdf [Accessed 15 January 2015].

UNAIDS. 2013b. *Informe nacional sobre los progresos realizados en la aplicacion del UNGASS, Chile, 2012.* Available at: www.unaids.org/en/dataanalysis/knowyourresponse/countryprogressreports/2012countries/ce_CL_Narrative_Report[1].pdf [Accessed 3 January 2013].

Valencia-Garcia, D., Starks, H., Strick, L. and Simoni, J. *et al.* 2008. After the fall from grace: Negotiation of new identities among HIV-positive women in Peru. *Culture, Health & Sexuality* 10(7): 739–752.

Villegas, N., Ferrer, L., Cianelli, R., Miner, S., Lara, L. and Peragallo, N. 2011. Conocimientos y autoeficacia asociados a VIH y SIDA en mujeres Chilenas. *Investigación y Educación en Enfermería* 29(2): 222–292.

Chapter 6

'What does it take to be a man? What is a real man?'

Ideologies of masculinity and HIV sexual risk among Black heterosexual men

Lisa Bowleg, Michelle Teti, Jenne S. Massie, Aditi Patel, David J. Malebranche and Jeanne M. Tschann

Introduction

In the USA, ideologies of masculinity, or culturally endorsed and internalised standards for how boys and men should behave (Pleck *et al.* 1993), include norms or rules for boys and men, such as: have sex with lots of women, endorse negative attitudes towards gay and bisexual men, and hold women responsible for contraception. An abundant theoretical literature posits that these specific ideologies are among those that many Black heterosexual men, particularly low-income young urban men, endorse and enact (Majors and Billson 1992; Whitehead 1997; Wolfe 2003). Although the relationship between gender role ideologies and sexual risk has been a core focus of much of the HIV prevention theory and research focused on women in general (Amaro 1995), and Black heterosexual women in particular (Fullilove *et al.* 1990; Wingood and Diclemente 1998a; Bowleg *et al.* 2000), research on gender ideologies and sexual risk among Black heterosexual men is relatively scarce.

Escalating rates of HIV/AIDS among Black men and women in the USA underscore the importance of understanding how masculinity ideologies may facilitate HIV-related risk in Black communities. Black men represent approximately 13 per cent of the US male population, but in 2006 accounted for 65 per cent of newly reported HIV cases among Blacks (Centers for Disease Control and Prevention [CDC] 2007). Black men also represent 64 per cent of the HIV cases among men attributed to 'high risk heterosexual contact' (CDC 2009: 7).

Advocacy for a greater emphasis on heterosexual men's ideologies of masculinity and sexual risk in general (Kippax *et al.* 1994; Campbell 1995), and those of Black men in particular (Wright 1993, 1997; Bowser 1994), is not new. Although there is a plethora of HIV-prevention-focused research and interventions on the ideologies of masculinity among men in countries such as Brazil, Ethiopia, India, Nicaragua, South Africa, Tanzania and Zimbabwe (Pulerwitz *et al.* 2010), considerable gaps exist in empirical knowledge about how the masculinity ideologies of Black heterosexual men in the USA are associated with increased or decreased HIV risk.

In the USA, Black (Kerrigan *et al.* 2007) and multi-ethnic (Pleck *et al.* 1993) adolescents (36 per cent of whom were Black) and White college students (Noar and Morokoff 2002; Shearer *et al.* 2005; O'Sullivan *et al.* 2006) have been the focus of most of the research on masculinity ideology and HIV risk. These studies document that endorsements of traditional ideologies of masculinity are related to having more sexual partners, less consistent condom use and less belief in male responsibility for contraception (Pleck *et al.* 1993;

O'Sullivan *et al.* 2006) and more negative attitudes towards condoms (Pleck *et al.* 1993; Noar and Morokoff 2002).

Although these studies have advanced knowledge about masculinity ideologies and HIV risk, they may have limited external validity for non-college men or minority ethnic men such as Black heterosexual men (Sue 1999). The few quantitative studies that have included Black heterosexual men have documented links between more traditional ideologies of masculinity and sexual risk (Shearer *et al.* 2005; Santana *et al.* 2006). Findings from qualitative research suggest that it is normative for many Black men to report multiple sex partners (Whitehead 1997; Bowleg 2004; Carey *et al.* 2008; Corneille *et al.* 2008).

To address the gap in empirical knowledge about ideologies of masculinity and sexual HIV risk among Black heterosexual men, we conducted six focus groups with a sample of Black heterosexual men to explore two research questions: (1) What are the explicit (i.e. directly stated) masculinity ideologies that Black heterosexual men express that have implications for sexual HIV risk behaviours?; and (2) What are the implicit (i.e. not directly stated but inferred from our analyses) masculinity ideologies that have implications for Black heterosexual men's sexual HIV risk?

Methods

Participants

Participants were 41 Black men who ranged in age from 19 to 51 years (M = 33.68, SD = 8.42). The sample was socio-economically diverse, with reported annual incomes ranging from less than US$10,000 to US$59,999. Of the 41 participants, 15 (37 per cent) reported annual incomes of less than US$9,999 and 18 (44 per cent) reported annual incomes at or greater than US$20,000. The majority (n = 35, 85 per cent) of the sample reported having at least a high school or General Education Degree (GED). Demographic characteristics of the total sample and by focus group are shown in Table 6.1.

Procedures

We recruited a convenience sample of participants from various venues (e.g. stores, street corners, etc.) in Philadelphia, PA. The venue sites were selected based on US Census block sites with a Black population of at least 50 per cent and as part of the development of a random sampling frame for the quantitative phase of the study focused on the effects of structural factors (e.g. unemployment, incarceration, poverty), sexual scripts and ideologies of masculinity on Black heterosexual men's sexual risk.

Trained recruiters approached Black men who appeared to be at least 18 years old. The study's recruitment postcards invited men to participate in a confidential study about the 'health and sexual experiences of Black men'. Prospective participants were screened by phone to determine whether or not they met the study's eligibility criteria of: identifying as Black/African American, being at least 18 years old and reporting heterosexual intercourse during the last two months. Two trained Black men conducted each of the six focus groups and served as note-takers during the groups. The groups, which were digitally recorded, ranged in length from 70 to 111 minutes and included, on average, seven men. Participants received a US$50 cash incentive. The Institutional Review Board at Drexel University, the primary author's former institution, approved all study procedures.

Table 6.1 Demographic characteristics of focus group (FG) participants

Characteristic	Total sample (n = 41)	FG 1 (n = 6)	FG 2 (n = 8)	FG 3 (n = 6)	FG 4 (n = 6)	FG 5 (n = 8)	FG 6 (n = 7)
	n (%)	n (%)	n (%)	n (%)	n (%)	n (%)	n (%)
Age range	19–51	21–44	19–40	21–44	24–39	26–51	33–44
Age mean	33.68	32.50	31.00	30.17	30.83	38.25	38.00
Age SD	8.42	10.39	8.00	10.27	6.18	8.68	4.40
Annual income range							
Less than $9,999	15(37%)	4(67%)	3(38%)	3(50%)	0(0%)	0(0%)	5(71%)
$10,000–19,999	7(17%)	0(0%)	1(12%)	1(17%)	0(0%)	5(63%)	0(0%)
$20,000–39,999	13(32%)	2(33%)	2(25%)	0(0%)	4(67%)	3(38%)	2(29%)
$40,000–59,999	5(12%)	0(0%)	2(25%)	2(33%)	1(17%)	0(0%)	0(0%)
Employment status							
Work full-time	12(29%)	2(33%)	1(12%)	2(33%)	5(83%)	2(25%)	0(0%)
Work part-time	11(27%)	3(50%)	1(12%)	2(33%)	1(17%)	3(38%)	1(14%)
Unemployed	12(29%)	1(17%)	2(25%)	1(17%)	0(0%)	3(38%)	5(71%)
Disability	5(12%)	0(0%)	3(38%)	1(17%)	0(0%)	0(0%)	1(14%)
Other			1(12%)				
Highest level of education							
Some high school	6(15%)	0(0%)	1(12%)	3(50%)	0(0%)	1(12%)	1(14%)
High school graduate/General Education Degree (GED)	16(39%)	5(83%)	4(50%)	1(17%)	1(17%)	3(38%)	2(29%)
Some college/professional training	15(37%)	1(17%)	2(25%)	2(33%)	3(50%)	3(38%)	4(57%)
College degree	3(7%)	0(0%)	1(12%)	0(0%)	2(33%)	0(0%)	0(0%)
Some Master's work						1(12%)	
Master's degree	1(2%)	0(0%)	0(0%)	0(0%)	0(0%)	0(0%)	0(0%)

Note: n = total number of cases; n = number of cases in a subsample; % = percentage.

Measures

We used the interview guide approach to elicit narratives about the men's lives and experiences, ideologies of masculinity for Black men and sexual risk behaviours. The interview guide approach provides for topics and issues to be outlined in advance and grants facilitators the flexibility to decide the sequence and phrasing of questions (Patton 2002). We chose this approach because we wanted to systematically collect comprehensive responses to specific questions across the study's six focus groups, even if this meant inadvertently missing important topics that participants may have spontaneously raised (Patton 2002).

To lead the discussion about ideologies of masculinity, a Black male facilitator provided each participant with a piece of paper divided into two columns. The first column read 'Black men should …' and the second read 'Black men should not …'. After participants listed their responses individually, the facilitator asked participants to share their responses with the group and wrote all responses on a whiteboard. Thereafter, he facilitated discussion about all of the items on the list, using prompts such as: 'Tell me more about this' and 'What things are not on this list, but should be?' Sample questions about sexual risk asked men to define sex, risky sexual behaviour and rules that Black men had about sex.

After reviewing the transcripts for the first four focus groups, the analysis team agreed that we had reached saturation about sexual risk behaviour. In qualitative research, saturation describes the point at which new themes or ideas cease to arise in the data (Charmaz 2006). It was still unclear, however, whether or not participants in the first four groups perceived the masculinity ideologies that they discussed to be relevant to Black men, a key focus of our research, or to men in general. Given our interest in Black men's ideologies of masculinity, we decided to conduct two additional focus groups to assess this. The guide for these groups included the identical format and sequence of questions about ideologies of masculinity that we had posed in the first four groups, but excluded questions about sexual risk. To be sure that we were capturing Black men's ideologies sufficiently well, after each key question we included the probe: 'Is this experience specific to Black men or men in general?'

Data analysis

Focus group discussions were professionally transcribed, edited for clarity and to remove personal identifiers and then imported into NVivo 8.0, a qualitative data analysis software package. The first and third authors used NVivo 8.0 to manage the data (i.e. import demographic data) and create analyst-generated topic and analytical codes. Topic coding refers to the assignation of labels to specific pieces of text; analytical coding focuses on meaning and interpretation (Richards 2009). To code analytically, analysts wrote memos in NVivo to record their interpretations of the topic codes and the relation of these codes to the study's main research questions. Finally, we created coding matrices, which highlighted codes per focus group, and allowed us to assess the depth and breadth of our topic and analytical codes and interpretations across all of the groups. We assessed the trustworthiness of our analysis as previously described (see Bowleg *et al.* 2004) and determined that our analyses demonstrated credibility, transferability and confirmability (Lincoln and Guba 1985).

Because group dynamics and interactions are a key feature of the focus group method (Seal *et al.* 1998; Krueger and Casey 2000), we highlight in the results specific verbal and non-verbal interactions between participants and between participants and the facilitator. We note when and how participants responded to other speakers verbally and non-verbally; highlight the discussion trail that produced reported findings; and indicate interactions that signalled agreement and disagreement with stated comments, including interruptions, side-talk and laughter.

Results

Across the six focus groups, men engaged in lively discussions about their lives and experiences and societal expectations for them as Black men. Participants reflected often on the many challenges of ideologies of masculinity for Black men, as this narrative from Joe, aged 51, highlights:

> How do we deal with the consequences of being a man in [the Black] community? Especially when it comes to the tough guy image – screwing [having sex with] all the women; all the different women. You know, knocking somebody upside the head when they so-call disrespect you kind of stuff. And sometimes, we fall into our own trap of what does it really mean to be a man. We get that really confused and distorted. And that is a good question: What does it take to be a man? What is a real man?

We present below our findings relevant to the study's two research questions about explicit and implicit ideologies of masculinity and implications for sexual risk behaviours.

Explicit masculinity ideologies and implications for sexual risk behaviours

Our analyses indicated that participants articulated two main ideologies of masculinity: that Black men should have sex with multiple women, often concurrently, and that Black men should not be gay or bisexual. Discussions about both themes were often spirited, with men speaking simultaneously and interrupting each other to make their points.

Sex with multiple women, often concurrently

Recurrent across the six focus groups were discussions about societal expectations for Black heterosexual men to have sex with multiple women, often concurrently. Demonstrating the perceived link between being a Black man and having multiple partners, Mike, aged 29, summarised the issue this way:

> Black men feel like you're not a man unless you have a whole lot of partners, multiple partners, and [that if you do not] have as many so-called freaky [sexually uninhibited] experiences as possible, you're not a man. That's society's expectations on us, and we of course [have] bought into those similar stereotypes.

Participants were especially vocal in endorsing the view that having sex with many women was intrinsic to being a Black heterosexual man. Typical of the conversation was one in which a participant declared emphatically that most Black men would disagree with the notion that 'you can't have no other women'. He, Larry, aged 43, stated: 'Every one of those men that you tell [you can't have no other women] is gonna go outside their circle; at least 99 per cent. What? Are you kiddin' me?' Another man in the group, Nate, aged 29, asked rhetorically: 'What Black heterosexual man don't want all the pussy he can get?' Other men in the group responded to this comment with laughter and general agreement, with Sam, aged 21, chiming in, 'I'll take [sex] in a heartbeat.'

In addition to noting that it was normative for Black men to have sex with many women, some men explained why they had sex with multiple women concurrently. Chris, aged 37, implied that sex ratios, the fact that Black women outnumber Black men, facilitated Black men's abilities to have sex with many different women: 'Bottom line, other women jockeyin' for your position. Remember: Black man is in fucking popular demand.'

Many men described being in emotionally committed relationships with one woman, but noted that they also had other 'jawns' on the side. Jawn is a Philadelphia slang term that can be used to describe a variety of things from inanimate objects to sex partners. Some participants shared their respect and admiration for Black men who had many women. Nate, aged 29, offered that 'the average Black man' who had lots of partners was admired because it suggested that he was a good lover. Will, aged 21, interrupted to challenge this statement by noting that he had 'been with one girl' since coming home from prison.

A similar discussion about respect and admiration for men with multiple female sex partners occurred in a group where Corey, aged 36, noted that Black men who did not have lots of women respected men who did: 'Most men that I know that are real men be like, "Damn, that's what's up! He gets a lot of jawns." Because real men don't hate … Real men look up to [that] dude and give them their props [respect].' Others countered that because sexual female partners were so readily available, the issue of respecting men with multiple sex partners was largely irrelevant. Tommy, aged 19, explained that getting sex was often as simple as placing a phone call:

> [A male friend will call another male friend and say]: 'I know a freak [woman who likes to have sex]. I'll drop her off at your house.' You know? Keep it moving. That's just how it is at our age. You don't look up to nobody [because he's having sex with lots of women]. It's just a phone call.

Black men should not be gay or bisexual: 'a man wasn't made for a man'

The second explicit ideology, articulated across the six focus groups, was that Black men should be heterosexual. Discussions about Black men who have sex with men centred around two key themes: real Black men are heterosexual, not men who have sex with men; and concerns that bisexual men, particularly those considered to be on the 'down low' (a term applied to men who have sex with men and women, but do not identify as gay or bisexual), were vectors of HIV transmission to Black heterosexual communities.

Black men who have sex with men are not real men

Demonstrating the perceived link between heterosexuality and Black masculinity, Richard, aged 38, summed up the norm this way:

> Us, as African-American, Black men, we macho! You know? Manly men. Forts and stuff like meat and potatoes. And for us … we don't want to be represented by some fairy … We talk about being Black men, and they're [gay and bisexual Black men] the antithesis of that. I don't have a problem.

Bisexual men as vectors of transmission

Several discussions focused specifically on bisexual men. Chief among these conversations was the fear that Black men who have sex with men, or as participants frequently referred to them, 'men on the DL [down low]', were vectors of HIV transmission to Black heterosexual communities. Typical were the sentiments of Phil, aged 27, who noted:

And then you have the switch hitters. That's what I call 'em: guys that like men and women. So when people are just having casual sex out here like that, it gets scary because you won't know what the switch got you. And you bringing it in, transmitting diseases and stuff over to the straight community.

'Dangerous' was how another man described Black men who have sex with men who were closeted about their sexual preferences. Echoing this theme, Lloyd, aged 24, said that he worried that he might have sex with a woman who might have had sex with a man who has sex with men:

Because I don't want them to transmit any potential diseases that they might have because of their homosexuality, or because they're promiscuous … I don't know if that's the case or not. But if that is, I just don't wanna be involved in any of that.

Perceptions that Black men who have sex with men were promiscuous were also common, as Floyd, aged 39, in the group opined: 'In terms of brothers on the DL, [they are] just out of control.'

Implicit masculinity ideologies and implications for sexual risk behaviours

To explore the more implicit ideologies of masculinity that have implications for Black heterosexual men's sexual HIV risk, we analysed narratives relevant to sex, sexual risk behaviours and condom use. Our analyses illustrated two key implicit masculinity ideologies: men's perceived inability to decline sex when confronted with their own or a female partner's sexual desire and that women should be responsible for condom use.

Inability to decline sex: sex and women as the 'most powerful thing[s] on Earth'

Across the focus groups, men described instances of being overpowered by their own sexual desire for women or the sexual desire of female partners. A discussion in which James, aged 32, posed this question to his group best exemplified participants' perspectives on this theme: 'What do you think is the most powerful weapon on Earth?' He answered: 'Woman. The most powerful thing on Earth is pussy' – a comment that Don, aged 40, affirmed with: 'A woman. A woman. Without a doubt, a woman.' This perception of perceived inability to overcome sexual desire was a core feature of narratives in which men discussed engaging in sex that they themselves perceived to be risky.

A recurrent theme throughout the focus groups was the notion that sexual desire could be so overpowering that it often robbed men of their agency to use condoms, even with a sexual partner that they perceived to be risky. Many participants noted that they were motivated to use condoms with casual partners to prevent STIs, and especially to prevent the transmission of STIs to their main partners, which would in essence confirm their infidelity. Although most of the men noted that their goal was 'for 100 per cent' condom use with casual partners, many admitted that they often fell short of this goal.

'Weakness' was the term that some men used to describe why they had sometimes engaged in sexual behaviours with casual partners that they knew to be risky; 'laziness' was the term that others invoked. Asked by the focus group facilitator whether the group perceived that 'a lot of Black men take risks [of not using condoms with casual partners]', some men laughed or uttered 'Mmm-hmms'. Andrew, aged 28, illustrated how a man's sexual arousal could readily thwart his best intentions to use a condom:

> Like, you could plan to use a Trojan. Like you could have a Trojan anything, or she could have one … You [get] … heated you know … and y'all whatever kissing and whatever … like grinding, whatever the situation is. And stuff … clothes start coming off, like – but your intention was to strap up [put on a condom], but you got heated! Like, shit happens.

Women should be responsible for condom use

The second implicit ideology that men across the groups articulated was the notion that women, rather than men, should be responsible for condom use. The flip side of this ideology was that men also blamed women for the lack of condom use. Across the groups, men discussed instances of not using condoms in ways that absolved them of their responsibility for condom use. As Mike, aged 29, explained, women sometimes requested that men not use condoms in casual encounters, a request with which some men unquestioningly complied:

> No, we don't talk about condoms much [with casual partners]. Not me. I never raise it. Before we had sex it's like [she says], 'Yo, take off the condom', or, 'You ain't gonna use the condom.' It's like, rarely do I ever have a girl that say, 'Here you go [use this condom]' before we even get down [start having sex].

Other men were unanimous in their assertion that 'A lot of [women] don't say nothin' [about using condoms]. They don't care,' chimed in Kevin, aged 26: 'They don't care and that could stop a lotta of the issues [in terms of the transmission of STIs].' High rates of pregnancy provided further proof, some men noted, of women's silent assent to not use condoms. For example, although Phil, aged 27, called using condoms a 'necessity for most [women]', Andrew, aged 28, refuted this comment by noting that, 'Well, basically the way I look at it right now, like, [women] ain't saying too much,' 'cause every time you turn around, they're pregnant.' Echoing this theme, Evan, aged 41, said that the topic of using condoms rarely arose: 'Nope [the topic of condoms] don't [come up]; it mostly, it's mostly everybody around the hood in South Philly … got a baby mom.'

Charles, aged 31, noted that a woman who did not ask about condoms made him anxious about STIs: 'If she don't wanna [use condoms, if] she just wants you to pound at her … now you cautious, you know what I'm saying. You don't know what to think now. You're like, "Dang. She ain't gonna ask [about condoms]?" ' This comment elicited what appeared to be nervous laughter from other men in the group, as if they too had found themselves faced with the option of having sex with a woman whom they suspected might be risky.

Some men said that they denied their HIV risk by hoping, as one man explained, 'that [contracting an STI] won't happen to me'. Men who had had these experiences described them as being fraught with anxiety. 'It bad to go to bed haunted' was the way that the same man described the aftermath of having unprotected sex with a woman he suspected might have an STI.

Some participants also perceived that women's use of substances or involvement in exchange sex also influenced women's lack of interest in using condoms, as Andrew, aged 28, opined:

A lot of these females today is about money. So, like, you could get girl for a couple of hours like sometimes, sometimes, you probably don't even got to put no Trojan on, she don't even care. Like real rap. And they get so high these days now, right? They taking all kinds of pills, smoking weed, dust, wet [PCP] – whatever. So they stuck already. Like, some of them don't even look at you, see if you got a Trojan on, you know what I mean?

Narratives of men leaving condom use to the women's volition were not unanimous, however. Some men noted that a woman's disinterest in condom use signalled danger either of the woman's desire for greater emotional intimacy, pregnancy or that she might have an STI. A handful of men discussed how they had declined to have sex with women who did not want to use condoms. Adam, aged 21, recounted how a woman had told him that she was allergic to condoms. His response: 'I never bopped [had sex with] her, man ... I just nipped it in the bud 'cause I couldn't trust it, know what I'm sayin'?'

Discussion

This study provides insights into both explicit and implicit masculinity ideologies that may be associated with sexual risk for a sample of Black heterosexual men in Philadelphia. Explicit ideologies of masculinity included that Black men should have sex with multiple women, often concurrently, and not be gay or bisexual. Implicit masculinity ideologies included the perception that Black men lack the agency to use condoms when confronted with their own or a female partner's sexual desire, and that women should be responsible for condom use.

The ideology of masculinity that men are socialised to have more non-relational attitudes to sex compared with women is not new (see Levant 1997). An abundant empirical base documents that men, regardless of race, ethnicity and nationality, affirm the masculinity ideology that men should have sex with multiple women (see Schwarz et al. 2008). Black men's endorsement of this ideology in the context of the HIV epidemic, however, has grave consequences for heterosexually transmitted HIV in Black communities. Several factors underscore the need to address this ideology in HIV prevention, including that: the virus is more efficiently transmitted from men to women (Nicolosi et al. 1994); Black men are disproportionately represented among men with HIV (CDC 2009); and that young Black men with three or more sexual partners are more likely than those with two or fewer partners to use condoms incorrectly (Crosby et al. 2008).

Participants' affirmation of the ideology that men should have multiple sexual partners echoes the findings of other qualitative HIV prevention research with Black heterosexual adolescents (Kerrigan et al. 2007), men (Whitehead 1997; Aronson et al. 2003; Bowleg 2004; Corneille et al. 2008) and women (Bowleg et al. 2004), as well as a recent study on sexual partner concurrency among urban Black men recruited from an STI clinic (Carey et al. 2008). Yet, theory and research on sexual concurrency with adult heterosexual men in the USA is relatively rare (for exceptions see Adimora et al. 2006, 2007; Carey et al. 2008) compared with the plethora of theory and research on heterosexual sexual concurrency among men in sub-Saharan Africa (e.g. Epstein 2010; Lurie and Rosenthal 2010a, 2010b; Mah and Halperin 2010a, 2010b).

There was also consensus across the focus groups regarding negative attitudes towards Black gay and bisexual men. This is a consistent finding in research on masculinity in general

(Levant and Fischer 1998; Levant et al. 2007), and on Black masculinity in particular (Lemelle and Battle 2004). Heterosexism is a defining element of masculinity for many heterosexual men (Herek 1986; Kimmel 1994). Some of our participants' narratives reinforce previous scholarship about how heterosexism functions to define who men are (and are not) in Black communities (Thomas 1996; Lemelle and Battle 2004; Ward 2005). The conflation of Black masculinity and heterosexuality has implications for HIV risk because it may motivate some Black men to have sex with multiple women to prove their heterosexuality (Ward 2005). It may also encourage some Black men to conceal their same-sex relationships for fear of stigmatisation (McKeown et al. 2010). Critically needed are interventions to change heterosexist norms that equate heterosexuality and masculinity for Black men.

Our study also underscores the importance of understanding implicit ideologies of masculinity, those that Black heterosexual men may not directly articulate, but that nonetheless may shape sexual HIV risk behaviours. The notion that sexual desire can overpower men's intentions to use condoms is empirically well documented with multi-ethnic populations of men who have sex with men (see Diaz and Ayala 1999; Malebranche et al. 2009) and heterosexual men (see Flood 2003; Bancroft et al. 2004; Bowleg 2004). A troubling finding in our research, however, was the tendency for some men to note that they persisted in having sex even when they perceived that doing so might increase their risk of HIV. This finding suggests numerous avenues for intervention, including, but not limited to, explicitly addressing and challenging this ideology in health and sexuality programmes and HIV prevention messages targeted to Black boys and men. The female sexual partners of men who persist in having sex despite perceived HIV risk would also benefit from interventions that educate them about this tendency, highlight their increased risk and teach them strategies to successfully negotiate and use condoms with such partners. Equally noteworthy was the tendency for many (and it is important to note, not all) men to eschew responsibility for condom use in casual sexual encounters, with no apparent sense of their own agency in using condoms. This finding underscores the need for interventions to emphasise men's responsibility for condom use.

Indeed, our research highlights several opportunities for intervention with Black heterosexual men using ideologies of masculinity as a theoretical framework. As we have already noted, changing ideologies of masculinity has been the central focus of global HIV prevention work for heterosexual male adolescents and men, but not for men in the USA (Seal and Ehrhardt 2004; Dworkin et al. 2009; Pulerwitz et al. 2010). Results from Project H, for example, a programme in Brazil, showed the promise of gender-based interventions for heterosexual men. Designed to change inequitable gender ideologies (e.g. that men should have multiple partners, control female partners) among young men between the ages of 14 and 25 in three low-income communities in Rio de Janeiro, Brazil, results demonstrated increases in men's endorsing equitable gender role norms, increases in condom use, increased communication about HIV with partners, and decreases in STI symptoms (Pulerwitz et al. 2006; Pulerwitz and Barker 2008).

Not only are HIV prevention interventions targeted specifically to Black heterosexual men in the USA rare (Darbes et al. 2008), we are aware of only two that incorporate some aspect of masculinity ideologies (see Kalichman et al. 1999; Operario et al. 2010) and none that feature changing ideologies of masculinity as a core element. In contrast, changing women's traditional gender ideologies is a key component in many HIV prevention interventions for Black women in the USA (Wingood and DiClemente 1998b, 2000; Dworkin et al. 2009).

Incorporating structural approaches to masculinity-focused interventions is also important. A recurrent theme in much of the theoretical (J.W. Wright 1993; Bowser 1994; J. Wright 1997) and some empirical work (Whitehead 1997) on Black heterosexual men's sexual HIV risk is that the structural context of Black men's lives may shape Black masculinity in ways that may increase HIV risk. Black men are disproportionately represented among men who are unemployed (Bureau of Labor Statistics 2009), poor (DeNavas-Walt *et al.* 2009) and incarcerated (Sabol *et al.* 2009). Denied access to the ideologies of masculinity that equate manliness with financial achievement, some Black low-income men may compensate instead by focusing on the norms that they can fulfil: masculinity through having sex with multiple women, concurrently (Whitehead 1997).

The contributions of our research to advancing knowledge about explicit and implicit Black ideologies of masculinity and implications for HIV risk notwithstanding, this study has several limitations. Among them are that the sampling and qualitative methods that we used do not allow generalisation beyond the study's sample. Another limitation is that the group setting may have motivated men to express more socially desirable norms, such as that Black men should have sex with multiple women or that Black men should not be gay or bisexual. Finally, although we draw inferences about the association between particular ideologies and the men's self-reported sexual risk behaviours, our focus group guide did not include specific questions about this link, something that future studies could do.

At the end of one focus group, Joe mused: 'That is a good question: What does it take to be a man? What is a real man?' The voices of the men in our study illustrate that the answer to this question is multifaceted, complex, dependent on structural context and dynamic. We echo the call of other scholars who advocate for heterosexual men to be partners in HIV prevention and for a focus on ideologies of masculinity to be integrated with HIV prevention research and interventions (Higgins *et al.* 2010; Pulerwitz *et al.* 2010). Preventing HIV in Black communities, our research suggests, may lie somewhere between understanding Black heterosexual men's explicit and implicit ideologies of masculinity and the structural contexts that shape these ideologies, and developing culturally grounded interventions that challenge and change ideologies that increase sexual risk in Black communities in the USA.

References

Adimora, A.A., Schoenbach, V.J. and Doherty, I.A. 2007. Concurrent sexual partnerships among men in the United States. *American Journal of Public Health* 97(12): 2230–2237.

Adimora, A.A., Schoenbach, V.J., Martinson, F.E., Coyne-Beasley, T., Doherty, I., Stancil, T.R. and Fullilove, R.E. 2006. Heterosexually transmitted HIV infection among African Americans in North Carolina. *Journal of Acquired Immune Deficiency Syndromes* 41(5): 616–623.

Amaro, H. 1995. Love, sex and power: Considering women's realities in HIV prevention. *American Psychologist* 50: 437–447.

Aronson, R.E., Whitehead, T.L. and Baber, W.L. 2003. Challenges to masculine transformation among urban low-income African American males. *American Journal of Public Health* 93(5): 732–741.

Bancroft, J., Janssen, E., Carnes, L., Goodrich, D., Strong, D. and Long, J.S. 2004. Sexual activity and risk taking in young heterosexual men: The relevance of sexual arousability, mood and sensation seeking. *Journal of Sex Research* 41(2): 181–192.

Bowleg, L. 2004. Love, sex and masculinity in sociocultural context: HIV concerns and condom use among African American men in heterosexual relationships. *Men & Masculinities* 7: 166–186.

Bowleg, L., Belgrave, F.Z. and Reisen, C.A. 2000. Gender roles, power strategies and precautionary sexual self-efficacy: Implications for Black and Latina women's HIV/AIDS protective behaviors. *Sex Roles* 42(7–8): 613–635.

Bowleg, L., Lucas, K.J. and Tschann, J.M. 2004. 'The ball was always in his court': An exploratory analysis of relationship scripts, sexual scripts and condom use among African American women. *Psychology of Women Quarterly* 28: 70–82.

Bowser, B.P. 1994. Black men and AIDS: Prevention and Black sexuality. In: R.G. Majors and J.U. Gordon (eds) *The American Black Male: His Present Status and his Future*. Chicago, IL: Nelson-Hall, 115–126.

Bureau of Labor Statistics. 2009. *The Employment Situation, November 2009*. Washington, DC: US Department of Labor.

Campbell, C.A. 1995. Male gender roles and sexuality: Implications for women's AIDS risk and prevention. *Social Science & Medicine* 41(2): 197–210.

Carey, M.P., Senn, T.E., Seward, D.X. and Vanable, P.A. 2008. Urban African-American men speak out on sexual partner concurrency: Findings from a qualitative study. *AIDS & Behavior* 14(1): 38–47.

Centers for Disease Control and Prevention (CDC). 2007. *CDC HIV/AIDS Fact Sheet: HIV/AIDS among African Americans*. Atlanta, GA: US Department of Health and Human Services, Centers for Disease Control and Prevention.

Centers for Disease Control and Prevention (CDC). 2009. *HIV/AIDS Surveillance Report, 2007*. Atlanta, GA: US Department of Health and Human Services, Centers for Disease Control and Prevention.

Charmaz, K. 2006. *Constructing Grounded Theory: A Practical Guide through Qualitative Analysis*. Thousand Oaks, CA: SAGE.

Corneille, M.A., Tademy, R.H., Reid, M.C., Belgrave, F.Z. and Nasim, A. 2008. Sexual safety and risk taking among African American men who have sex with women: A qualitative study. *Psychology of Men & Masculinity* 9(4): 207–220.

Crosby, R.A., Diclemente, R.J., Yarber, W.L., Snow, G. and Troutman, A. 2008. Young African American men having sex with multiple partners are more likely to use condoms incorrectly: A clinic-based study. *American Journal of Men's Health* 2(4): 340–343.

Darbes, L., Crepaz, N., Lyles, C., Kennedy, G. and Rutherford, G. 2008. The efficacy of behavioral interventions in reducing HIV risk behaviors and incident sexually transmitted diseases in heterosexual African Americans. *AIDS* 22(10): 1177–1194.

DeNavas-Walt, C., Proctor, B.D. and Smith, J.C. 2009. *Income, Poverty and Health Insurance Coverage in the United States, 2008*. US Census Bureau. Washington, DC: US Government Printing Office.

Diaz, R.M. and Ayala, G. 1999. Love, passion and rebellion: Ideologies of HIV risk among Latino gay men in the USA. *Culture, Health & Sexuality* 1(3): 277–293.

Dworkin, S.L., Fullilove, R.E. and Peacock, D. 2009. Are HIV/AIDS prevention interventions for heterosexually active men in the United States gender-specific? *American Journal of Public Health* 99(6): 981–984.

Epstein, H. 2010. The mathematics of concurrent partnerships and HIV: A commentary on Lurie and Rosenthal, 2009. *AIDS & Behavior* 14(1): 29–30.

Flood, M. 2003. Lust, trust and latex: Why young heterosexual men do not use condoms. *Culture, Health & Sexuality* 5(4): 353–369.

Fullilove, M.T., Fullilove, R.E., Haynes, K. and Gross, S. 1990. Black women and AIDS prevention: A view towards understanding the gender rules. *Journal of Sex Research* 27: 47–64.

Herek, G.M. 1986. On heterosexual masculinity: Some psychical consequences of the social construction of gender and sexuality. *American Behavioral Scientist* 29: 563–577.

Higgins, J.A., Hoffman, S. and Dworkin, S.L. 2010. Rethinking gender, heterosexual men and women's vulnerability to HIV/AIDS. *American Journal of Public Health* 100(3): 435–445.

Kalichman, S.C., Cherry, C. and Browne-Sperling, F. 1999. Effectiveness of a video-based motivational skills-building HIV risk-reduction intervention for inner-city African American men. *Journal of Consulting and Clinical Psychology* 67(6): 959–966.

Kerrigan, D., Andrinopoulos, K., Johnson, R., Parham, P., Thomas, T. and Ellen, J.M. 2007. Staying strong: Gender ideologies among African-American adolescents and the implications for HIV/STI prevention. *Journal of Sex Research* 44(2): 172–180.

Kimmel, M.S. 1994. Masculinity as homophobia: Fear, shame and silence in the construction of gender identity. In: H. Broad and M. Kaufman (eds) *Theorizing Masculinities*. Thousand Oaks, CA: SAGE, 119–141.

Kippax, S., Crawford, J. and Waldby, C. 1994. Heterosexuality, masculinity and HIV. *AIDS* 8: S315–323.

Krueger, R. and Casey, M.A. 2000. *Focus Groups: A Practical Guide for Applied Research*. 3rd ed. Thousand Oaks, CA: SAGE.

Lemelle, A.J. and Battle, J. 2004. Black masculinity matters in attitudes toward gay males. *Journal of Homosexuality* 47(1): 39–51.

Levant, R.F. 1997. Non-relational sexuality in men. In: F. Levant and G.R. Brooks (eds) *Men and Sex: New Psychological Perspectives*. New York: John Wiley & Sons, 9–27.

Levant, R.F. and Fischer, J. 1998. The Male Role Norms Inventory. In: M. Davis, W.H. Yarber, R. Bauserman, G. Schreer and S.L. Davis (eds) *Sexuality-related Measures: A Compendium*. Newbury Park, CA: SAGE, 469–472.

Levant, R.F., Smalley, K., Aupont, M., House, A., Richmond, K. and Noronha, D. 2007. Initial validation of the Male Role Norms Inventory-revised (MRNI-r). *Journal of Men's Studies* 15(1): 83–100.

Lincoln, Y.S. and Guba, E.G. 1985. *Naturalistic Inquiry*. Beverly Hills, CA: SAGE.

Lurie, M.N. and Rosenthal, S. 2010a. The concurrency hypothesis in sub-Saharan Africa: Convincing empirical evidence is still lacking. Response to Mah and Halperin, Epstein and Morris. *AIDS & Behavior* 14(1): 34–37.

Lurie, M.N. and Rosenthal, S. 2010b. Concurrent partnerships as a driver of the HIV epidemic in sub-Saharan Africa? The evidence is limited. *AIDS & Behavior* 14(1): 17–24.

Mah, T.L. and Halperin, D.T. 2010a. Concurrent sexual partnerships and the HIV epidemics in Africa: Evidence to move forward. *AIDS & Behavior* 14(1): 11–16.

Mah, T.L. and Halperin, D.T. 2010b. The evidence for the role of concurrent partnerships in Africa's HIV epidemics: A response to Lurie and Rosenthal. *AIDS & Behavior* 14(1): 25–28.

Majors, R. and Billson, J.M. 1992. *Cool Pose: The Dilemmas of Black Manhood in America*. New York: Lexington Books.

Malebranche, D.J., Fields, E.L., Bryant, L.O. and Harper, S.R. 2009. Masculine socialization and sexual risk behaviors among Black men who have sex with men: A qualitative exploration. *Men and Masculinities* 12(1): 90–112.

McKeown, E., Nelson, S., Anderson, J., Low, N. and Elford, J. 2010. Disclosure, discrimination and desire: Experiences of Black and South Asian gay men in Britain. *Culture, Health & Sexuality* 12(7): 843–856.

Nicolosi, A., Correa Leite, M.L., Musicco, M., Arici, C., Gavazzeni, G. and Lazzarin, A. 1994. The efficiency of male-to-female and female-to-male sexual transmission of the human immunodeficiency virus: A study of 730 stable couples. Italian study group on HIV heterosexual transmission. *Epidemiology* 5(6): 570–575.

Noar, S.M. and Morokoff, P.J. 2002. The relationship between masculinity ideology, condom attitudes and condom use stage of change: A structural equation modeling approach. *International Journal of Men's Health* 1(1): 43–58.

O'Sullivan, L.F., Hoffman, S., Harrison, A. and Dolezal, C. 2006. Men, multiple sexual partners and young adults' sexual relationships: Understanding the role of gender in the study of risk. *Journal of Urban Health* 83(4): 695–708.

Operario, D., Smith, C.D., Arnold, E. and Kegeles, S. 2010. The Bruthas Project: Evaluation of a community-based HIV prevention intervention for African American men who have sex with men and women. *AIDS Education and Prevention* 22(1): 37–48.

Patton, M.Q. 2002. *Qualitative Research and Evaluation Methods*. 3rd ed. Thousand Oaks, CA: SAGE.

Pleck, J.H., Sonenstein, F.L. and Ku, L.C. 1993. Masculinity ideology: Its impact on adolescent males' heterosexual relationships. *Journal of Social Issues* 49(3): 11–29.

Pulerwitz, J. and Barker, G. 2008. Measuring attitudes toward gender norms among young men in Brazil: Development and psychometric evaluation of the GEM scale. *Men and Masculinities* 10: 322–338.

Pulerwitz, J., Barker, G., Segundo, M. and Nascimento, M. 2006. Promoting gender-equity among young Brazilian men as an HIV prevention strategy. In: *Horizons Research Summary*. Washington, DC: Population Council/Horizons, 1–8.

Pulerwitz, J., Michaelis, A., Verma, R. and Weiss, E. 2010. Addressing gender dynamics and engaging men in HIV programs: Lessons learned from horizons research. *Public Health Reports* 125: 282–292.

Richards, L. 2009. *Handling Qualitative Data: A Practical Guide*. 2nd ed. Los Angeles, CA: SAGE.

Sabol, W.J., West, H.C. and Cooper, M. 2009. *Prisoners in 2008. Bureau of Justice Statistics Bulletin*. Washington, DC: US Department of Justice.

Santana, M.C., Raj, A., Decker, M.R., La Marche, A. and Silverman, J.G. 2006. Masculine gender roles associated with increased sexual risk and intimate partner violence perpetration among young adult men. *Journal of Urban Health* 83(4): 575–585.

Schwarz, D., Feyler, N., Cella, J. and Brady, K. 2008. *HIV/AIDS in the City of Philadelphia, 2008 Report*. Philadelphia, PA: AIDS Activities Coordinating Office, Philadelphia Department of Public Health.

Seal, D.W. and Ehrhardt, A.A. 2004. HIV-prevention-related sexual health promotion for heterosexual men in the United States: Pitfalls and recommendations. *Archives of Sexual Behavior* 33(3): 211–222.

Seal, D.W., Bogart, L.M. and Ehrhardt, A.A. 1998. Small group dynamics: The utility of focus group discussions as a research method. *Group Dynamics. Special Research Methods* 2(4): 253–266.

Shearer, C.L., Hosterman, S.J., Gillen, M.M. and Lefkowitz, E.S. 2005. Are traditional gender role attitudes associated with risky sexual behavior and condom-related beliefs? *Sex Roles* 52(5–6): 311–324.

Sue, S. 1999. Science, ethnicity and bias: Where have we gone wrong? *American Psychologist* 54(12): 1070–1077.

Thomas, K. 1996. Ain't nothin' like the real thing: Black masculinity, gay sexuality and the jargon of authenticity. In: M. Blount and G.P. Cunningham (eds) *Representing Black Men*. New York: Routledge, 55–69.

Ward, E.G. 2005. Homophobia, hypermasculinity and the US Black church. *Culture, Health & Sexuality* 7(5): 493–504.

Whitehead, T.L. 1997. Urban low-income African American men, HIV/AIDS and gender identity. *Medical Anthropology Quarterly* 11(4): 411–447.

Wingood, G.M. and Diclemente, R.J. 1998a. Gender-related correlates and predictors of consistent condom use among young adult African-American women: A prospective analysis. *International Journal of STD and AIDS* 9(3): 139–145.

Wingood, G.M. and Diclemente, R.J. 1998b. Partner influences and gender-related factors associated with non-condom use among young adult African American women. *American Journal of Community Psychology* 26(1): 29–51.

Wingood, G.M. and Diclemente, R.J. 2000. Application of the theory of gender and power to examine HIV-related exposures, risk factors and effective interventions for women. *Health Education & Behavior* 27(5): 539–565.

Wolfe, W.A. 2003. Overlooked role of African-American males' hypermasculinity in the epidemic of unintended pregnancies and HIV/AIDS cases with young African-American women. *Journal of the National Medical Association* 95(9): 846–852.

Wright, J. 1997. African American males and HIV: The challenge of the AIDS epidemic. *Medical Anthropology Quarterly* 11(4): 454–455.

Wright, J.W. 1993. African-American male sexual behavior and the risk for HIV infection. *Human Organization* 52(4): 421–431.

Chapter 7

'I just need to be flashy on campus'

Female students and transactional sex at a university in Zimbabwe

Tsitsi B. Masvawure

Introduction

On 15 July 2007, the Zimbabwean government-owned daily press, *The Herald*, carried a story with the headline, 'When love turns sour', of a sugar daddy whose car was set alight by University of Zimbabwe (UZ) students. Here is a short excerpt from the article:

> 'When love turns sour, it is like buttermilk. The more you shake it, it spills out of the churn and the more it gets sour' [*sic*], a philosopher once said. This is what a sugar daddy, a respectable member of his church, recently experienced at the University of Zimbabwe, after his Toyota Camry was reduced to a shell by unruly students, following a dispute that he had with his young varsity girlfriend [*sic*]. The sugar daddy is believed to be in his 40s and has been a headmaster of several schools while his lover, young enough to be his daughter, was a final year student.

An eyewitness is quoted as saying: 'The girl's room … was the most beautifully furnished room on the UZ campus. She had gadgets like a microwave, television and DVD player while she wore trendy clothes bought by her "old" boyfriend.' This dramatic incident was also reported on national TV (ZTV), on the main 8 pm news, a day after the event. The manner in which the incident was reported encapsulates how many people view these relationships. In the press report, the focus is on the age and wealth disparities between the sugar daddy and the female student, as well as on the material resources that are said to have flowed from the man to the young woman.

In this chapter, I argue that the 'transactions' that constitute transactional sex are complex and involve more than just straightforward exchanges in which 'women give men sex' and 'men give women money'. My intention is twofold: first, to examine what is transacted (or exchanged) in transactional sex, other than – or in addition to – sex and money; and second, to examine how the transacting parties manage the 'exchange' relationship. Existing scholarship on transactional sex in Africa links the practice almost exclusively to economic survival (Chatterji *et al.* 2004; Luke and Kurz 2002) and, in doing so, often portrays the women involved as victims. However, as I will show, young women sometimes enter into transactional sex for reasons that have very little to do with survival or subsistence. In this study, for instance, female students from lower middle-class backgrounds used transactional sex to attain an otherwise elusive modern lifestyle, while those from upper middle-class backgrounds used it to maintain an already privileged class position. For yet others, transactional sex spared them from having to manage the usual encumbrances of emotional commitment and sexual exclusiveness associated with standard boyfriend/girlfriend relationships. Ultimately, many exercised considerable agency and employed a variety of strategies to benefit maximally from transactional sex.

Literature review

The existing literature on transactional sex (e.g. Dunkle *et al.* 2004; Longfield *et al.* 2004; Machel 2001) is based on a number of problematic assumptions. The first is the simplistic view that money and sex are the only objects exchanged in transactional sex. Here, it is useful to refer back to Luise White's (1986) influential work on female prostitution in 1980s Nairobi. White showed that even a seemingly straightforward practice like prostitution often entailed much more than the simple exchange of money and sex. '[I]n addition to providing sexual services,' White argued, 'prostitutes in Nairobi also routinely provid[ed] bedspace, cooking, cleaning, bath water, companionship, hot meals, cold meals and tea' (256). She famously termed these non-sexual services 'the comforts of home' in the title of her book (White 1990), and argued that these non-sexual services were usually just as important, to the men concerned, as the actual sex itself.

The second assumption is that intimate relationships that entail monetary and/or material exchanges are necessarily exploitative (Maganja *et al.* 2007). In reality, the 'intimate' and the 'material' straddle each other in ways that make it impossible (if not meaningless) to separate the two. Anthropologists Hunter (2002) and Wojcicki (2002), both writing on sex-for-money relationships in South Africa, argue, for instance, that the exchange of material goods is commonly used as an indicator of partner commitment in much of Africa. The transfer of material goods from a man to a woman is therefore crucial rather than inimical to many intimate relations.

A clear example of this are bridewealth payments, which can be argued to be, in part, a test of a prospective groom's ability to provide materially for his future wife and family, as much as they also facilitate the transfer of uxorial and genetricial rights between the parties involved. In a study of transactional sex among women fish traders in Malawi, Swidler and Watkins (2006) argue that these relationships are part of broader 'systems of interdependence that characterize African societies' and in which 'women need patrons to provide for them [while] men need clients who provide them with an outlet for the display of power, prestige and social dominance' (12). The authors suggest that transactional sex is therefore a corrupted form of such patron–client relationships, which they insist are of much greater importance to most Malawians than the monetary and sexual exchanges themselves. Transactional sex for the women fish traders thus acts as a much-needed social safety net. In fact, despite a long theoretical tradition of dividing intimate and material spheres (Zelizer 2005), their entanglement is not unique to Africa or to so-called developing country contexts (see Poulin 2007).

The third assumption views transactional sex through a single, narrow lens: as a survival strategy of economically disadvantaged women (Meekers and Calves 1997; Pettifor *et al.* 2000). While this is certainly true in many Zimbabwean cases (see Matshalaga 1999; Muparamoto and Chigwenya 2009; Muzvidziwa 2002), especially given the country's incessantly shrinking economy, it does not explain why relatively well-off young women – such as the university students in question – engage in the practice. For them, and indeed for many women, decisions are often motivated by the desire for conspicuous consumption, not subsistence. A comparative study conducted by Moore *et al.* (2007) in four African countries, namely Malawi, Uganda, Ghana and Burkina Faso, found no significant differences by household economic status, orphan status or level of education with regards to which young women were more likely to receive money in exchange for sex in any of these countries (see also Iversen 2005; Kaufman and Stavros 2004). Hunter (2002: 114) identifies two main types of transactional sex in South Africa: 'sex linked to subsistence' (for which poverty is a key factor) and 'sex linked to consumption' (for which poverty is not a key factor). Wojcicki (2002) makes a similar distinction, but adopts the terms informal sex and survival sex to differentiate between sex-for-money exchanges that are culturally acceptable and those that are linked to poverty, respectively.

A paper by Bene and Merten (2008) further illustrates these multiple meanings of transactional sex in Africa. The authors focus on women fish traders in different African countries and show how 'fish-for-sex' is resorted to both as a short-term survival strategy in times of economic crisis and as a longer-term business strategy for profit maximisation. The women fish traders in question establish temporary marriages with fishermen as a way of assuring themselves of an uninterrupted supply of fish, particularly during periods when fish are scarce and competition among traders is extremely high. These temporary marriages are not confined to periods of economic hardship, but are incorporated into the women fish traders' long-term business strategies (cf. Muzvidziwa 2002). This suggests that in some cases, even after subsistence needs have been met, these relationships will not necessarily be terminated but will be maintained in order to fulfil other, non-survival needs.

Methodology

This chapter is based on ethnographic fieldwork conducted at the UZ campus over a 16-month period from August 2006 to December 2007. In-depth interviews were conducted with ten female students, six of whom were involved in transactional sex relationships at the time of the interview and three of whom were not in a transactional sex relationship at the time of the interview, but had been since joining the university. The last had never been involved in transactional sex, but had close friends who had. In-depth interviews were also conducted with four male students who were actively involved in facilitating the formation of transactional sex relationships between female students and wealthy non-university men. Through these interviews, insights were obtained into some of the reasons why men engage in transactional sex.

During fieldwork, I was hosted by an HIV-prevention organisation, SHAPE Zimbabwe Trust, which is based at the campus. SHAPE Zimbabwe Trust has been implementing its HIV-prevention programme at UZ since 2001 and, at the time of the fieldwork, it had a large student following of 500 registered students, known as 'SHAPE Members'. I spent my first 6 months of fieldwork operating from the SHAPE offices and interacting closely with SHAPE Members, including attending SHAPE Club events and meetings. The remaining 9 months I spent operating from students' residences and the other social spaces of the university campus (e.g. the bus terminus, sports fields, common rooms, etc.). This gave me access to other students who were not part of the SHAPE programme. I thus relied on students I already knew to refer me to their friends and classmates.

Zimbabwe's economic crisis and the University of Zimbabwe

UZ is the oldest university in the country and was established in 1955. After independence in 1980, UZ opened its doors to accommodate more Black students (see Gaidzanwa 2007). In 2005, there were approximately 14,000 undergraduate students enrolled, of whom 30 per cent were female (Terry *et al.* 2006). UZ is a residential campus and is located in an affluent area of the capital city Harare. As a public institution, UZ has largely attracted students from poor urban working-class and poor rural backgrounds (Bennell and Ncube 1994). Like most Zimbabweans, UZ students have been deeply affected by the country's ongoing economic crisis. For instance, prior to 1998 all students could apply for full government funding, of which 75 per cent was given as a loan to be paid back upon securing employment. In 1998, the government decided to privatise certain aspects of university education. It thus introduced a policy whereby students had to meet 50 per cent of their university expenses. By late 2006, the situation had become worse. Many students could not afford to take care of their subsistence needs for a whole semester and so the university authorities decided that they should be made to pay for their meals in advance, at the start of each semester. In August 2006, resident students were charged Z$40 million (then the equivalent of USD27) for accommodation and food per semester (16 weeks). By February 2007, this amount had shot up to Z$365 million (USD19 at the new prevailing rate), again due to inflation. Most students, however, had received government grants of just Z$1 million for the same semester. In June 2007, dining halls on campus ran out of food – the result of a combination of hyperinflation and price-control-induced shortages. Lecturers fared no better, with professors taking home salaries of USD50 a month (Gaidzanwa 2007). Nevertheless, even in this dire economic context, many individuals thrived by playing into the possibilities opened up by the parallel market, such as trading in scarce foreign currency and fuel. One student I knew sold mobile phone airtime vouchers, converted the money he made into foreign currency and saved enough to pay for his tuition and accommodation fees. Access to foreign currency – however obtained – opened up unforeseen avenues for accumulation and ensured that one was cushioned from the negative effects of hyperinflation. The ability to thrive in an economic crisis in these ways is not unusual, as in times of economic crisis money can often be easily made by being in the right place and at the right time, rather than through hard work.

Study findings

Transactional sex, NABAs and Big Dharas at the University of Zimbabwe

Transactional sex at UZ is popularly referred to as Big *Dhara* or NABA relationships. The term *dhara* is a slang derivative from the Shona word *mudhara*, which is used to refer to elderly men. The term 'Big *Dhara*', as used by most Zimbabweans, draws attention to the ages of these men, on the one hand, and to their socio-economic status and physical attributes, on the other. Most Big *Dharas* are quite portly and seem literally to carry their wealth on their persons. Often, the 'portliest' Big *Dharas* often drive the latest 'Mercs' (Mercedes Benz) and are chauffeured around. The use of the term Big *Dhara* to refer to sugar daddies has only recently entered the general parlance, while the term sugar daddy has been in use since the mid-1990s.

In contrast, the acronym NABA (which stands for Non-Academic Bachelor's Association) is a UZ-specific term that is used by students to refer to any man who is not a university student. Although the term encompasses male alumni from UZ (hence a recent 20-something graduate is also referred to as a NABA), it is usually used scathingly to refer to all 'outside' men who visit the university. Therefore, while a NABA is also typically constructed as an older and wealthy man, of dubious intellectual capacity and who dates female students, the term is not synonymous with Big *Dhara*. The latter is reserved for politicians, government ministers, businessmen and directors of non-governmental organisations (NGOs), who are viewed as being considerably wealthier than NABAs. This distinction is usually contained in the question 'Is her NABA a Big *Dhara*?', which students use often during conversations on the topic.

'Flashiness' and prestige-making

> I can't really say it was financial 'cos my parents can provide. It's just this thing, you know. It's whereby you tell yourself like I've got money but I can't use it to buy takeaways. I've got better things to buy … So, if somebody is there, who will buy the takeaway for me, why not?
>
> (Samantha, 19 years old)

> I don't even know what drove me to be in that relationship, 'cos my mother's sister has got a salon. She always says if you want to have a new hairstyle, come to me. If you have got something you need, come to me. My brother works for some NGOs [and he too says] 'I'll give you anything that you need'. My mother is a teacher, of course, but she's [also] a florist. She always sends me money. Of course, I just need to be flashy on campus. That's what I wanted.
>
> (Tendai, 20 years old)

These were the responses I got from two friends I interviewed separately. Although they acknowledged that some students are pushed into such relationships out of economic need, and gave examples of their friends and other female students in such situations, they insisted that this was not the case with them. As the quotes show, Tendai and Samantha have other people to whom they can turn for financial and material support and thus appear to have no reason to be in Big *Dhara* relationships. The fact that they are, however, suggests that these relationships are not always just about financial need – even though money and material resources are a key feature. These relationships must therefore hold other attractions for the young women concerned. The notion of being 'flashy on campus', mentioned in the second quote, appears to be central. All ten female students, as well as the male students I interviewed, alluded to this notion of 'flashiness'. I soon realised that the term referred to the desire to be seen and to be visible on campus through the conspicuous consumption of particular luxury goods, as highlighted in the newspaper story cited earlier. Conspicuous consumption of luxury goods, in turn, enabled female students to fashion themselves as 'more sophisticated', 'more successful' and even as 'more sexually appealing' than their peers.

While a common-sense view of transactional sex views it as a market relation, it is also worthwhile to consider its relation to other forms of exchange. In the anthropological literature, the association of gifts with prestige is common. For instance, in his classic analysis, Paul Bohannan (1959) identified three spheres of exchange among the Tiv. Bohannan described the Tiv as 'a pagan people numbering over 800,000 who live in the middle Benue Valley of Northern Nigeria' (Bohannan 1955: 60). In the first, exchanges served a subsistence function and involved foodstuffs, household utensils and some tools. The second sphere was associated with prestige and involved the exchange of brass rods and slaves. The last sphere entailed 'rights in dependent persons', such as wives and children. Bohannan noted that even though brass rods and slaves had an economic value for the Tiv, they were primarily exchanged for their prestige rather than their utilitarian value. Much the same can be said of exchanges between female students and Big *Dharas* and NABAs: while the money and gifts transacted surely have 'use-value', the attraction lies more in the prestige value of these relationships rather than in the contribution they make to subsistence. Being 'flashy' is therefore about competing with one's peers, asserting one's superiority over one's rivals, and carving out a niche for oneself as a high status individual. To reduce all of this to mere utility would be to miss a great deal.

Food and 'flashiness'

The constant consumption of prestigious food is particularly important to the concept of 'flashiness'. Female students involved in Big *Dhara* and NABA relationships were proud of the fact that they ate out for most of the semester and were thus shielded from the supposed indignity of campus meals. The latter were often described to me, by both female and male students, as consisting of 'watery soup' and 'a few pieces of meat or beans'. Besides the obvious fact that campus meals were of terrible quality and insufficient quantity, many students considered it a mark of extreme poverty if one was solely dependent on campus meals. Eating out was therefore greatly valued by both female and male students. In addition, for the female students in question, avoiding campus meals – especially those from the dining halls – suggested that they were not as ordinary as their peers, especially given that conspicuous consumption in food was ongoing (one has to eat daily) and required a constant supply of cash and tremendous resources to sustain. As one female student impressed upon me: 'Imagine going through a whole semester without going to the DH [dining hall]!' Tendai, a second-year Arts student, for instance, had 'dated' a 50-something Big *Dhara* in her first year. She narrated, at length, how she and her friends 'ate out all the time' and gave details about the various food items they bought. She explained that on the days that she did not eat out, she only purchased her meals from the campus supermarket and the Senior Common Room. These were both expensive options for the average student. The Senior Common Room was reserved for lecturers and non-academic staff and meals were not as highly subsidised as they were in the student dining halls. However, the meals there were of a much higher quality. The campus supermarket, in turn, was the most expensive meal option on campus and was referred to by students in the vernacular as '*Ende muno dhura*', that is, 'You are So Expensive!' Meals at the supermarket cost twice as much as they did at the dining halls. Taking one's meals from these two places therefore counted as 'being flashy', albeit not as much as eating out did.

Although in our discussions, Tendai appeared to describe her Big *Dhara* relationship in utilitarian terms: 'I think about that man when I was just broke [*sic*]. That's the only time I think of him. And I think, "Oh, I have only money to buy bread. What about these things? I need something like pie, like takeaways, like [a Kentucky Fried Chicken, KFC] twister ..." '; when further analysed, it is clear that Tendai is not talking about absolute levels of poverty. She could still afford to buy bread at a time when the latter was beyond the reach of most students and many civil servants. Bread is not typically the kind of consumption that UZ students associate with 'flashiness', but its general unavailability in the country and consequent unaffordability at the time of the interview (July 2007) had catapulted it into the category of a prestige-conferring food item. Not so for Tendai, however. She preferred to dine on 'twisters' – a supposedly low-fat wrap sold at KFC – and 'pies'. These are clearly non-subsistence foods and required tremendous financial resources in the Zimbabwean context – hence the prestige attached to them. As Leclerc-Madlala (2004) notes with regard to university students in KwaZulu-Natal (South Africa), perceptions of 'need', rather than actual 'need', are often some of the factors behind female university students' participation in transactional sex. This is why many young women readily classify mobile phones, fancy clothes and luxury transportation as needs, rather than as wants.

Among the female students I interviewed, pizza and cerevita (a type of cereal) were the most coveted foods. Again, it is no coincidence that these particular food items are also quite expensive. Even those students who are not involved in Big *Dhara* or NABA relationships described satisfactory 'dates' as those that entailed 'going out for pizza' and a good boyfriend as one who 'brings you pizza when he visits'. Male students generally agreed. As one explained, 'It makes a lot of difference if someone brings you pizza, Chicken Inn, that sort of thing.' Consequently, female students often snub advances from male students by asking them '*Unondipei?*', which literally means 'What can you give me?' and figuratively 'What can you do for me?'

Food seems best suited for showing off to one's immediate circle of friends and classmates and allows one to assert oneself as being of a higher status than one's peers. This is because it is mostly these individuals that one invites to one's room and who get to see the empty pizza and the cerevita boxes. Close friends and people in one's residence (especially those in the same corridor) also know which students eat out and never dine on campus. One female student shared the story of a girl on her corridor who threw out her empty pizza boxes only at the weekend. She would deliberately walk very slowly to the trash can (which was in the foyer, a very public space) holding a huge pile of large pizza boxes accumulated during the week so that everyone would see her. Then she would speak disparagingly about campus meals, declaring that she could not stand campus meals! My informant admitted to feeling very envious and said that she had contemplated finding a boyfriend of her own who would provide her with the same gifts. Through the consumption of expensive food, female students thus construct themselves not only as different from their peers, but also as successful, desirable, middle-class subjects.

'Flashy' fashions and 'flashy' hairdos

Aside from food, female students also use their relationships with Big *Dharas* and NABAs to purchase gadgets, fashionable clothes and trendy hairdos, and to have facials, pedicures and manicures done. Samantha, 19 years old, explained:

> The pressure is there, like right now you go into campus and you see the other girls are flashy and all that … so you get the pressure that 'Oh! I'm wearing these clothes. I've had them for so long' … Basically, it's all about clothes. With girls it's about looking nice. Getting your hair done. I know most girls, some go out with ministers and all that, who are doing it just to get their hair done or something.

In contrast to food, these items of consumption are used to achieve flashiness at a broader level. They are quite visible and enable female students to be noticed by everybody on campus. As the pizza story shows, female students particularly want to stand out from other female students, and their competitiveness and rivalry is directed at each other. The goal with clothing is to show more skin and curves, thus emphasising the visual aspect of flashiness. Female students consider body-hugging clothes, such as 'hipsters' and 'tank tops',[1] especially trendy, even more so if they happen to be imports from the UK.

Hair plays a similar role and is equally visible. Especially esteemed are weaves, that is, artificial hairpieces sewn into one's own hair. They are often modelled along 'Caucasian' hairdos and look and feel like Caucasian hair. It was not uncommon to see female students on campus in 2006 and 2007 with waist-length, super straight hair topped off with a perfect fringe. Again, images from the media helped create these particular fashion ideals. For instance, the heroine in the local soap, *Studio 263*, and her onscreen 'sister' both wore their hair in long, ostentatious and expensive-looking weaves, which many female students tried to emulate with different levels of success depending on one's access to capital. In one student discussion forum, almost half of the 30 female students in attendance had their hair in different varieties of weaves. So-called '100 per cent natural' weaves were preferred to synthetic ones because they look less artificial. However, the more natural looking a weave is, the more expensive it is and hence the status attached to particular weaves. Much advice circulates among female students on which salons to avoid when having a weave done, as social status is also contingent on having the 'perfect' weave. The latter is determined by the quality of the weave and the skill with which it is sewn on. I got a clue of just how expensive some of these weaves could be when Tendai remarked that she had only ever thought of buying a particular brand of weave known as *Sangika* after she had 'worked for ages'. Luckily, she did not have to wait that long, as her Big *Dhara* purchased one for her. After having her weave done, Tendai's friend wanted one too, so Tendai called him for more money.

Sihle, a first-year female student, kept a one-week diary at my request and in it she captured the level of competition among female students to acquire the various trappings of modernity (cf. Leichty 2003). She described an afternoon spent engaging in 'girl talk' with her female classmates. 'Girl talk,' she wrote, 'usually revolves around five topics [which she numbered as follows]: hairstyles (1), fashion (2), movies (3), music (4) and boyfriends (5).' The pressure to be fashionable, and to appear a certain way, is not unique to these female university students, nor is the self-image that they are trying to create. If anything, it has come to be synonymous with female youth culture across the globe (see Luke and Kurz's [2002] review of transactional sex in 12 countries in sub-Saharan Africa). Jennifer Cole's (2004) study of transactional sex in Madagascar is illustrative. She demonstrates how teenage girls are pressured by their peers, and even by their parents, to enter into sexual exchange relationships with *vazaha* (i.e. foreign men from Europe) so that they can access foreign consumption goods, of which fashionable hairdos and clothes are part. Consumerism, as Mike Featherstone (2000) pointed out, 'is a form of *stylistic self-consciousness*, which allows everyone, regardless of age and class position, to create a lifestyle of their choice through the assemblage of goods, clothes, experiences, appearance and bodily disposition' (95; emphasis in original). Featherstone's notion of stylistic self-consciousness suggests that the adoption of particular lifestyles is a deliberate decision that individuals make and not something individuals 'unreflectively adopt through tradition or habit' (95). Furthermore, as Thorstein Veblen (in Lee 2000: 31–47) argued, the consumption of unproductive goods, in particular, is often considered much more honorific and reputable and is a defining feature of middle-classness.

Managing reciprocity in Big Dhara/NABA relationships

A gift is always a provocation to reply (Mauss 1954). It is therefore fitting at this point to attend to the question of what female students give in return for the money they receive from Big *Dharas* and NABAs, which money they in turn use for prestige-making. Do they, as the literature suggests, reciprocate sexually? Or do they find ways of wriggling out of this obligation to reciprocate (Sahlins 1965)? If they do, what strategies do they employ and with what outcomes? Do they even consider it to be 'reciprocation'? In attempting to answer these questions, the complexity of transactional sex as a practice and the inadequacy of the sex–money dichotomy become very clear. Clearly, transactional sex is not prostitution in the sense of selling sex at a predetermined price communicated to men, who are the buyers (see Hyde 2007; Odzer 1994). Neither can one conclude that it is definitively sex work either. The UNAIDS Inter-Agency Task Team on Gender and HIV/AIDS (2005), for instance, defines sex workers as 'female, male and transgender adults and young people who receive money or goods in exchange for sexual services, either regularly or occasionally, and who may or may not consciously define those activities as income-generating'. This definition makes any material exchange in the context of a sexual relationship evidence of sex work, thus occluding the phenomena in question. In fact, female students – and many young women in general – actively exploit these ambiguities to their advantage, resulting in a situation of negative reciprocity (Sahlins 1965) in which one party benefits at the expense of the other.

There were two types of female students in the sample: those who preferred to date older men for emotional reasons and those who did so for prestige-making purposes. These different goals influenced how they managed reciprocity in their relationships. For instance, one student, who I will refer to as Tari, insisted that she found older men attractive as sexual partners. At the time of the research she was in an on-off-on-again relationship with a senior politician in his late sixties. She had also dated a company director in his early forties. Tari was 23 and in her final year of a physical sciences degree. Her reasons for entering these relationships were partly emotional (she loved them), partly sexual (she found them good in bed) and partly prestige-related. But unlike the female students I discussed earlier who use these relationships to attain high social status on campus, Tari used her relationships with these influential men to maintain her already high social class position. Tari was from a privileged background: her father was a former high-level university administrator, her family had strong political links, and they lived in an affluent neighbourhood in the capital. Tari therefore did not consider sexual relations with her Big *Dharas* as a form of payback for the material goods they lavished on her. As far as she was concerned, gift-giving was a normal feature of any relationship. It is difficult to say how representative Tari's experiences are, given that most research on transactional sex focuses on economically disadvantaged women. However, her case does draw attention to the fact that transactional sex has many different meanings for different women.

In contrast to Tari, the rest of the female students I interviewed engaged in transactional sex primarily for prestige-making reasons, rather than emotional ones. As such, they were not as keen to reciprocate sexually. All had also devised ingenious strategies aimed at escaping any perceived obligation to reciprocate sexually. One almost foolproof strategy (according to them) was to pretend to be menstruating each time they went out on an evening date with a Big *Dhara* or NABA. Neria, a first-year female student, narrated an incident in which her 'date' with a NABA went awry and she found herself trapped in a dingy motel, 10 km away from campus, at 4 am. Neria explained that when the NABA made sexual advances towards her, she informed him that she was having her period. When he did not believe her, she invited him to feel her pad. As intended, the man turned away in disgust and did not bother her again that evening. He did, however, threaten to confiscate her mobile phone as payment for the money he had spent on her at the club. Neria conceded that this had been a very 'close call' and that next time she might not be as lucky.

Another strategy entails drawing attention to the age disparities between themselves and the Big *Dharas*. Samantha, a second-year student, claimed to have successfully avoided physical intimacy by using 'embarrassment' as a strategy. Once, when her Big *Dhara* tried to kiss her, she spurned his advances by 'playfully' yelling out 'Child abuse! Child abuse!' Apparently, the Big *Dhara* found this jest to be in bad taste and he did not pursue the matter any further. Samantha also took advantage of the fact that they were in a public place and in the company of a third person. Her friend, Tendai, had also used a similar strategy successfully. Each time her Big *Dhara* made sexual advances towards her, she would remind him that he was old enough to be her father. This seemed to put him off, and he settled for other forms of physical intimacy with her, such as kissing. Ultimately, she was able to maintain a month-long relationship with him without ever reciprocating sexually, although he had spent considerable money on her and had even left his BMW in her care at one point. Finally, many students terminated their relationships before sexual demands were translated into action, a common female strategy (see Longfield *et al.* 2004). By acting creatively, many could successfully stall relationships from becoming sexual for a month or more (as in Tendai's case) and then terminate them when the demands became too persistent. However, these strategies did not always work. Female students explained that when they found themselves in situations where it was impossible to avoid reciprocating sexually, they often tried to regulate sexual encounters instead:

> You have to weigh up if a blouse is worth giving him sex. Obviously, it is not. So if a guy wants sex just because he bought me a blouse I will tell him to take it back!
>
> (Saru, 19 years old)

Sometimes sexual access was thus conceived almost entirely in terms of a gift threshold, and while this material calculation appears to conform to the standard model of transactional sex, the fact is that not every gift is equal, nor do women easily accept that a gift should automatically lead to sex. For these young women, therefore, transactions are always negotiable.

What's in it for the Big **Dharas** and **NABAs** then?

If female students' interests in transactional sex are more complicated than often conceded, what of men? Is it safe to say that what Big *Dharas* and NABAs seek to acquire is sex, pure and simple? In fact, even here, interests and desires are a good deal more complex than the standard model allows. For instance, in those situations where female students avoid reciprocating sexually, Big *Dharas* and NABAs still benefit in other ways. For instance, they deliberately take female students out to those public places that afford the greatest visibility, such as fancy restaurants that are patronised by other wealthy and influential men. They also invite female students to social outings organised by their companies and business associates. Many female students described how some Big *Dharas* tried to control their physical appearance by sponsoring elaborate 'makeovers'. Tendai's Big *Dhara*, for instance, informed her that he did not like her hairdo and had consequently purchased a synthetic hairpiece for her. He had even financed a wardrobe 'upgrade' for her and had also suggested that she get a facial, manicure and pedicure done. By so doing, he was able to transform her physical appearance to fit into a specific look that he desired, seemingly not just for his pleasure alone but also so that he could show her off in his peer group, as such makeovers often preceded outings.

Again, a parallel can be drawn to economic anthropology. In his classic study of the *kula* system of gift exchange among the Trobriand Islanders, anthropologist Bronislav Malinowski (1922) noted that the two main exchange items, the *soulava* (armshells) and the *mwali* (necklaces), were so highly valued that ownership of either, even if just for a few minutes, brought 'a great deal of renown' and enabled one 'to exhibit his article [and] tell how he obtained it' (94). Likewise, Big *Dharas* and NABAs appear to accrue considerable social status in their peer groups when seen in the company of young university women, just as these women in turn accrue social status through such relationships. Hunter's (2002) study of men in KwaZulu-Natal (South Africa) makes a similar point: it is those men who are always seen in the company of attractive young women who are envied by their peers and regarded as *isoka*, that is, sexually successful men. It is the prestige that comes with dating young women, over and above the actual sex itself, that I suggest informs the particular type of transactional sex that I describe in this chapter. This is not to say that sex is not important for the Big *Dharas* and NABAs, but rather to draw specific attention to the multifaceted meanings of transactional sex.

Conclusion: transactional sex and multiple concurrent sexual partnerships

Although the study focuses on the experiences of a small and specific group of young women – female university students – it raises a number of important issues regarding transactional sex: first, the phenomenon takes multiple forms; second, transactional sex is not always confined to economically disadvantaged young women; third, young women have various strategies that they employ, often with great success, in order to avoid having to reciprocate sexually in these relationships; and finally, both women and men use transactional sex to elevate their social status within their peer groups. As with most studies on transactional sex and sex work in general, the actual voices of the men involved are missing in this chapter, although they are captured indirectly through the experiences of the male students who were mediating some of these relationships. Further research, with men, is thus needed to better understand the intricate processes involved in transactional sex. In conclusion, I will now briefly look at the intersections between transactional sex and the topical issue of multiple concurrent partnerships.

All ten female students interviewed had men that they considered to be 'boyfriends': four were dating non-university men, while the remaining six were dating male students on campus. Furthermore, with the exception of one, all female students were sexually active with their boyfriends, even though they actively avoided sex with their Big *Dharas* and NABAs. Saru, a first-year female student, for instance, was involved in transactional sex relationships with two NABAs and she had devised ways of ensuring that they never ran into each other on campus. She explained that one would visit her between 5 pm and 7 pm and they would go out for supper. She would lie to him that she had a discussion to attend at 7 pm so that she could be available for the second NABA. Upon returning to campus, she would wait for the second NABA to show up and then spend the next couple of hours at an off-campus bar with him. Again, she would use the 'class discussion' or something school-related to convince the NABA to return her to campus by 9 pm. She would then spend the remaining hours (9–10.30 pm) with her campus boyfriend. Saru's best friend, Neria, often accompanied her on these excursions, even though she was in a steady relationship with a young man who worked in a bank and whom she had been dating since high school. She described her boyfriend as the love of her life and hoped that they would one day marry. Both Saru and Neria's boyfriends were, as expected, unaware of this aspect of their lives. Saru acknowledged that her campus boyfriend would be devastated if he ever found out, but she justified her actions with the statement: 'I don't have sex with any of these guys. They are not my boyfriends, even though I'm sure that some of them see me as their girlfriend.' These female students were therefore juggling, rather successfully, relationships with multiple men and exercising some control with regards to which of these relationships became sexual and which did not – a perspective which needs to be highlighted a lot more in future research on transactional sex and multiple concurrent partnerships.

Note

1 Hipsters are basically any type of denim jeans worn at the hips rather than the waist and, at the time of the research, the 'skinny leg' and the 'bootleg' were the most popular designs on campus. Tank tops, on the other hand, encompass a whole range of tight-fitting blouses, often made from fabric that stretches. They can be completely sleeveless, halter-necked or short-sleeved. Female students' fashion sense appeared to be influenced by two TV shows that they all watched regularly – a local soap called *Studio 263* and the so-called *African Movie*. Ironically, neither comes directly from the 'West' (Leichty 2003). *Studio 263* is screened daily and is filmed in and around the capital, while *African Movie* movies are screened on the national television station and normally come from Nigeria and Ghana. In both, young women are depicted as highly fashion conscious and wear tight-fitting jeans and skimpy tops.

References

Bene, C. and Merten, S. 2008. Women and fish-for-sex: Transactional sex, HIV/AIDS and gender in African fisheries. *World Development* 31(5): 875–899.

Bennell, P. and Ncube, M. 1994. A university for the Povo? The socioeconomic background of African university students in Zimbabwe since independence. *Journal of Southern African Studies* 20(4): 587–601.

Bohannan, P. 1955. Some principles of exchange and investment among the Tiv. *American Anthropologist* 57(1): 60–70.

Bohannan, P. 1959. The impact of money on an African subsistence economy. *Journal of Economic History* 19(4): 491–503.

Chatterji, M., Murray, N., London, D. and Anglewicz, P. 2004. *The Factors Influencing Transactional Sex Among Young Men and Women in 12 Sub-Saharan African Countries*. The Policy Project. Available at: www.policyproject.com/pubs/countryreports/Trans_Sex.pdf [Accessed 12 May 2010].

Cole, J. 2004. Fresh contact in Tamatave, Madagascar: Sex, money and intergenerational transformation. *American Ethnologist* 31(4): 573–588.

Dunkle, K.L., Jewkes, R.K., Brown, H.C., Gray, G.E., McIntyre, J.A. and Harlow, S.D. 2004. Transactional sex among women in Soweto, South Africa: Prevalence, risk factors and association with HIV infection. *Social Science & Medicine* 59: 1581–1592.

Featherstone, M. 2000. Lifestyle and consumer culture. In: M.J. Lee (ed.) *The Consumer Society Reader*. Malden, MA: Blackwell Publishers, 92–105.

Gaidzanwa, R. 2007. Alienation, gender and institutional culture at the University of Zimbabwe. *Feminist Africa* 8: 60–82.

Hunter, M. 2002. The materiality of everyday sex: Thinking beyond prostitution. *Africa Studies* 61(1): 99–120.

Hyde, T. 2007. *Eating Spring Rice: The Cultural Politics of AIDS in Southwest China*. Berkeley, CA: University of California Press.

Iversen, A.B. 2005. Transactional aspects of sexual relations in Francistown, Botswana. *Norwegian Journal of Geography* 59: 48–54.

Kaufman, C. and Stavros, E. 2004. 'Bus fare please': The economics of sex and gifts among young people in urban South Africa. *Culture, Health & Sexuality* 6(5): 377–391.

Leclerc-Madlala, S. 2004. Transactional sex and the pursuit of modernity. *Social Dynamics* 29(2): 1–21.

Lee, M.J. (ed.) 2000. *The Consumer Society Reader*. Malden, MA: Blackwell Publishers.

Leichty, M. 2003. *Suitably Modern: Making Middle-class Culture in a New Consumer Society*. Princeton, NJ, and Oxfordshire: Princeton University Press.

Longfield, K., Glick, A., Waithaka, M. and Berman, J. 2004. Relationships between older men and younger women: Implications for STIs/HIV in Kenya. *Studies of Family Planning* 34(2): 124–134.

Luke, N. and Kurz, K.M. 2002. *Cross Generational and Transactional Sex Relations in Sub-Saharan Africa: Prevalence of Behavior and Implications for Negotiating Safer Sex Practices*. ICRW. Available at: www.icrw.org/files/publications/Cross-generational-and-Transactional-Sexual-Relations-in-Sub-Saharan-Africa-Prevalence-of-Behavior-and-Implications-for-Negotiating-Safer-Sexual-Practices.pdf [Accessed 12 May 2010].

Machel, J. 2001. Unsafe sexual behaviour among schoolgirls in Mozambique: A matter of gender and class. *Reproductive Health Matters* 9(17): 82–90.

Maganja, R.K., Maman, S., Groves, A. and Mbwambo, J.K. 2007. Skinning the goat and pulling the load: Transactional sex among the youth in Dar es Salaam, Tanzania. *AIDS Care* 19(8): 974–981.

Malinowski, B. 1922. *Argonauts of the Western Pacific: An Account of Native Enterprise and Adventure in the Archipelagoes of Melanesian New Guinea*. London: Routledge and Kegan Paul.

Matshalaga, N. 1999. Gender issues in STIs/HIV/AIDS prevention and control: The case of four private sector organisations in Zimbabwe. *African Journal of Reproductive Health* 3(2): 87–96.

Mauss, M. 1954. *The Gift: Forms and Functions in Archaic Societies*. Glencoe, IL: The Free Press.

Meekers, D. and Calves, A. 1997. 'Main' girlfriends, girlfriends, marriage, and money: The social context of HIV risk behaviour in sub-Saharan Africa. *Health Transition Review*, Supplement 7: 361–375.

Moore, A., Biddlecom, A.E. and Zulu, E. 2007. Prevalence and meanings of exchange of money or gifts for sex in unmarried adolescents' sexual relationships in sub-Saharan Africa. *African Journal of Reproductive Health* 11(3): 44–61.

Muparamoto, N. and Chigwenya, A. 2009. Adolescents' perceptions on sexuality, HIV and AIDS in selected schools of Kwekwe District, Zimbabwe. *Journal of Sustainable Development in Africa* 10(4): 31–58.

Muzvidziwa, V.N. 2002. An alternative to patriarchal marriage: Mapoto unions. *Nordic Journal of African Studies* 11(1): 138–155.

Odzer, C. 1994. *The Patpong Sisters: An American Woman's View of the Bangkok Sex World*. New York: Arcade Publishing.

Pettifor, E., Beksinska, M.E. and Rees, H.V. 2000. High knowledge and high risk behaviour: A profile of hotel-based sex workers in inner-city Johannesburg. *African Journal of Reproductive Health* 4(2): 35–43.

Poulin, M. 2007. Sex, money and pre-marital partnerships in Southern Africa. *Social Science and Medicine* 65: 2383–2393.

Sahlins, M. 1965. On the sociology of primitive exchange. In: S. Gudeman (ed.) *Economic Anthropology*. Northampton: Elgar Publications, Chapter 6.

Swidler, A. and Watkins, S.C. 2006. *Ties of dependence: AIDS and transactional sex in rural Malawi. Online Working Paper Series*. California Center for Population Research.

Terry, P., Mhloyi, M., Masvaure, T. and Adlis, S. 2006. An examination of knowledge, attitudes and beliefs related to HIV/AIDS prevention in Zimbabwean university students: Comparing intervention programme participants and non-participants. *International Journal of Infectious Diseases* 10: 38–46.

UNAIDS Inter-Agency Task Team on Gender and HIV/AIDS. 2005. *UNAIDS. HIV/AIDS, Gender and Sex Work*. Available at: http://prostitution.procon.org/viewanswers.asp?questionID=849 [Accessed 11 May 2010].

White, L. 1986. Prostitution, identity and class consciousness in Nairobi during World War II. *Signs* 11(2): 255–273.

White, L. 1990. *The Comforts of Home: Prostitution in Colonial Nairobi*. Chicago, IL: University of Chicago Press.

Wojcicki, M. 2002. 'She drank his money': Survival sex and the problem of violence in taverns in Gauteng Province, South Africa. *Medical Anthropological Quarterly* 16(3): 267–293.

Zelizer, V.A. 2005. *The Purchase of Intimacy*. Princeton, NJ: Princeton University Press.

Section 3

Sexual diversity and practice

Explorations of sexual diversity have been centrally important in much recent research on sexuality. The complex social and historical construction of lesbian, gay, bisexual and transgender identities and cultures has been especially significant in shaping understandings of sexuality more generally, and the investigation of diverse sexual practices and meanings has been at the forefront of the field. The three chapters in this section explore these issues in a range of different settings, emphasizing the complex interrelationship between sexual identities, sexual practices and sexual communities. They highlight the often contradictory meanings and values associated with struggles to express diversity and resist dominant and oppressive normative systems, and they call attention to the difficult challenges that must constantly be faced by individuals as well as communities that seek to affirm difference and diversity as central to their understandings of themselves and their ways of being in the world.

The chapter by Paul Willis focuses on constructions of lesbian, gay, bisexual and queer (LGBQ) identities among young people in contemporary Australia. Drawing on the perspectives of young people themselves, it seeks to explore their understandings of LGBQ identities, and to position these understandings in relation to theoretical and empirical debates about the significance of these identity frames. Willis draws on the narratives of young people who discussed their experiences of identifying as LGBQ in online, face-to-face and telephone interviews. He emphasizes the ways in which diverse elements of LGBQ identities are important for these youth, and examines how they adopt and utilize these categories in practice. This is contrasted with an assessment of the limitations of LGBQ identity categories, and of the homophobic attitudes and discourses that sometimes inform these same subjectivities. Willis argues that health and social welfare professionals have a key role to play in supporting LGBQ youth, working in partnership with them (in what he describes as a process of co-authorship) in order to construct narratives that enable them to transcend the restrictions of identity frames.

The second chapter, by Rita M. Melendez and Rogério Pinto, explores the intersections of gender, love and HIV-related risk among male-to-female (MTF) transgender persons. It highlights findings from multiple studies that report high rates of HIV infection among MTF transgender individuals, and that suggest that stigma and discrimination heighten their risk of HIV infection. But it emphasizes that there is relatively little research that explores how gender roles may contribute to HIV risk. Melendez and Pinto draw on in-depth interviews with 20 MTF persons attending a community clinic, and argue that the experience of stigma and discrimination can create a heightened need for feeling safe, accepted and loved by their male companions, which can in turn place them at a higher risk of HIV.

They emphasize that MTF transgender women may rely on their relationships with men in order to feel loved and affirmed as women. Their heightened HIV risk then results from their interactions with these sexual partners, who provide both love and acceptance, but who may also request unsafe sexual practices, pointing toward an analytic model in which HIV risk is generated primarily as a result of the experience of stigma and discrimination.

The third chapter in this section, by Bianca D.M. Wilson, focuses on gender and sexual culture among Black lesbians in the USA. Wilson argues that gender expression is a persistent theme in writing about lesbian culture, yet little empirical research has actually examined the ways in which gender functions within the sexual culture of lesbian communities, especially in ethnic minority communities. She seeks to document and analyse the role and function of gender as it is understood among African American lesbians. Drawing on a range of ethnographic methods, including focus group discussions, individual interviews and participant observation, she documents how lesbian gender roles often translate into distinct sexual roles and expectations that appear to both parallel yet simultaneously reject heterosexual norms. The analysis emphasizes the central importance that gender roles play in this community, yet also highlights important forms of resistance to dominant, heteronormative sexual scripts.

Chapter 8

Constructions of lesbian, gay, bisexual and queer identities among young people in contemporary Australia

Paul Willis

Introduction

Sexual identities can simultaneously operate as sources of affirmation and social connection as well as foundations for systems of social division. In Australian communities, social divisions on the basis of sexual identity are acutely evident. National and local health and well-being surveys have highlighted the prevalence of discriminatory treatment against lesbian, gay and bisexual-identifying people living in rural and urban environments (Attorney General's Department of NSW 2003; Leonard *et al.* 2012) and the pervasiveness of homophobic attitudes across states and territories (Flood and Hamilton 2005). For many young lesbian, gay, bisexual and queer (LGBQ)-identifying Australians, homophobic violence and bullying continues to be experienced as an everyday reality (Hillier *et al.* 2010). Social research from Australia and other Western nations has shown how coping with anti-homosexual attitudes can generate mental and emotional stressors for young LGBQ people. Young LGBQ people have reported numerous psychosocial stressors, including increased risks of homelessness (Dunne *et al.* 2002), mental health effects such as lowered self-esteem and heightened psychological distress (Poteat and Espelage 2007) and excessive alcohol and other drugs misuse (Hillier *et al.* 2010; Smith *et al.* 1999). On a symbolic level, homophobic expressions can reinforce oppressive messages about LGBQ identities as representations of 'illness, evil and abnormality' (Hillier and Harrison 2004: 89).

Despite the impact of homophobia, young people are not deflected from constructing affirmative subject positions as LGBQ-identifying individuals. In this chapter, I examine the identity frames deployed and discussed by a group of 28 young Australians (aged 18–26 years) to communicate their understanding about their sexual selves to others. The purpose of this discussion is to give voice to the ways in which young people construct LGBQ identity frames. The phrase LGBQ captures the identity descriptors consistently referred to by young people participating in the research. For health and social-care workers, professional competence in supporting LGBQ youth requires an understanding of the interpersonal lenses through which young people construct perceptions of self and sexuality. The literature in this field suggests polarised positions between the recognition of lesbian and gay identities as significant to LGBQ youth and contrasting standpoints that suggest these identity frames are no longer central to their everyday lives. The qualitative findings presented in this chapter show how LGBQ identity frames continue to be meaningful for this group of young people but with variations in the social significance attributed to these different identity frames. In the following section, I outline the theoretical framework for this discussion. I then examine other knowledge claims about youth and LGBQ identities, before turning to the perspectives of young people gathered through qualitative interviews.

Background literature

Theoretical perspectives informing the research

This discussion is informed by social constructionist and post-structural perspectives about self and sexuality. Within sociology, human sexuality has been conceptualised as a contested field of cultural meanings, language and power relations (Weeks 2003a). Social constructionist perspectives emergent in 1960s sociology were pivotal in shifting focus away from natural-ised explanations to rethinking sexuality as a social phenomenon (Jackson and Scott 2010). While varied in perspective, sociological writers give emphasis to the social and historical contexts that shape modern understanding about sexuality and intimate relationships. In contrast, essentialist perspectives primarily locate sexuality as a naturalised, innate and fixed human quality (Weeks 2003a). Understanding sexuality as a social product requires analysis of the historical discourses that inform contemporary knowledge bases. Michel Foucault (1978) examined how medical and legal discourses in the nineteenth century informed modern knowledge about sexuality as an innate human drive and as a subject of enquiry, classification and regulation. Locating sexuality as a naturalised quality masks how power is produced and exercised through the interrelated concepts of sexuality and identity (Foucault 1978).

Through a post-structural lens, notions of identity and self are constructed through dis-course and language. From this standpoint, discourse refers to a series of shared meaning systems about self and identity (Sullivan 2003). Following post-structural trends, queer theory represents a critical approach for troubling taken-for-granted ideas about gender and sexual identity categories. This includes questioning the social and cultural divisions main-tained between heterosexual and homosexual subjectivities (Sullivan 2003). According to Gamson (2003), 'queer' represents 'a marker of the instability of identity' (543), echoing post-structuralist attempts to destabilise the notion of a stable and unified self. In the wake of the HIV/AIDS crisis, 'queer' has also been reclaimed as an identity label by activists seek-ing to demonstrate the power of counter-discourse by 'turning a repertoire of regulation into a category of resistance' (Mort 1994: 207).

The present research diverges from queer perspectives and is more closely aligned with lesbian and gay studies, as the primary focus is on young people's affiliation with LGBQ identities rather than a critical deconstruction of these subject positions. While this remains a theoretical tension running throughout the chapter, this does not inhibit incorporating queer perspectives on the limitations of identity categories within social research (Gamson 2003). In the present discussion, I seek to incorporate a critical reading of identity catego-ries as historically situated constructs by being mindful of the confines and constraints of LGBQ categories as well as recognising the personal and social significance attached to these identity frames.

Theorising sexual identities: functions and limitations

With emphasis on the lived experience of sexuality, sociological authors assert that sexual identity categories matter on both a personal and collective level. Seidman (2002) defines identities as the 'ways we think of ourselves and the self-image we publicly project' (9), while Hammack (2005) likens the adoption of identity categories to a 'cultural press' in which individuals identify with available social categories that match their sexual desires. Weeks (2003b: 129) identifies identity categories as 'necessary fictions', recognising sexual identities as social constructs, while equally acknowledging how identity categories bolster notions of individual agency. On a collective level, lesbian and gay identities provide a social conduit for individuals to express values shared with others, while functioning as a basis for political resistance to anti-homosexual practices (Weeks 2003b), as witnessed in gay liberation movements during the 1970s.

In developmental psychology, stage models on identity formation have provided frameworks for making sense of how young people acquire LGBQ identities. Two well-cited models include the work of Cass (1979) and Troiden (1988) – both authors have sought to provide more positive models about sexual identity development. One critique of these models is the tendency to universalise lesbians' and gay men's experiences of identity construction and to overshadow differences in how LGBQ youth experience sexual desires and relationships (Harwood and Rasmussen 2004). Harwood and Rasmussen maintain that knowing about sexual identity within psychological discourse is part of a cultural imperative to glean 'truths' about sexuality as a naturalised phenomenon. In addition, Harwood (2004) asserts that knowledge claims about LGBQ sexualities tend to privilege discussions about homosexual victimhood over other sexual discourses, such as the experience of sexual pleasure.

Queer theorists have raised important questions about the limitations of LGBQ identities as master narratives about lesbian and gay lives. Sedgwick (1990) suggests that sexual identities can operate as totalising frameworks through which individual experiences of sexuality are distilled and interpreted. Butler (1990) has argued against the notion of an authentic self and alternatively emphasised the performative dimensions of identity construction through which gender and sexual identities are constituted. More recently, Harwood and Rasmussen (2004: 399) have argued that while 'identity matters', it is highly problematic to think of sexual identities as fixed indicators of sexual behaviours and characteristics.

Constructing affirmative sexual identities in homophobic environments

Living in homophobic environments can complicate young people's attempts to construct affirmative notions of self and identity. McDermott *et al.* (2008) describe homophobia as a form of punishment for transgressing heterosexual norms. Homophobic discourses are conveyed through verbal and physical abuse to evoke shame and position young LGBQ people as 'abnormal, dirty and disgusting' (821). In relation to women's experiences, Mason (2002) discusses how gendered and sexual discourses sustain negative representations of lesbian bodies as disruptive to heterosexual relations. Lesbian identities disturb the assumed heterosex bond between men and women and therefore upset the implicit social order established on the basis of gender and heterosexuality (Mason 2002). In parallel, bisexual identities undermine both systems of cultural logic that separate and associate male and female bodies and heterosexual and homosexual identities (McLean 2008). This can result in the expression of biphobic attitudes by straight and gay individuals alike, for example questioning individuals about the legitimacy of bisexual identities (McLean 2008).

A more recent stream of research has emphasised young people's agency in speaking back to homophobia, and presented evidence on how young LGBQ people refute negative subject positions. Hillier and Harrison (2004) propose that lesbian and gay youth are well versed in locating the 'fault lines' in homophobic discourse – the contradictions and inconsistencies running through homophobic beliefs. Their national research illustrates how young LGBQ people reframe homophobia as a societal problem rather than an individual deficiency. Similarly, McDermott et al. (2008) have highlighted how LGBQ youth in the UK construct pride identities as a buffer against homophobic expressions. However, they also recognise that it would be difficult for young people to constantly adhere to these subject positions as the distress and pain felt by the impact of homophobia is not easily alleviated.

Contemporary youth and LGBQ identities: reclaiming or redefining?

Within the literature, there are mixed debates about the continuing significance of LGBQ identities for same-sex attracted youth. One notable trend in Australian and US research is the increased likelihood of young people identifying as LGBQ earlier in their teens (Hillier et al. 2010; Savin-Williams 2005). Hillier et al. (2010) suggest this is a result of multiple social and cultural changes, including the introduction of equality policies in political, health and educational institutions and expanding representation in popular media and public life. Alongside these changes, some authors contend that lesbian and gay identities have lost their currency in contemporary Western societies. In the USA, Seidman (2002) has proposed that many lesbian and gay individuals are now living 'beyond the closet' and that the concealment of LGBQ identities is no longer a central preoccupation. The significance of the 'closet' as a symbolic space of shelter from homosexual oppression has dwindled as lesbian and gay identities have entered everyday vernacular and popular culture (Seidman 2002).

In a similar vein, Savin-Williams (2005: 222) argues that we are entering a 'post-gay' era in which LGBQ youth are no longer reliant on lesbian and gay identities. Alternatively, the 'new gay teenager' is 'coming out' earlier in their teens and redefining a new vocabulary of sexual description (Savin-Williams 2005). Contrary to this argument, Russell and others' (2009) survey of US secondary school students indicates that a high proportion of same-sex attracted students continue to affiliate themselves with lesbian, gay and bisexual identities (70 per cent). Russell et al. contend that contemporary lesbian and gay youth still embrace, rather than reject, these labels as personally significant.

Within Australian communities, individual affiliations with lesbian and gay identity-based communities have rapidly changed since the height of the HIV/AIDS crisis in the 1980s. Based on gay men's stories of urban community life, Holt (2011) argues that gay communities in Australia have become increasingly fragmented as gay men report stronger ties within friendship and familial networks. In similar qualitative research, Fraser (2008) highlights a problematic tension between young gay men's desire for cohesive gay communities and their experiences of exclusion and disenchantment within commercialised environments. Balanced alongside these tensions, younger men within this sample continued to gravitate towards gay identities and reject the more sexually ambiguous label 'queer' – for these young men, 'queer' identities still conveyed homophobic connotations (Fraser 2008). While public health research into young women's construction of LGBQ identities is less prominent, survey research from the USA and Australia suggests that while lesbian and bisexual identities are both meaningful for same-sex attracted young women, these identity frames do not necessarily align with reported sexual attractions or relationships

(Diamond 2008; Hillier 2006). This suggests that LGBQ identities should not be treated as definitive dimensions of young women's sexual biographies. Together, these debates and findings provide the background context to the present research that further explores how young Australians construct and frame LGBQ identities.

Approach to the research

Findings reported in this chapter have been extracted from a qualitative study exploring how young people negotiate LGBQ identities in their places of paid employment in Australia (see Willis 2009). The research received institutional approval through the Tasmanian Social Sciences Human Ethics Research Committee (University of Tasmania). This chapter focuses on the stories shared by 28 young people about their sexual selves through interviews conducted in 2005–2006. The approach to interviewing followed a similar method of questioning deployed by Stein (1997) when inviting lesbian women to share their sexual narratives. Stein describes these narratives as 'self stories' (7) – stories about how individuals perceive the sexual self, which are informed by wider discourses about sexual identities and communities.

Participation was open to young people who were between 16 and 26 years of age and identified as non-heterosexual/not straight. When advertising, references to lesbian and gay identities were avoided to ensure that young people who did not identify with these labels were not excluded. The minimum age requirement was 16 years, in line with ethical requirements for young people to be able to give informed consent. The maximum age was set at 26 years to allow participation of young people who had completed tertiary education and entered paid employment in their early twenties. This rationale was based on the study's primary focus on workplace experiences. Following a purposive sampling approach, the project was advertised through online and on-site sources. Online sites included lesbian and gay youth-related websites, for example group email lists, and youth and health service providers. On-site sources included hard copy advertisements displayed in LGBQ venues and student services on university campuses. Interested parties were directed to a research website that outlined the project.

The sample group was located between the ages of 18 and 26 years, with a mean age of 23, reflecting an 'older' post-adolescent group. There were no participants under 18. This gap could reflect their reluctance to discuss sexuality with an unfamiliar party or their limited experience in employment. Participants were located across all Australian states, with no responses from the two territories. Within the sample there were 17 men and 11 women, and the majority of participants identified their current location as 'urban'. Over half the participants (15) had either completed or were currently studying for higher education degrees. Table 8.1 lists participants' first name (pseudonym selected by participants), age at time of participation, gender and self-description of sexuality. While transgender individuals were not excluded from participating, no participants identified as transgender or gender questioning. Information was not routinely gathered about participants' ethnic identity – this is a limitation to the present study. Some participants elected to discuss pertinent aspects of their ethnicity during the course of the interviews.

Interview methods and analysis

Young people participated through one of three methods: online interviews (15), face-to-face interviews (12) or telephone interview (1). These approaches yielded equally detailed

Table 8.1 Participants' pseudonym, age, gender and self-description of sexuality (n = 28)

Self-selected pseudonym	Age	Gender	Self-description of sexuality
Nick	18	Male	Bisexual, 'nearly gay'
Bubbles	19	Female	Bisexual
Luke	19	Male	Gay
Franky	20	Male	Gay
Michael	20	Male	Gay
Diego	20	Male	Gay
Madeleine	20	Female	Gay
Trent	21	Male	Gay
Aiden	21	Male	Queer, bisexual, gay
Sam	22	Female	Homosexual, gay
Pearson	22	Male	Gay
Peggie	23	Female	Gay
Ingrid	23	Female	Gay
Moskoe	23	Male	Gay
Kheva	23	Male	Gay
Chester	23	Male	Gay
Alex	24	Female	Queer, dyke, lesbian
Mia	24	Female	Queer, lesbian
Steven	24	Male	Gay
Ruby	24	Female	Queer, lesbian
Jack	25	Male	Gay
Joseph	25	Male	Gay, queer
Tobias	25	Male	Bisexual
Shirley	25	Female	Bisexual, lesbian
Bruce	26	Male	Gay
Nadi	26	Female	Bisexual
Maree	26	Female	Gay, lesbian
Jacob	26	Male	Gay

accounts about the meanings participants attributed to LGBQ identities. Online interviews required longer periods of engagement because of the requirement to respond through type-written text. Online interviews ranged from two to four meetings for an average of 2.5 hours per meeting. This method assisted in accessing young people who could not meet due to geographical distance or because participants preferred online communication.

Interviews were facilitated through an instant messaging program that provided a free platform to meet participants in real time (see Willis 2012). Face-to-face interviews ran for

1–2 hours and in some cases extended across several meetings; this culminated in approximately 30 hours of recorded data. Face-to-face interviews were facilitated by participants living in the researcher's home-state in private venues nominated by the participant. One person requested to participate by telephone interview, and the same interview format was followed. Across all interviews, questions similar to Stein's (1997) approach were asked; for example: 'How would you describe your sexuality?', 'What do these words mean to you?' and 'At what point in your life did you come to call yourself that?' (208).

Transcripts were returned to each participant for their review before data analysis. Thematic coding techniques were applied through the qualitative analysis software NVivo7 and followed the constructivist ground theory method outlined by Charmaz (2006). Charmaz draws on Glaser and Straus' (as cited in Charmaz 2006: 4) approach and adopts a more reflexive standpoint that acknowledges the subjective presence of the researcher in data generation. However, this analysis did not adhere to the cyclical approach advocated by grounded theorists. Initial codes were formulated through a line-by-line analysis and clustered into axial codes that contained subthemes. More detailed axial codes were selected as core themes that conveyed a shared narrative about young people's sexual experiences, self-perceptions and meanings. In the following section, findings are presented thematically to decrease the risk of identification.

Findings

Framing lesbian and gay identities – from negative representation to individual affirmation

Throughout their self stories, participants discussed lesbian and gay identities as familiar reference points for framing their sexual selves. Bisexual and queer categories were also discussed as significant identity frames in participants' everyday lives – these stories are discussed in the second core theme. Participants reflected on how they were introduced to the meanings associated with lesbian and gay identities through family members, exposure to popular media or interaction with peers. During primary and secondary school, lesbian and gay identities were discussed by peers as a subject of derogation and ridicule. Within the family home, lesbian and gay identities were framed as a subject of disgust, religious disapproval or moral danger. During his childhood, Jack (25 years) remembered hearing his father express hostile views about gay individuals:

> Probably early childhood … I suppose that's probably the first time I heard it, through my father, because my father had quite strong anti-gay sentiments … So that's the first time I was introduced to this concept of 'being gay' … but then you go into this huge internal struggle saying 'Oh shit! This is who I am and that's really bad' because all you've heard up until then is that it's wrong and it's bad and you shouldn't do it and you shouldn't be like that …

Ingrid (23 years) recalled overhearing how 'lesbian' identities were negatively portrayed in the news media and discussed between family members:

> … just watching the news when I was a kid probably 5 or 6 even, because I've known quite a long time, and just hearing other people say the word and usually hearing it

come up with negative connotations as well, especially we're talking about a bit over well, almost 20 years ago ... Also hearing my parents relay that as well, 'There's another thing about lesbians on the news!'

There were occasional stories in which family members conveyed positive messages about same-sex relationships and homosexual identities. Chester (23 years) shared his first conversations with his parents about gay relationships when he was 11:

I remember hearing the term 'homosexual' on *The 7.30 Report* [current affairs programme] and I remember asking my parents what a homosexual person was and my mother described a homosexual person as two men who loved each other, so I remember referring to my father and my grandfather as homosexuals in that context, not completely understanding it.

These stories were the exception to the norm. Despite predominantly negative first encounters, this did not prevent male and female participants from later constructing gay identities as core dimensions of their sexual selves and as an inner source of pride, strength and affirmation. For Trent (21 years), the term 'gay' was an empowering expression for distinguishing his sexuality from the more clinical term 'homosexual': 'The word gay to me is a respectful way and a more dignified label than "homosexual", far less clinical. And more meaningful than queer or queen.' Trent discussed 'coming out' as a reservoir of strength:

I draw on the strength when I'm faced with stressful situations, when I doubt myself whether I can do a certain task, I can think back and say this is easy, it's immaterial, you have done something much bigger, that I have come to terms with who and what I am and are proud of it.

Alongside their discussions about pride and personal strength, participants spoke at length about their first 'coming out' experiences during their mid- to late teens. These stories represented significant turning points in which they consolidated lesbian and gay identities in parallel with other important life transitions, such as commencing university studies or leaving the family home. For Jacob (26 years), 'coming out' was associated with his transition to university. This was a 'liberating' change as he began to connect with other gay youth and construct a 'gay' identity:

Going to university was kind of liberating, not just with regard to exploring your sexuality, but a chance to explore a personal identity, without the cliques that were common at my high school. I came out to my best friend during second year when I was 19. During my first year, I went to a couple of gay youth support group outings without telling anyone I knew. Then soon after I told my first friend, my other close friends also were told.

For several young women their 'coming out' stories were synonymous with entering intimate relationships with other women that confirmed their sexual feelings. Maree (26 years) recounted her first relationship with a work colleague during her late teens:

... we really started talking a lot more, and she actually disclosed to me and said to me 'I'm a lesbian' and I said 'Ok yeah', and I think it was like maybe the second time I'd heard that word and was like 'Ok – wow' … just in hearing that and talking about that with her something was happening for me where I was going – 'Yep, I know what you're talking about.'

While Maree discussed lesbian identities in a positive light, other young women expressed a greater sense of ambivalence.

Problematic identity frames – identifying as lesbian and bisexual

Within this subgroup, lesbian and bisexual identities were discussed as primarily problematic and difficult to communicate to others. While seven young women referred to the word 'lesbian', there were varying degrees of ambivalence expressed about this label. Ingrid (23 years) perceived the term lesbian as implying an interpersonal barrier between herself and other gay men and women:

> Generally I classify myself as 'gay', I don't like – I hate the word 'lesbian'. I've always hated that, it's one of those ones that makes my skin crawl a bit, and I feel that it makes other people a little more uncomfortable sometimes as well. So if I just say 'gay', it's broad and then I've got more people on my side if you know what I mean, I've got men in my group as well as just women.

Madeleine (20 years) had studied feminism and sociology at university and had felt aggrieved by some of the debates held with her lecturers about feminist standpoints and lesbian identities:

> To say 'Look, we don't need men. Ha-ha.' Some rad fem writers even talk about the 'lesbian continuum', referring to women–women relationships of various degrees … so for them, the ideal is for all women to be complete 'lesbians', meaning that they think women are wonderful and men are scum. And I hate that for two reasons, one is that it implies choice – that women choose to be lesbian/bi – and the other that it means that girls are with girls because they hate men, which is just bullshit.

Madeleine's story suggests an over-simplified reading of feminist politics and lesbian subjectivities. However, her reflections do highlight her initial impressions of lesbian and, to a lesser extent, feminist identities as conflicting, more so than self-affirming.

Bisexual identities were discussed by both women and men with uncertainty and were not perceived in the same affirming light as gay identities. Five participants referred to bisexuality as a signifier of their attractions to both genders and their experiences of sexual relationships with men and women. Nadi (26 years) described herself as bisexual out of habit: 'Well I use the word bisexual out of habit, because that's something other people (sometimes!) understand … but personally I don't really think about it … I just don't prefer one sex over the other.' Simultaneously, Nadi had felt that her lesbian friends and ex-girlfriends had dismissed her bisexual identity as a phase and as unacceptable. Other popular misconceptions expressed by both heterosexual and homosexual peers and friends included conflating bisexuality with promiscuity or misperceiving bisexuality as a transitory condition. Tobias (25 years) had experienced similar challenges from heterosexual and lesbian and gay acquaintances to renounce his bisexual identity and identify as either gay or straight:

> I have had conversations where I have been challenged, or in some instances told, that I am either gay and don't want to admit it, or straight and looking for controversy; neither is particularly accurate and I have found myself quite hurt after having these discussions. Being bi has different challenges to being gay, and it involves being slightly ostracised by both gay and straight groups.

These responses position bisexual identities as illegitimate and incomplete in comparison to lesbian and gay identities. While identifying as bisexual, Shirley (25 years) had found it difficult to discuss this among her circle of lesbian friends:

> And it's much easier to sort of identify as one particular type as in lesbian or gay [emphasis], when you're hanging out with a lot of other lesbian women ... I know that these women are incredibly gay and they think of themselves as gay, and because they do so to have somebody in their midst who's suddenly switching back and forth would cause a lot of concern and discomfort.

Equally, Shirley's story illustrates how lesbian identities generated a point of entry into a friendship network that provided close social connections with other women. Participation in this network needs to be balanced alongside the interpersonal tensions signalled by Shirley and by other young women earlier in this theme.

Multiple identity frames – shifting identities across social audiences

LGBQ identities were not always discussed as mutually exclusive categories, as some participants referred to lesbian and gay identity frames in tandem with queer identities. The terms they used to communicate their sexual self to others shifted across audiences and social settings and were referred to interchangeably rather than one term being assigned higher social value or meaning over another. In addition, some participants conveyed a reflexive awareness of the social and political connotations attached to LGBQ identities and the limitations of these frames for conveying elements of their personal and sexual lives to others. Participants reflected on the language that would be considered more acceptable when communicating LGBQ identities to others, and in several instances deployed a combination of terms. Most importantly, they selected labels that would not provoke negative responses. The term 'gay' was perceived as a familiar expression that required minimal explanation from the speaker, as discussed by Aiden (21 years):

> I don't really like giving myself a label, I believe sexuality is fluid and not fixed – clearly I know I'm not heterosexual; however, I don't really have a specific term to describe my sexuality. I suppose gay 'works' best because that's what most people are familiar with and it doesn't require a lot of explaining.

Six participants reflected on how lesbian and gay identities sometimes felt restrictive and inadequate for communicating their self and sexuality to others. Jack reflected on the informal codes of conduct which accompanied the performance of gay identities in urban gay male communities:

> … especially I suppose since I was out and I started to become part of the gay community, I could see this new set of social rules that were 'OK. If you're gay you have to behave like this and have to dress like this and you should do this and you should do that', and then I think, 'Well, I don't like that. [Laughs] I don't want to be part of that. That's not me!'

Five participants had gravitated towards the term 'queer' as an alternative label that denoted fluid sexual attractions that were non-gender-specific. However, these participants did not dispense with lesbian and gay identities – queer identities were discussed in parallel with lesbian, gay and bisexual identities and with varying personal and political significance. For this group of young people, there were no identified difficulties in using these contrasting labels in tandem or interchangeably. However, the social context shaped when and how they referred to these identity frames. This subgroup had encountered the term 'queer' during their university studies. On a personal and political level, elements of this term had resonated with facets of their sexual biography. One appealing aspect was the sexual ambiguity conveyed through the expression 'queer' that made participants feel that they were not locked into a singular category or read by others as exclusively gay or straight. According to Ruby (24 years), the term 'queer' was a political marker that contravened normative understandings about gender and sexual identities: 'To me being queer is about challenging sexuality and gender norms … It's about confronting people, systems and ideals that hold heterosexuality and the gender binary as the ultimate.' For Ruby, 'queer' identities challenged conventional binary divisions between straight/gay identities and male/female genders:

> My sexuality is not just about who I have sex with, it's about who I love, how I live and what I believe in. I believe that by being queer you don't necessarily have to be 'not straight' – you just have to believe and live a life that supports the notion that heterosexuality is not the only way and that gender binaries should be abolished.

Participants were mindful of the historical connotations attached to 'queer' as a homophobic expression as well as its more contemporary theoretical and political synergies. Joseph (25 years) discussed queer as a familiar label within university networks; however, he had used this word sparingly in reference to himself:

> Queer is a term that I'd never quite felt comfortable with, but is good at creating instant rapport with politically active and university types … I grew up in a very rural area. Queer is an insult there. I accommodated the term because of its ubiquity in university circles, but won't use it off my own bat.

For this group of participants, LGBQ identities were not experienced as fixed or mutually exclusive frames – their stories highlight their awareness of the varied social and political meanings attached to these identity frames and their capacity to deploy different terms across different social networks. Furthermore, their stories show insight about how lesbian, gay and bisexual identity frames can be experienced as constraining as well as affirming subject positions.

Discussion

This chapter has set out to examine the ways in which a group of 28 young Australians construct and frame LGBQ identities. The literature on this topic indicates polarised positions. One argument suggests that for many young LGBQ people, lesbian and gay identities continue to be meaningful and inform their sense of self, while other authors propose that the individual and social significance attached to lesbian and gay identities is diminishing. The findings show how LGBQ identities continue to be meaningful within the biographies of this group, with variations in the social significance attributed to these identity frames.

In response to Savin-Williams's (2005) proposal, the young people in this research do not appear to be refashioning new identity labels and they continue to frame their sexual selves through LGBQ identities. Across the group, gay identities continued to function as positive anchorage points that brought affirmation to their sense of self and, like participants in Fraser (2008) and Russell et al.'s (2009) research, still mattered to young women and men alike. This finding further illustrates young people's capacity to reframe lesbian and gay identities as points of affirmation and pride and to reject homophobic discourses that often accompany their first encounters with these identity frames.

Lesbian and gay identities were not always discussed as cohesive or comfortable subject positions as some participants conveyed a reflexive awareness of the constraints of these identity frames. This finding resonates with elements of Hillier et al.'s (2010) survey of same-sex attracted youth, in which respondents likewise identified lesbian and gay categories as restrictive and ill-fitting. Moreover, this finding emphasises young people's capacity to critique the apparent usefulness of sexual categories. It shows young people participating in a wider questioning about the utility of existing sexual 'taxonomies' (Sedgwick 1990) for framing their individual lives, sexual attractions and relationships.

In contrast to Fraser's (2008) participants, several participants had gravitated towards 'queer' as an alternative frame that transcended the identified restrictions accompanying lesbian and gay identities. However, like Fraser's participants, they were mindful of the homophobic connotations that accompanied this identity frame. Some participants indicated an awareness of the historical and political tensions inherent with the use of queer as an identity position, but this did not hinder them from adopting queer identities alongside lesbian and gay identities. The conceptual tensions that exist between queer perspectives and politics and lesbian and gay identities do not prevent these young people from appropriating queer as a marker of sexual difference. These young people locate their sexual biographies both outside and within identity frames that challenge and consolidate the divide between heterosexual/homosexual subjectivities. While their self stories bring these subject positions together, how participants deploy these terms frequently depends on the social setting and audience.

The shifting between identity frames is an equally important finding as it highlights how gay identity frames are perceived as more socially acceptable than other identities in the LGBQ spectrum. Following Harwood and Rasmussen's (2004) argument, participants in this research are not only engaged in a process of 'truth telling' about their sexual selves, but feel compelled to present sexual truths in an acceptable language. The term gay is framed as a neutral term that does not evoke disapproval. In parallel, gay identities are discussed in parallel with notions of pride. While elements of this resonate with McDermott et al.'s (2008) discussion of 'proud identities', more importantly, this finding indicates that lesbian and bisexual identities do not appear to be affiliated with notions of pride. Lesbian identities were perceived by participants to hinder relationships with men and create barriers to a cohesive community shared with gay men. In line with Mason's (2002) arguments, discussions about lesbian identities were primarily framed in the context of the disruptions generated to heterosex relations and how this subject position hindered connections with men. This suggests that these young women's perceptions of lesbian identities are overshadowed by wider sexist and heterosexist discourse. These are dominant discourses that complicate attempts to associate lesbian identities with pride identities, which limits the potential for more enabling discussions about lesbian identities, self and social connectivity.

Participants identifying as bisexual had received challenging responses from gay and straight individuals in which bisexuality was positioned by others as an illegitimate identity. This finding chimes with the accounts of bisexual adults living in Australia who have shared similar experiences of community exclusion and isolation (McLean 2008). Arguably, bisexuality is the most difficult identity to disclose to others because of its invisible status within the heterosexual/homosexual divide. Consequently, bisexual identities are confounded by stereotypes of bisexuality as a symptom of psychological instability and indecision (McLean 2008), representing bisexuality as a null identity. This status is compounded by a deficit of more nuanced research into young bisexual people's experiences of identity construction.

Implications for health and social-care professionals

The themes discussed suggest a number of areas for future consideration by health and social-care professionals working with LGBQ-identifying youth. The findings show how LGBQ identity frames continue to serve important functions in signalling points of affiliation for some young people. Equally, it is important to consider how young people may associate elements of their sexual lives with several identities along the LGBQ spectrum – these categories are not mutually exclusive. This complicates public health strategies that seek a singular reference point for targeting sexual-health campaigns. It highlights the need for a plurality of language when discussing homosexual identities and seeking to target a diverse population of young people.

The findings highlight that young people not only require permission to discuss their sexual history and health-related outcomes, but also encouragement to discuss their sexuality outside the familiar templates of lesbian and gay. Helping professionals have a pivotal role to play in supporting young LGBQ people through a process of co-authorship – to work in partnership to construct more enabling self stories that transcend restrictive or ill-fitting identity frames. This approach begins and ends with the individual's understanding of self and sexuality, requiring a person-centred approach that privileges the self stories of service users and carers. It also requires a process of evaluating with young people the utility of existing beliefs and discourses about LGBQ identities when seeking to construct positive representations of their self and identity. This is particularly fundamental for young people whose attempts to identify with lesbian and bisexual identities are overshadowed by homophobic, sexist and biphobic discourses.

Conclusion

This research is one of a small number of Australian studies to examine how young people construct LGBQ identities. Through the perspectives of young people, this chapter has sought to position their understanding of LGBQ identities alongside theoretical and empirical debates about the individual and social significance attached to these identity frames. Findings highlight how varying elements of LGBQ identities continue to bear currency with this group. This is balanced alongside an awareness of the limitations of identity categories and experiential knowledge of the homophobic discourse that can inform these subject positions. Queer identities are not discussed in isolation, but in tandem with lesbian and gay identities, highlighting young people's interchangeable use of these frames dependent on the social context.

The findings provide a snapshot of participants' perceptions of LGBQ identities, and as such it is difficult to capture the identity transitions experienced between early adolescence and adulthood. Furthermore, this discussion has not considered ethnicity as a social lens for interrogating the findings. For young people from some minority ethnic backgrounds, LGBQ identities may be in conflict with cultural and familial identities and affiliations. Further research is required with same-sex attracted young people who do not associate their lives with LGBQ identities to explore the ways in which they make sense of their sexual selves outside of these familiar frames.

References

Attorney General's Department of NSW. 2003. *'You Shouldn't Have to Hide to be Safe': A Report on Homophobic Hostilities and Violence Against Gay Men and Lesbians in New South Wales*. Sydney: Attorney General's Department.

Butler, J. 1990. *Gender Trouble: Feminism and the Subversion of Identity*. New York: Routledge.

Cass, V. 1979. Homosexual identity formation: A theoretical model. *Journal of Homosexuality* 4: 219–235.

Charmaz, K. 2006. *Constructing Grounded Theory: A Practical Guide Through Qualitative Analysis*. London: SAGE.

Diamond, L. 2008. Female bisexuality from adolescence to adulthood: Results from a 10-year longitudinal study. *Developmental Psychology* 44: 5–14.

Dunne, G.A., Prendergast, S. and Telford, D. 2002. Young, gay, homeless and invisible: A growing population? *Culture, Health & Sexuality* 4: 103–115.

Flood, M. and Hamilton, C. 2005. *Mapping Homophobia in Australia*. Canberra: Australia Institute.

Foucault, M. 1978. *The History of Sexuality, Volume 1: An Introduction*. Harmondsworth: Penguin.

Fraser, S. 2008. Getting out in the 'real world': Young men, queer and theories of gay community. *Journal of Homosexuality* 55: 245–264.

Gamson, J. 2003. Sexualities, queer theory, and qualitative research. In: N.K. Denzin and Y.S. Lincoln (eds) *The Landscape of Qualitative Research: Theories and Issues*. 2nd ed. Thousand Oaks, CA: SAGE, 540–568.

Hammack, P.L. 2005. The life course development of human sexual orientation: An integrative paradigm. *Human Development* 48: 267–290.

Harwood, V. 2004. Telling truths: Wounded truths and the activity of truth telling. *Discourse: Studies in the Cultural Politics of Education* 25: 467–476.

Harwood, V. and Rasmussen, M.L. 2004. Problematising gender and sexual identities. In: D. Riggs and G. Walker (eds) *Out in the Antipodes: Australian and New Zealand Perspectives on Gay and Lesbian Issues in Psychology*. Perth: Brightfire, 392–415.

Hillier, L. 2006. Mix or match? Sexual attraction, identity and behaviour in same-sex attracted young women in Australia: An update. *Redress* 15: 10–15.

Hillier, L. and Harrison, L. 2004. Homophobia and the production of shame: Young people and same-sex attraction. *Culture, Health & Sexuality* 6: 79–94.

Hillier, L., Jones, T., Monagle, M., Overton, N., Gahan, L., Blackman, J. and Mitchell, A. 2010. *Writing Themselves In 3: The Third National Study on the Sexual Health and Wellbeing of Same-Sex Attracted and Gender Questioning Young People.* Melbourne: Australian Research Centre in Sex, Health and Society, La Trobe University.

Holt, M. 2011. Gay men and ambivalence about 'gay community': From gay community attachment to personal communities. *Culture, Health & Sexuality* 13: 857–871.

Jackson, S. and Scott, S. 2010. *Theorizing Sexuality.* Maidenhead: Open University Press.

Leonard, W., Pitts, M., Mitchell, A., Lyons, A., Smith, A., Patel, S., Couch, M. and Barrett, A. 2012. *Private Lives 2: The Second National Survey of the Health and Wellbeing of GLBT Australians.* Melbourne: Australian Research Centre in Sex, Health and Society, La Trobe University.

Mason, G. 2002. *The Spectacle of Violence: Homophobia, Gender and Knowledge.* London: Routledge.

McDermott, E., Roen, K. and Scourfield, J. 2008. Avoiding shame: Young LGBT people, homophobia and self-destructive behaviours. *Culture, Health and Sexuality* 10: 815–829.

McLean, K. 2008. Silences and stereotypes: The impact of (mis)constructions of bisexuality on Australian bisexual men and women. *Gay and Lesbian Issues and Psychology Review* 4: 158–165.

Mort, F. 1994. Essentialism revisited? Identity politics and late-twentieth-century discourses of homosexuality. In: J. Weeks (ed.) *The Lesser Evil and the Greater Good: The Theory and Politics of Social Diversity.* London: Rivers Oram Press, 201–221.

Poteat, V.P. and Espelage, D.L. 2007. Predicting psychosocial consequences of homophobic victimization in middle school students. *Journal of Early Adolescence* 27: 175–191.

Russell, S.T., Clarke, T.J. and Clary, J. 2009. Are teens 'post-gay'? Contemporary adolescents' sexual identity labels. *Journal of Youth and Adolescence* 38: 884–890.

Savin-Williams, R.C. 2005. *The New Gay Teenager.* Cambridge, MA: Harvard University Press.

Sedgwick, E.K. 1990. *Epistemology of the Closet.* Berkeley, CA: University of California Press.

Seidman, S. 2002. *Beyond the Closet: The Transformation of Gay and Lesbian Life.* New York: Routledge.

Smith, A.M.A., Lindsay, J. and Rosenthal, D.A. 1999. Same-sex attraction, drug injection and binge drinking among Australian adolescents. *Australian and New Zealand Journal of Public Health* 23: 643–646.

Stein, A. 1997. *Sex and Sensibility: Stories of a Lesbian Generation.* Berkeley, CA: University of California Press.

Sullivan, N. 2003. *A Critical Introduction to Queer Theory.* Melbourne: Circa Books.

Troiden, R.R. 1988. Homosexual identity development. *Journal of Adolescent Health Care* 9: 105–113.

Weeks, J. 2003a. *Sexuality.* 2nd ed. London: Routledge.

Weeks, J. 2003b. Necessary fictions: Sexual identities and the politics of diversity. In: J. Weeks, J. Holland and M. Waites (eds) *Sexualities and Society: A Reader.* Cambridge: Polity Press, 122–131.

Willis, P. 2009. From exclusion to inclusion: Young queer workers' negotiations of sexually exclusive and inclusive spaces in Australian workplaces. *Journal of Youth Studies* 12: 629–651.

Willis, P. 2012. Talking sexuality online: Technical, methodological and ethical considerations of online research with sexual minority youth. *Qualitative Social Work* 11: 141–155.

Chapter 9

'It's really a hard life'

Love, gender and HIV risk among male-to-female transgender persons

Rita M. Melendez and Rogério Pinto

Introduction

The term transgender refers to individuals whose sexual assignment at birth does not correspond with their current gender identity. Transgender individuals represent a diverse spectrum of gender expressions. The limited data on transgender persons and HIV point to high rates of infection (Kenagy and Hsieh 2005). Reports of HIV rates among male-to-females (MTFs) range from 19 to 47 per cent (Nemoto *et al.* 1999; Simon *et al.* 2000; Clements-Nolle *et al.* 2001; Kenagy and Bostwick 2001; Kenagy 2002; Risser and Shelton 2002; Nemoto *et al.* 2004a). A study conducted in San Francisco on MTFs (n = 392) and female-to-male (FTM) individuals (n = 123) found that 35 per cent of MTFs in the study were HIV-positive; FTMs had a lower rate of 2 per cent (Clements-Nolle *et al.* 2001).

Researchers have outlined a number of processes relating to stigma and discrimination that may increase the risk of HIV infection (Herek and Capitanio 1999), specifically among MTFs (Green 1994; Nemoto *et al.* 1999). Stigma generally refers to an adverse reaction to individuals who are perceived to be 'different' based on one or more characteristics (Susman 1994). Discrimination is often conceived as a concrete outcome of stigma (Link and Phelan 2001) and prevents stigmatised individuals from engaging in social and economic opportunities (Link and Phelan 2001). This chapter explores how MTFs experience stigma and discrimination and how those experiences increase their need to feel wanted, loved and accepted by male partners, which may in turn place them at increased risk of HIV.

HIV, stigma and discrimination among male-to-females

In a sample of 402 transgender individuals, over half reported some form of harassment or violence at some time in their lives; 25 per cent report experiencing a violent incident (Lombardi *et al.* 2002). Although all MTFs face discrimination, there is evidence suggesting that transgender individuals of colour are at increased risk of HIV infection (Nemoto *et al.* 1999; Clements-Nolle *et al.* 2001). This may indicate that multiple layers of stigma and discrimination increase risk of HIV among MTFs of colour.

Economic discrimination is a common outcome of stigma that may indirectly lead to increased HIV rates for MTFs. A study found that 37 per cent of transgender individuals experienced some form of economic discrimination in their lives (Asthana and Oostvogels 1993). Some MTFs turn to sex work because they lack employment options (Garber 1992; Clements-Nolle *et al.* 2001), and sex work provides an opportunity to earn money to pay for sex reassignment surgery (Pang *et al.* 1994; Bockting *et al.* 1998). The desire to undergo sex reassignment surgery may also lead some MTFs to engage in particularly risky sex work as some clients pay extra for barrier-free sex (Boles and Elifson 1995; Nemoto et al. 1999; Nemoto et al. 2004a). Higher rates of HIV-seropositivity for MTFs compared to other groups of sex workers has been documented in a number of studies (Elifson et al. 1993; Clements-Nolle et al. 2001; Reback et al. 2001).

Studies report that many MTFs turn to substance abuse as a means of dealing with their transgender identity or in easing their ability to reveal their transgender identity to others (Bockting et al. 1998). Among the 392 MTF participants in the San Francisco study, 34 per cent had injected drugs in the past 6 months and drug use was highly predictive of a positive HIV serostatus (Clements-Nolle et al. 2001).

Gender roles

Researchers have yet to understand the relationship between stigma and discrimination and gender roles for MTFs. Gender roles refer to the culturally prescribed norms, ways of being and acting particular to men and women (Gagnon and Parker 1995). Gender roles are socially constructed and, as transgender individuals demonstrate, they can be transgressed, combined or even ignored. Over the years, gender roles have changed for both men and women, but research indicates that traditional gender roles, where women are passive and men active, still prevail in sexual relationships (Williams et al. 2001). Men actively seek out sexual relations with women, and women await men's actions. Researchers have discussed how female gender roles place (non-transgender) women at risk of HIV (DeBruyn 1992; Felmlee 1994; Amaro 1995; Gomez and Marin 1996; Zierler and Krieger 1997). Men decide whether and if to use protection, leaving many women vulnerable. This body of literature describes how social relations and expectations of women and men are played out in interpersonal relations. Although MTFs face very distinct issues surrounding HIV risk to non-transgender women, many of the same issues are relevant when examining MTFs' HIV risk. Gender roles that interfere with safer sex may be practised, including roles whereby women are expected to cater to men's sexual pleasure. In focus group research, Bockting et al. (1998) found that many MTFs reported that not using condoms with their partners served as an affirmation of trust in the relationship. Similar to research findings on women (Margillo and Imahori 1998), Bockting and colleagues (1998) found that MTFs also encountered difficulties negotiating condom use with their partners.

Sexual relations are an essential component of gender roles. The desire to be affirmed as a woman may contribute to HIV risk (Kammerer et al. 2001; Nemoto et al. 2004b). Bockting and colleagues (1998) found that engaging in sex work with men served as gender affirmation for MTFs. Moreover, MTFs were more likely to engage in safer sex with clients as opposed to sex with a relational partner (Nemoto et al. 2004b). Other research has revealed that the pursuit of a feminine body and the desire to be affirmed as female contributed to HIV risk when MTFs engaged in sexual activity with relational partners (Kammerer et al. 2001). Bockting et al. (1998) state that MTFs discussed how their quest for affirmation of their gender identity led to unsafe sex. Rodriguez-Madera and Toro-Alfonso (2005) found that MTFs' construct of feminine gender identity interferes with condom negotiation and is a major factor to consider in HIV prevention for MTFs. While a number of researchers describe how stigma and discrimination place MTFs at increased risk of HIV, there is less research examining how gender roles and the desire to feel loved contribute to HIV risk for MTFs. This chapter examines how stigma and discrimination interact with gender roles to place MTFs in a unique position with regards to HIV risk.

Methods

Qualitative research methods were utilised to engage 20 MTF participants in discussion about their lives, relationships and health-care needs. Data were collected using semi-structured in-depth interviews from clients of a community clinic in a major urban centre. The study was approved by the New York State Psychiatric Institute and Columbia University's Institutional Review Board. Details of the study location and design are described in detail in the following sections. Interviews were conducted between November and December 2003.

Study location

The health clinic where the study was conducted is located in a low-income area. The clinic does not cater to lesbian, gay, bisexual or transgender (LGBT) individuals but, rather, sets out to serve the low-income community where it is located, which by and large does not identify as LGBT. Through word-of-mouth, several MTFs came to learn of the clinic, where they receive hormone therapy, HIV counselling, testing and treatment, and general health care. The clinic also provides social services to all its clients. Staff have been trained and are accustomed to working with MTFs. The clinic serves mainly Latinos (the majority of which are Puerto Rican) and African Americans; the transgender clientele reflects the ethnic make-up of the non-transgender clinic clients. At last count, there were approximately 80 MTFs who were receiving care at the clinic.

Recruitment

Two medical doctors from the clinic recruited all participants. Transgender individuals were approached by the doctors and asked whether they would like to participate in an interview. They were informed that the interview was informal and that they would be asked questions about their lives including HIV health concerns and needs. Patients were told that service access at the clinic would not be affected in any way if they chose not to participate in the study.

Participants

All participants were clients of the clinic and 18 years of age or older. All but four of the 20 participants were Latina. The four non-Latina participants identified as African American, with one African-American participant describing herself as Caribbean. Of the 16 Latina participants, one was from Central America, another from South America and the remaining participants were from Puerto Rico or of Puerto Rican descent. The mean age of the participants was 30.7 years (range = 18–53, standard deviation = 9.8). Four of the 20 participants identified themselves as HIV-positive. To ensure respondents were comfortable discussing their sexual relationships with male, female and transgender individuals, only gender-neutral terms were utilised to enquire about sexual partners; however, all participants expressed desire and sexual activity only with men.

The average monthly income for this sample was US$525, although one participant earned as little as US$136 and another as much as US$1,200. Six participants had completed high school (age 18), seven had one or two years of high school (ages 15 or 16), five had finished junior high school (age 14) and one had a fourth grade education (age 10). The majority of respondents (16) lived in apartments or houses, two lived in a shelter for homeless individuals and one lived on the street. Almost half of the sample (nine) lived alone. All others lived with family (six), a partner (four) or friends (one).

None of the MTFs in this sample had undergone genital reconstruction surgery and only a handful had had breast augmentation. However, all were currently taking female hormones (with the exception of two participants who had recently lost the ability to pay for their hormones). To protect the confidentiality of participants, pseudonyms replace actual names in the excerpts presented in the following sections. This sample represents a unique opportunity for addressing issues that particularly concern ethnic and racial minority MTFs who may have limited resources. It is not known how representative this sample is of MTFs in urban cities in the USA.

Interviews

All interviews were conducted by the first author and were tape-recorded. Since the first author is bilingual, participants could select Spanish or English in which to conduct the interview; seven interviews were conducted primarily in Spanish. Occasionally, participants used Spanish words to describe certain feelings or material objects even though the interview was conducted primarily in English, or vice versa. Quotations taken from the Spanish interviews will appear first in Spanish and then in English to preserve the voice of the participant.

Interviews were conducted in the clinic on the day of recruitment. After a participant told the doctor that she wished to participate in the interview, the doctor would introduce the participant to the interviewer. All interviews were conducted in a private doctor's office. On occasion, participants were asked by the medical doctors to wait until an interview was concluded. In these instances, participants introduced themselves to the interviewer.

Most interviews lasted about an hour, with three interviews extending to 2 hours. Before the interview commenced there was a careful consenting process. Participants were instructed that they were under no obligation to participate and that their services at the clinic would in no way be affected if they decided not to participate. Participants were given a consent form to complete, the content of which was explained carefully by the interviewer. At several times during this process participants were asked if they had any questions.

An interview protocol was developed which covered broad areas of life such as discrimination, gender roles, stigma, relationships and health care, including medical procedures and hormone usage. The interview protocol was not used as a formal interview guideline; participants were never read questions directly from the protocol. The purpose of the interview protocol was to ensure that the same type of question was asked to all participants and that the same themes would be covered among all the participants. The interviews maintained the feeling of a conversation with pointed questions. An example of a typical question asked during the interview is: 'Can you tell me about a past relationship?' Typical follow-up questions include: 'What did you like about this partner?' and 'What did you dislike about this partner?'

Upon commencing the interview, each participant was asked: 'Is there anything on your mind you would like to discuss?' This question allowed some participants to ask questions or to discuss concerns regarding their visit to the clinic. Since the location of the study was a health clinic, there were many possible reasons why participants could have been at the clinic (e.g. receiving results of a medical test or coming in for HIV treatment), and it was important to give participants an opportunity to discuss anything that may be on their minds. On occasion, this question led to a discussion surrounding participants' concerns. For example, one participant described seeking shelter from an abusive relationship, which led to a discussion surrounding her abusive relationship, moved into a discussion of her relationships in general and proceeded to other topics such as health-care needs and concerns.

At the end of the interview, each participant was thanked and asked if she would like to receive a list of referrals for HIV services in their area. She was also asked if she would like to receive a safer sex packet containing a number of products including lubricant, male condom, female condom, finger cot and dental dam. Each participant also received $35 cash for their time and transportation costs.

Analysis

Interviews were transcribed verbatim. A modified form of grounded theory (Strauss and Corbin 1990) was used to guide the coding of the interviews. Unlike traditional grounded theory, the approach utilised here does not assume an inexperienced orientation to the data on the part of the investigator. It embraces the idea that the researcher's background, including theoretical orientations, analytic training, skill and experience with the data, is a necessary and important part of the analysis (Lincoln and Guba 1985).

Three researchers coded the transcripts. To commence analyses, three interviews were randomly selected. From these three interviews a coding schema was developed that included themes relevant to the aims of the study and the focus on gender roles. After establishing a thematic schema, the remaining interviews were read and coded for themes. If new themes emerged, they were added to the thematic schema. To enhance reliability, the authors met to discuss the themes coded and discrepancies with codes. All discrepancies were discussed and agreement was reached. The themes reported here are those relating to gender and HIV risk. These themes are in line with what the authors found to be an overarching story told by participants – that of stigma and discrimination leading to feeling unwanted and desiring to have a partner in order to feel loved, resulting in HIV risk.

Results

Within the public sphere, stigma and discrimination is prevalent in the lives of MTFs; their experiences of stigma and discrimination create a heightened need to feel safe and loved – and they turn to men in an attempt to feel loved, desired and affirmed as women.

'It's really a hard life'

All participants discussed the difficulties they experienced because they were transgender. Several participants used the phrase 'the life' and 'the hard life' to refer to being transgender. Yolanda, a 24-year-old Puerto Rican participant, says:

> It's really a hard life. It's really hard. See, it's easier for like two guys that are like two thugs and they're tough and gay and they'll be together for years, because nobody can tell and they like to keep it that way, but when it's a transgender, I don't care how pretty you may be, it's always going to be somebody can tell you're a man.

Respondents discussed how the threat of discovery was stressful to them. Walking down the street could invoke anger and violence if others recognise they are transgender.

Participants reported a tremendous amount of violence in their lives. All described being verbally attacked in the streets, and many described being physically attacked by strangers: several had been stabbed, one had been shot and another had had a gun put to her back. Many said they called the police; however, no action was taken on their behalf. Going outside the home was perceived as dangerous by many. Isabel, a 28-year-old Puerto Rican participant, was asked whether she went out with friends, and she replied, 'No. I'm not going out with people, I don't go out.' She then described being attacked by people on the street: 'See I walk in the street [alone], nobody tells who I am, [that] I'm a transvestite.' Isabel felt that going out with other MTFs makes it easier for people on the street to recognise her as transgender and therefore increases her chances of harassment and violence. When people recognise Isabel as transgender, she says, 'They start "Oohh"…and they start calling me "faggot", "you homo" and hit [us] with bottles, brick[s], stuff like that.' Many felt threatened and scared to go out in public, and staying home served as a means of dealing with this threat. Home was the place where they could escape these stresses – a place they could feel safe.

In contrast to her description of being in public and having people harass and be violent towards her, Isabel describes coming home at night:

> I'm in my house already by 8 tonight and [by] 10 o'clock that's it. Once I lock the doors behind me they are staying locked. Yeah, because I don't like to open, once I'm in my house, cluck cluck and that's it…I'm not going back out and if I did forget something, it's going to stay for tomorrow. I'm just going to stay in my house.

Isabel took time to describe the locking of the door, insisting that the door stayed locked once she is in her house. Her use of the onomatopoeia 'cluck cluck' corresponds to hand movements where she mimed someone turning a knob in vertical space. Her insistence that she will not leave the house, even if she had forgotten something, represents a sense of protection from danger.

Mirasol, a Puerto Rican respondent, was 53 years old and the oldest person interviewed. She felt vulnerable leaving the house because she feared men in her neighbourhood would realise she was not a biological woman. She was concerned they would hurt her and cause problems for her in her apartment complex by telling others she was transgender. She described leaving the house covering her face and timing her movements to avoid men – only leaving her home to come to the clinic where she was interviewed. She says:

> No, no, yo no puedo trabajar porque es que yo le tengo miedo a la calle. No puedo tener un trabajo porque yo tengo terror…yo quiero estar en la casa, como te dije, fue algo increíble que llegue aquí, porque yo tengo terror a la calle.

> No, no, I cannot work because I am scared of the street. I can't have a job because I am terrified…I want to stay in the house [to the clinic], like I said it was incredible that I came here, because I am fearful of the street.

Many respondents associate the world outside their homes with danger. The inside world of their homes was associated with safety. Home for most respondents took on the significant characteristic of protecting them from harassment they might encounter when going outside and being seen.

Domestic gender roles

Participants clearly described their preferred gender roles in relation to their homes and partners. They described taking on roles equivalent to what people often describe as traditional women's roles as homemakers and caretakers. Perhaps because public places were seen as dangerous, many respondents spoke eloquently about how they saw themselves inside their homes. Mirasol, for example, described herself in relation to her home:

> Así, casera, tú sabes, yo quiero, quisiera ser una mujer pero mujer de mi casa…es el 'look' que yo quiero dar, mujer de mi casa…Me da por limpiar, cocinar, ir a lavar cosas, me las paso en la casa y sí, viendo novellas.

> Oh yes, housewife, you know, I want to be a woman but a woman of my house…that is the 'look' I want to give, woman of my house…I have an inclination to clean, cook and to wash things, I pass my time in the house and, yes, I watch soap operas.

Mirasol's sense of self is tied to her home. The 'look' she chooses is one of a housewife. She also described herself as having an inclination to clean and take care of the house.

Ana, who lived with her partner and is a 33-year-old Puerto Rican, described herself in her relationship and the duties she performs at home:

> I cook for him, I do things for him. Everything a wife will do. Stay in the house, cook, clean, wash clothes, you know what I'm saying…I made that yesterday and I have an avocado and I'm going to open it today and I'm going to make him some pork chops. That's food today.

Ana actively sets out to care for her home and partner. She takes on the traditional female role vis-à-vis her partner. Her demeanour and discussion of her home highlight the importance of the domestic life as a place to be the woman she wants to be and the freedom to do so without worry of harassment or violence.

'They've always got a girl on the side'

Respondents who did not have a partner discussed the importance of finding one. Isabel said, 'It's like, oh my God, I need somebody. C'mon, I'm 28 now and I live my life this way for 6 years. It's time for me to get someone that's gonna help me.' Isabel denotes a sense that a man can help her with her life.

Although having a male partner was valued, many participants discussed the difficulties of finding a man who wanted to be with them for a long-term relationship. Respondents described living in a world where men want to have sex with them but few wanted committed relationships. Jasmine, a 22-year-old participant, provided her perspective on relationships with men and summed up what many respondents said about men:

> You run into a lot of relationships where guys just want you for sex. You know what I'm saying? You have a girl, I'm 22. I have met so many men that promised me the earth, moon and stars and I really thought they was going to give it to me and they turned out to be shit. You know what I'm saying? And it's because a lot of men are insecure about their own sexuality, so you will always be [on] the backburner. You will always be the

person that if they…they're always…I don't care, any transgender that don't know this by this age is stupid. Every man that deals with a transgender always has a girl on the side. Always. Believe me. I've been in the life a long time; they've always got a girl on the side.

Among study participants, only four were currently with a partner who they described as their committed partner or husband. Yet, all respondents wanted to have a loving and committed relationship with a man. Another participant, Maria, who was 35 years old and Puerto Rican, also reported that it was hard to find a man who will accept MTFs as they are. She said:

I mean my whole life I've always been with men that only want you for sex. You know, the majority of men…the reason they like transsexuals is that they resemble females, but, how can I put [it], when it comes to relationships it is very hard for us transsexuals to find a man who's proud of you, who wants you for you and walk down the street with you and don't care who knows you're a transsexual. It's really hard to find a man like that.

Maria describes a nuance that is not well explored in the research literature. She says men like MTFs because they look like women but also because they are not women. While the intersection between female and male is highly desirable for some men, many MTFs fear that their partners will leave them for a non-transgender male or female person. Joy, a 32-year-old African-American respondent, shed light on the importance of her partner in her life. She says her partner helped her deal with the difficulties she faced due to being HIV-positive:

My current relationship now is good. He's aware of all my medical problems and he's there for me. He's there for me. He's a wonderful human being. He loves me for me. He helps me with whatever, whenever I have…doctor's appointments…he's there. If he has to take off from what he has to do, he always is there. If I'm – if it's days that I don't feel good or I don't feel like doing anything, he steps in and does whatever has to be done. He's a good support system. He's a very good support system and I wouldn't trade him for nothing in the world.

Joy's partner keeps her spirits high and this in turn helps her stay hopeful and focused on taking care of herself. Joy states that her partner 'loves her for her'. The sentiment of being loved and accepted was discussed by other respondents as ideal, but few reported currently having a partner who accepted them. MTFs who did not have a partner stated that finding someone who accepted them for being transgender was a major hurdle.

Love, gender roles and HIV risk

Although there was a desire to have a committed relationship with a man, respondents discussed the difficulties of having a long-term relationship. Jasmine, a 22-year-old African-American respondent who was HIV-positive, offered her perspectives on the relationship between the need for an intimate relationship and HIV risk. At one point in the interview, she leaned into the microphone and said:

We know how hard the life is so when you meet a guy it's like you go through all means to keep this man, because you really want to be with him, you know what I'm saying? So it's really hard. You just want to be loved, that's it. Being ridiculed so much, called this, called that, being used…It's just like after a certain point in your life you just…you get needy, I guess…And a lot of people don't want to admit it, but a lot of people settle. A lot of us settle…I really think that it's so many of us that are getting this [HIV] because we want to be loved and you know…and a lot of times you meet somebody and you feel as though that this person's going to love you, so you…you risk a lot of things that…you know what I'm saying? To make this person happy, you know, you feel as though if you don't use it [condom] it's going to be closer, it's going to make him love you even more.

Perhaps because Jasmine was in the midst of dealing with her newly discovered HIV status, she reflected on how relationships may lead some MTFs to become infected with HIV. For participants who described the difficulties they face, being put down and made to feel like they are worth less than others, relationships take on added meaning and value. The need to feel loved, to feel 'closer' to someone, can trump the knowledge that one needs to be protected against disease.

Jasmine linked her experiences of being discriminated with those of finding a partner and feeling accepted; she said:

You meet a guy and he's attractive and, you know, you feel like oh, he really likes me, he walks down the street with me, he knows what I am, he holds my hand and then here you go caught in that ploy, now here it is, he wants to have sex with you, and the first couple of times you might use a condom, but then he want[s] to stop, because you feel like he really cares about you, and I mean part of us being transgender, we feel like we're women, so I guess that woman side of us wants to please our man, so it's a lot of things that we would do to just to please our man.

This description of wanting to be accepted and loved was common to other respondents in the sample. As with the importance of the home as safety from the outside world, intimate relationships were emotional locations in which participants could be themselves, be accepted for who they were and feel free from the discrimination they faced outside their homes. Jasmine wanted to be accepted as a transgender person. Beyond being accepted as transgender, Jasmine's sense of being a woman could place her at risk. Jasmine discussed the importance of wanting to please a man. She stated that she wants to please her partner – this is her sense of what it means to be a woman.

Another participant, Clara, also discussed the relationship between gender and HIV risk for MTFs. Clara had undergone several operations to enhance both her face and body and reported that she receives much attention from men. However, she also reported that no man is capable of truly loving her. She noted that men want to be with her for sex, but stated that as she gets older and presumably less attractive, she will surely be alone. She talks here about the possibility of contracting HIV in the future:

Claro que no me gustaría tener el SIDA ahora porque soy joven pero quizás en unos años…no me asustaría el hecho de contraerlo porque yo creo que no me gustaría vivir una vida en después de los 40 años, es una etapa muy dura para una y es muy triste quedarse sola y el sentir que nadie va a estar contigo por el hecho de no verte bonita o verte joven como ahora lo estoy.

Of course I would not like to have HIV now because I am young, but maybe in a few years…I wouldn't be scared to get infected because I do not think I would like to live a life, after 40, which is a hard stage for you, and it is very sad to be alone and to feel that no one wants to be with you because you are not being attractive and young like I am now.

Clara associated HIV with death and saw an early death as a possible escape from her life. She felt that getting HIV could help prevent a life where no man would want to be with her and where she would feel alone and unloved. Clara's sense of self-worth, interestingly enough, comes from her sense of beauty and youth. She feels that once these are lost, she will not have men's attention. Although Clara describes having various men in her life and often mentions that some men pay for her hormones and have paid for her surgery, she does not believe that a man could actually love her. Like other respondents, such as Jasmine and Maria, Clara feels that men want to be with her primarily for sex.

Discussion

In the book *Gender Play* (1993), Thorne discusses her observations of young boys and girls. She describes a 'heterosexual market' where girls receive an added sense of self-worth when involved in a relationship with a boy. Thorne describes a context where adolescent girls experience a diminished sense of self, self-esteem and self-worth at the same time that they begin to enter into heterosexual relationships. Although relationships appear to provide a sense of self-worth for these girls, in actuality, it is a false sense of worth. Because girls enter into relationships on unequal terms, they often experience relationships where they are unable to partake equally. Relationships are about keeping a boy rather than finding a mutually beneficial companionship. Rather than finding themselves, girls lose themselves in a false sense of security.

The experiences of MTFs in this study resemble aspects of Thorne's 'heterosexual market'. Because MTFs experienced stigma and discrimination, their own sense of self-worth had been greatly diminished. While the diminishment of self-worth for young girls can be difficult to locate in complex social processes involving gender, for MTFs this phenomenon is clearly located in the verbal and physical harassment they experience in the public sphere. Having a male partner was one way that they could regain a sense of self-worth and protection. Gender within the lives of MTFs plays a complicated role that interacts greatly with stigma and discrimination and together increases HIV risk for them. The interview data reveal a process of risk that emerges from stigma and discrimination. Stigma and discrimination create a context whereby the private sphere becomes a place where they can escape from the dangers present in the public sphere. The home is where MTFs are free to live according to their desired gender roles. The presence of a man adds to the feeling of being accepted and loved.

HIV risk emerged in two ways. First, MTFs wanted to find a male partner who would accept them for being transgender. Because all MTFs in the sample experienced severe forms of stigma and discrimination, a partner would provide them with one person in their lives who loved and accepted them for who they are. The need to have such a person may make safer sex a distant priority for them. Second, because many MTFs felt that they would not find a partner, they also felt doomed to lead a lonely and difficult life. Because their lives were filled with stigma, discrimination and an inability to find a partner who loved them, many felt their lives were very hard. Some, like Clara, may feel that becoming infected with HIV would provide an escape from this life. Figure 9.1 represents a model of how stigma and discrimination lead to HIV risk through the need to feel loved and accepted by a male partner.

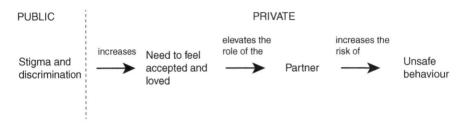

Figure 9.1 Stigma and discrimination lead to increased risk of unsafe behaviour by increasing the need to feel accepted and loved, which elevates the role of the partner and places MTFs at risk of HIV

The quest for a home and a romantic partner are common in society; however, among MTFs in this study, these needs were heightened. The need for someone to accept and love participants was important and understandable given the difficulties they encountered in their everyday lives. Although gender roles are important and do play a role in HIV risk, it is important to place gender roles and their relation to HIV risk within the larger context of the stigma and discrimination experienced by MTFs.

The concept of a 'heterosexual market' is important to consider for MTFs. Evidence suggests that MTFs' experience in the public sphere severely limits their abilities to enter into relationships in terms where they are able to demand equal power from their male partners. Because the relationship is more meaningful and valuable for them, many MTFs may feel compelled to give in to their male partners not only with regard to condom use but with a whole range of behaviours that may lead to increased emotional and physical vulnerability. HIV-prevention efforts for MTFs may need to take into account how stigma and discrimination influence MTFs' romantic relationships.

References

Amaro, H. 1995. Love, sex and power: Considering women's realities in HIV prevention. *American Psychologist* 50: 437–447.

Asthana, S. and Oostvogels, R. 1993. Communication participation in HIV prevention: Problems and prospects for community-based strategies among female sex workers in Madras. *Social Science and Medicine* 43: 133–148.

Bockting, W.O., Robinson, E. and Rosser, B.R.S. 1998. Transgender HIV prevention: A qualitative needs assessment. *AIDS Care* 10: 505–526.

Boles, J. and Elifson, K.W. 1995. The social organization of transvestite prostitution and AIDS. *Social Science and Medicine* 39: 85–93.

Clements-Nolle, K., Marx, R., Guzman, R. and Katz, M. 2001. HIV prevalence, risk behaviors, health-care use and mental health status of transgender persons: Implications for public health intervention. *American Journal of Public Health* 91: 915–921.

DeBruyn, M. 1992. Women and AIDS in developing countries. *Social Science and Medicine* 34: 249–262.

Elifson, K.W., Boles, J., Posey, E., Sweat, M., Darrow, W. and Elsea, W. 1993. Male transvestite prostitutes and HIV risk. *American Journal of Public Health* 83: 260–262.

Felmlee, D.H. 1994. Who's on top? Power dynamics in romantic relationships. *Sex Roles* 31: 275–295.

Gagnon, J.H. and Parker, R.G. (eds) 1995. *Conceiving Sexuality: Approaches to Sex Research in a Postmodern World*. New York: Routledge.

Garber, M. 1992. *Vested Interests: Cross-Dressing and Cultural Anxiety*. New York: Routledge.

Gomez, C.A. and Marin, B.V. 1996. Gender, culture and power: Barriers to HIV-prevention strategies for women. *Journal of Sex Research* 33: 355–362.

Green, J. 1994. *Investigation into Discrimination Against Transgendered People: A Report by the Human Rights Commission*. San Francisco, CA: City and County of San Francisco.

Herek, G.M. and Capitanio, J.P. 1999. AIDS stigma and sexual prejudice. *American Behavioral Scientist* 42: 1130–1147.

Kammerer, N., Mason, T., Connors, M. and Durkee, R. 2001. Transgender health and social service needs in the context of HIV risk. In: W. Bockting and S. Kirk (eds) *Transgender and HIV: Risks, Prevention and Care*. Binghamton, NY: Haworth Press.

Kenagy, G. 2002. HIV among transgender people. *AIDS Care* 14: 127–134.

Kenagy, G. and Bostwick, W. 2001. *Health and Social Service Needs of Transgendered People in Chicago*. Chicago, IL: Jane Addams College of Social Work, University of Illinois at Chicago.

Kenagy, G. and Hsieh, C. 2005. The risk less known: Female-to-male transgender persons' vulnerability to HIV infection. *AIDS Care* 17: 195–207.

Lincoln, Y.S. and Guba, E.G. 1985. *Naturalistic Inquiry*. Beverly Hills, CA: SAGE.

Link, B.G. and Phelan, J.C. 2001. Conceptualizing stigma. *Annual Review of Sociology* 27: 363–385.

Lombardi, E., Wilchens, R.A., Priesing, D. and Malouf, D. 2002. Gender violence: Transgender experiences with violence and discrimination. *Journal of Homosexuality* 42: 89–101.

Margillo, G.A. and Imahori, T.T. 1998. Understanding safer sex negotiation in a group of low-income African-American women. In: N.L. Roth and L.K. Fuller (eds) *Women and AIDS: Negotiating Safer Practices, Care, and Representation*. Binghamton, NY: Harrington Park Press/Haworth Press, 43–69.

Nemoto, T., Luke, D., Mamo, L., Ching, A. and Patria, J. 1999. HIV risk behaviors among male-to-female transgenders in comparison with homosexual or bisexual males and heterosexual females. *AIDS Care* 11: 297–312.

Nemoto, T., Operario, D., Keatley, J., Han, L. and Soma, T. 2004a. HIV risk behaviors among male-to-female transgender persons of color in San Francisco. *American Journal of Public Health* 94: 1193–1199.

Nemoto, T., Operario, D., Keatley, J. and Villegas, D. 2004b. Social context of HIV risk behaviours among male-to-female transgenders of colour. *AIDS Care* 16: 724–735.

Pang, H., Pugh, K. and Catalan, J. 1994. Gender identity disorder and HIV disease. *International Journal of STDs* 5: 130–132.

Reback, C., Simon, P., Bemis, C. and Gatson, B. 2001. *The Los Angeles Transgender Health Study: Community Report*. Los Angeles, CA: University of California at Los Angeles.

Risser, J. and Shelton, A. 2002. *Behavioral Assessment of the Transgender Population, Houston, Texas*. Galveston, TX: University of Texas School of Public Health.

Rodriguez-Madera, S. and Toro-Alfonso, J. 2005. Gender as an obstacle in HIV/AIDS prevention: Considerations for the development of HIV/AIDS prevention efforts for male-to-female transgenders. *International Journal of Transgenderism* 8: 113–122.

Simon, P., Reback, C.J. and Bemis, C. 2000. HIV prevalence and incidence among male-to-female transsexuals receiving HIV prevention services in Los Angeles County. *AIDS* 14: 2953–2955.

Strauss, A.L. and Corbin, J. 1990. *Basics of Qualitative Research: Grounded Theory Procedures and Techniques*. Newbury Park: SAGE.

Susman, J. 1994. Disability, stigma and deviance. *Social Science and Medicine* 38: 15–22.

Thorne, B. 1993. *Gender Play*. New Brunswick, NJ: Rutgers University Press.

Williams, S.P., Gardos, P.S., Ortiz-Torres, B., Tross, S. and Ehrhardt, A.A. 2001. Urban women's negotiation strategies for safer sex with their male partners. *Women and Health* 33: 133–148.

Zierler, S. and Krieger, N. 1997. Reframing women's risk: Social inequalities and HIV infection. *Annual Review of Public Health* 18: 401–436.

Chapter 10

Black lesbian gender and sexual culture

Celebration and resistance

Bianca D.M. Wilson

Introduction

> It is clear … that rather than a lesbian community per se, there exists now a whole lesbian society comprised of different lesbian communities.
>
> (Rothblum and Sablove 2005: xvi)

The notion that there are several forms of lesbian communities in the USA, distinguished by racial, ethnic, socio-economic class and regional diversity, has been reflected in multiple studies of communities of same-gender loving women[1] (Lapovsky-Kennedy and Davis 1993; Morris 2005; Rabin and Slater 2005). While there are few studies that have attempted to examine cultural systems within lesbian communities, empirical research (see, for example, Lapovsky-Kennedy and Davis 1993) and published personal narratives (see, for example, Hampton 1981; Nestle 1984) on the way lesbian community life has been organized reveal lesbian gender expression as a persistent and core feature of lesbian sexual culture.

Sexual culture is a group's world view regarding normative sexual behaviour and sexuality (Herdt 1997). In an effort to examine sexual culture as a dynamic construct, I used sexual discourse theory as delineated by Schifter and Madrigal (2001), who studied sexual health risks among Costa Rican youth. Sexual discourse theory holds that one way to understand a group's sexual culture is to examine the ways people speak about sex and sexuality, as well as the messages they report hearing from various institutions (e.g. family, school, religion). Within this framework, a researcher approaches the study of sexual culture as a dynamic construct by purposively examining both dominant and less dominant discourses regarding sex and through the expectation that cultures do not remain the same across time (Schifter and Madrigal 2001).

Within lesbian sexual culture, gendered sexual discourses have illuminated the myriad ways that lesbian women have used and expected one another to identify with labels along masculine and feminine continua; terms like 'femme' and 'butch' are among the labels that lesbians have used to describe where they fall along these continua. Gayle Rubin (1992) describes butch and femme as 'ways of coding identities and behaviours that are both connected to and distinct from standard societal roles for men and women' (467). Contrasting these forms of lesbian gender, Taylor and Rupp argue that one of the most significant forms of US second-wave feminist ritual that has characterized contemporary lesbian culture is the androgynous or 'neither masculine nor feminine' mode of self-presentation. These ways of dressing and behaving have been presented as an oppositional stance against the mainstream dominant view of appropriate feminine expression. However, women of colour and working class women have also asserted that these androgynous modes of expression are a cultural artefact of White middle class lesbians, not necessarily all lesbians (Burch 1998; Crawley 2001; Taylor and Rupp 1993).

Black lesbian gender expression

Historians have noted gender non-conforming modes of expression as core features of sexual life among Black same-gender loving women in the USA since the 1920s (Garber 1989; Walker 2001). African American blues and jazz singers during the Harlem Renaissance, such as Ma Rainey in her song 'Prove it On Me', asserted that they did not hang around 'no men' and that they 'talk to the gals just like any old man' while wearing suits and ties (Davis 1998). Black women who partnered with women and adopted masculine gender-scripted dress and behaviours have used the term 'butch' (Lorde 1983), but also used racially specific terms such as 'stud' (Hampton 1981). More recently, terms like 'aggressive' (Peddle 2005) and 'dominant' have also been used by Black same-gender loving women and girls who identify as masculine in appearance, behaviour, erotic expression and/or relationship role (Wilson 2003). The term 'femme' continues to be used in Black same-gender loving communities to denote women who identify as feminine in appearance, behaviour, erotic expression and/or relationship roles (Chisholm and Stark 2006). Black lesbians' personal narratives illustrate the ways that dress and hair styles have been important markers of Black lesbian gender roles (see, for example, Blackman and Perry 1990; Lorde 1983; Smith 1992), and contemporary representations of style differ dramatically depending on age, geography and interests, ranging from hip-hop to sportswear to business attire.

There is relatively little empirical research on lesbian gender expression. The few researchers who study lesbian gender have focused on varying topics, from butch and femme identity development processes (Hiestand and Levitt 2005; Levitt et al. 2003) to biological factors associated with lesbian gender identification (Brown et al. 2002; Singh et al. 1999). Among them, even fewer have focused on the role lesbian gender plays in organizing sexual or romantic life (see Crawley 2001 and Pitman 2000 for examples of exceptions). In a small qualitative study of lesbian body image issues, Pitman (2000) found that, for her Black participant, butch identity and Black identity were central to her body image. However, the ways in which butch or masculine identities played a role in Black lesbian culture was not further examined, as it was not the central focus of the study.

Most studies on lesbian gender expression focus solely or primarily on White lesbians. The social sciences have devoted little attention to documenting and examining the role of lesbian gender in the sexual cultures of African American lesbians, possibly reflecting what Hammond (2002) describes as the absence of Black queer women's experiences from dominant sexual discourses and the silencing of Black female subjectivity. One exception is an in-depth qualitative study of a community of Black lesbians in New York City (Moore 2006) that identified three categorizations of gender among Black lesbians, including femme, transgressive and gender blender. Trangressive referred to more masculine identified women, including masculine identified women who did not like the terms butch and stud, whereas gender blender referred to the mixing of explicitly feminine and masculine characteristics. Moore's study was an important step in the direction of documenting an often ignored segment of US culture, Black lesbians. The current study is aimed at adding to this body of research by specifically examining dimensions of Black lesbian sexual cultures. Additionally, this study aims to expand the use of sexual discourse theory to a multiple minority group. In doing so, I seek to demonstrate the complex relationships Black lesbians have to sexual messages that are generated within primarily Black lesbian spaces, as well as those from the multiple oppressed communities in which they may participate (e.g. women, African American, lesbian) or through the dominant mainstream (i.e. patriarchal, European American, heterosexual) US society.

Current study

The current study on lesbian gender roles within African American lesbian communities is part of a larger study, the Black Lesbians' Ideas about Sex and Sexuality (BLISS) study. The BLISS study was designed to document the defining features of African American lesbian sexual culture in Chicago, including the beliefs, values and perspectives about sex and sexuality. Using sexual discourse theory as a framework for studying sexual culture (Schifter and Madrigal 2001), the BLISS data were analysed for the current study to address the following research questions: (1) what function, if any, does lesbian gender play in Black lesbian sexual life?; (2) how is lesbian gender constructed and understood?; and (3) what are the range of perspectives regarding lesbian gender in Black lesbian communities?

Methods

Setting

The manifestations of racism and heterosexism in Chicago and their impacts on the lives of African American lesbians and gays are well known by sexual minorities of colour in the USA. Chicago is highly residentially segregated, in part because of its history of entrenched racist housing policies (Massey and Denton 1998). Paralleling the racism of the larger White community, racism within the gay communities in Chicago that are predominantly White has marginalized many African American lesbians and gays. African American lesbians and gays in Chicago cannot easily access support for their sexuality and a community based on their sexual identity. Additionally, heterosexism within African American communities isolates many African American lesbians and gays from support and resources as racial minorities. No predominantly Black lesbian, gay, bisexual and transgender (LGBT) neighbourhood in Chicago exists.

However, several Black LGBT organizations and groups exist, suggesting a continued resistance against multiple oppressions and an effort to create empowering, affirmative and culturally specific spaces and institutions for LGBT people of colour. Yet most of the organizational resources for Black gay people in Chicago are through health institutions, which tend to focus mostly on HIV services for gay and bisexual men, leaving a dearth of places for Black gay people that are not focused on issues of disease, especially for women. Only one of the city's organizations that solely focused on Black lesbians and bisexual women has its own physical space separate from other organizations, Affinity Community Services, which is a 13-year-old advocacy and service organization for Black lesbian and bisexual women. Prior to beginning this study, I had worked with several gay organizations that included Black gay and bisexual men as part of a university-based HIV-prevention team. I was also involved with Affinity Community Services, first as a youth programme chair and then later as a Board of Directors member.

Participants and procedures

I employed a rapid ethnographic assessment methodology (Kluwin *et al.* 2004), including three data collection methods: focus groups (FG), individual interviews and participant observations. Each method offered a unique lens through which to examine African American lesbian sexual culture. The study involved focus groups (n = 9; 26 participants) with African American lesbians (see Table 10.1 for demographics), individual interviews (n = 5) with community leaders,[2] and participant observations (n = 10 across 4 months) at a weekly open mike night for African American lesbians. Focus group participants were recruited through snowball sampling techniques. I conducted the focus groups using a protocol that was composed of five domains: attitudes toward Black lesbian community; defining sexuality; defining sex; butch and femme; and the influence of various communities (African American, lesbian and women) on their views about sex. The open mike events were important because they provided an opportunity to see how sex and sexuality were talked about outside of the research-directed setting. I listened to the open mike performances and noted characteristics of the audience, how and when performers talked about sex, what kinds of people were referred to in sexual poetry (e.g. perceived lesbian identity labels, sexual identities or race), the reactions of the audience, and the topics of other non-sexual poetry. The individual interviews with community leaders served as an opportunity to validate and expand upon the findings from the focus groups and observations.

Sampling issues

I sought to recruit a diverse group of participants for the focus group and individual interviews. However, I was unable to enrol more than two women who had never been to college. The findings therefore primarily represent the perspectives of women who have attended some college or technical school and those that have graduated college with undergraduate and graduate degrees. Additionally, I used convenience sampling and recruited through established LGBT institutions and media, such as agency listservs and community newspapers. Therefore, the respondents represent a population of lesbian-identified women that are relatively well connected to gay and lesbian communities. Though this sampling was useful for the primary aim of the study, which was to document lesbian community beliefs and norms, the absence of the perspectives of African American lesbians who were no longer or had never been connected to the community may limit the representation of other subgroups within the community. Finally, because the primary goal was to document sexual discourses more broadly and the prominence of the lesbian gender theme in this study was emergent, I had not anticipated the need to purposively sample participants that represent various lesbian gender categories. As such, the sample is composed primarily of lesbians who reported that they did not currently have a strong or salient lesbian gender identity, and the findings should be contextualized by the sample composition.

Analyses

I followed a coding process endorsed by many qualitative researchers (Vaughn *et al.* 1996; Wolcott 1994) and used NVivo software to organize the data. In short, the analyses followed a five-step process that began with identifying initial themes of the interview transcripts and observation notes. Then, I unitized the data into smaller units (i.e. coding) and examined

Table 10.1 Focus group participants

Focus group	Education level	Age	Years in Chicago
FG1	Some college	35	17
	Some college	40	16
	College graduate	44	14
		M = 39.7	M = 15.7
FG2	College graduate	40	40
	Some college	20	20
	Some college	37	37
		M = 32.3	M = 32.3
FG3	College graduate	50	50
	College graduate	30	30
		M = 40.0	M = 40.0
FG4	College graduate	40	2
	College graduate	53	25
		M = 46.5	M = 13.5
FG5	Some college	34	5
	Some college	38	17
	Some college	35	35
		M = 35.7	M = 19.0
FG6	Some college	20	20
	High school graduate	22	22
	Some college	19	19
	High school graduate	20	20
		M = 20.3	M = 20.3
FG7	College graduate	41	41
	College graduate	30	30
	College graduate	25	25
		M = 32.0	M = 32.0
FG8	Some college	65	65
	Some college	46	10
	Some college	39	20
		M = 50.0	M = 31.7
FG9	Some college	40	40
	Some college	44	2
	Some college	32	32
		M = 38.7	M = 24.7

Note: All participants identified as African American and as lesbian. M is the mean age for that group.

patterns among codes across data sources. Following these steps, I negotiated the coding structure with a second coder to increase code consistency and interpretation validity. I conducted these first four steps for the focus groups and observations prior to conducting the community leader interviews, which were used primarily as a way to help further negotiate my interpretation of the coding structure and identify themes that may have been missed in the focus groups and observations. Finally, the fifth step in the analysis process was identifying final themes and uses for theory.

Results and discussion

Overview

Using the analytic process described previously, I identified several aspects of the beliefs and practices regarding lesbian gender roles within African American lesbian sexual culture in Chicago. The results section is divided into three main parts that represent the dimensions of lesbian gender discussed by participants. First, I present how specific lesbian gender labels were constructed to create a stud–femme gender role dichotomy that functioned to organize sexual life. Then I discuss current debates among Black lesbians in this community about the prominence of the roles and labels, including evidence of resistance to the polarized dichotomy of these roles. Finally, I discuss my interpretations of how lesbian gender was given meaning in sexual situations to produce a radical interpretation of gender sex roles. Quotes from focus group participants and community leaders and observation notes are included as evidence of key themes, and relevant literature is included to illustrate connections to contemporary theory and research on lesbian gender expression. Pseudonyms are used for focus group participants and community leader interviewees.

One of the main questions of the focus group protocol was, 'Are roles or labels like butch or femme or aggressive or passive important in sex and sexuality? How so or why not?' This question was eventually rephrased to include the term stud as another term for butch since this was the term most often used by participants to describe masculine gender identities, reflecting ethnic differences in masculine identity terminology in the city. Every focus group chose to devote significant time and energy to answering this question. Participants consistently highlighted lesbian gender roles as a key organizing construct of African American lesbian sexual life. Four participants claimed these labels for themselves. Several other participants supported women's adoption of these roles. The ways in which participants spoke about stud and femme categories indicated that these ways of constructing lesbian gender were part of an overarching sexual cultural norm of which all were aware. Within every focus group, participants conveyed a sense that the expectation to adopt a label and to operate within the category was a strong message throughout the Black lesbian community. Hence, expectations to be a femme or stud appeared to be a sexual cultural script for this Black lesbian community. Participants indicated that this cultural script was communicated in several contexts, including romantic relationships and community settings.

In addition to lovers, participants reported being encouraged strongly to take on these labels by friends or acquaintances. In response to my question about who was trying to ascribe these labels, one participant, Pat, who was in FG3, said, 'I've been asked the most questions by Black lesbians. Not that they try to ascribe a label to me, but truly try to figure out where I fit and where I belong from other Black lesbians.' Community leaders who were interviewed testified to the strong presence of these labels and expectations within African American lesbian communities. Some focus group participants also suggested that although they do not use labels such as stud, butch or femme to describe themselves, they nonetheless yield to expectations around choosing a role within relationships in order to find dates or to satisfy a current partner.

The deep roots of the social pressure to date within these roles were also evident within my observations at the open mikes. Most women that appeared to be coupled off, as evidenced by them kissing or cuddling with each other, were a clear butch and femme couple. Using the language suggested by Moore (2006), only one couple was a 'gender-blender' couple. They were a younger couple, maybe in their early twenties, and were each dressed in both feminine and masculine clothing. I did not observe any couple that was composed of two women who were traditionally feminine and observed only one couple in which both were dressed and acted in traditionally masculine ways. An inherent aspect of sexual discourse and cultural scripts are the potential disconnects between expected norms and individual transgressions against those norms (Parker 1991; Schifter and Madrigal 2001). This one masculine–masculine couple appeared to be participating in this type of transgression. Recognizing the discrepancy between their coupling and the coupling expectations set forth by the cultural sexual scripts, I asked them whether they had experienced negative reactions to their being a couple in which both women appeared masculine identified. They explained that they had received harsh reactions and lack of understanding from other African American lesbians. However, they felt that they were no longer into labels and loved each other. They had been together for over 8 years and people knew them as an established couple, so left them alone.

Constructing the dichotomous stud–femme label system

With regard to non-sexual roles within romantic relationships, the extreme stud and femme labels carried expectations around partner choices. In particular, femmes are supposed to date studs and vice versa. Focus group participants and my participant observations suggest that there is little tolerance for femmes or studs dating one another. Once choosing a partner of the other lesbian gender, participants mentioned a few relationship roles that each person was expected to fill. Participants within several groups talked about being with a stud or femme partner who was disappointed that they would not follow the 'rules' of lesbian gendering. For example, Dalia indicated that she was expected to act more 'mannish' in her gestures when she was with a femme partner (FG3). Another participant, who was partnered with someone who identified as a hard stud, in turn expected her partner not to cry in order to live up to the masculine image (FG4, Cynthia). Similarly, participants who were with partners who were studs were expected to act in certain ways to be considered good femmes, such as in the case of Bré, who reported that she was expected to sleep on the inside of the bed in order to be protected (FG7). The expectations and tendencies to date within a stud–femme dyad that participants reported were very similar to those reported in Moore's (2006) study of New York Black lesbians, suggesting a Black lesbian cultural script that spans the boundaries of one city.

Specific to sexual practice, participants within groups and individual community leader interviews, as well as my participant observations, provided a rich description of how these labels translated to the sexual lives of Black lesbians in the community. The data indicated unique expectations and norms around sexual expression for feminine and masculine identified lesbians.

Masculine expression

Lesbians who expressed a highly masculinized gender were labelled 'hard studs', and hard studs had relatively strict guidelines for sexual practice. For example, participants talked about the 'hard studs that will come out and say, "I don't want my woman to touch me. I want to be the total pleaser" ' (FG2, Leslie). Contrasting femmes and hard studs, another participant claims:

... because studs mostly in traditional situations, they're usually the one who initiates, they're usually the one who, if you have oral sex, they usually the one who would initi- ate having oral sex on that particular person, when they want, on a femme. I know a lot of studs. They don't like to be touched to a certain point, you know, you can touch them in certain places, but you know, you can't really touch them like on, on their, you know, vagina or so things that may make them feel feminine. (FG5, Jay)

These participants' descriptions of the hard stud with which they were familiar is similar to the stone butch described in the fictional autobiography of Feinberg's (1993) *Stone Butch Blues* and discussed in Halberstam's (1998) critique of the tendency to pathologize the stone butch in her book *Female Masculinity*. As such, it is possible that the language of hard stud is an ethnic-specific term that denotes a lesbian gender category identified in other ethnic com- munities. While a few participants who identified themselves as either aggressive, tomboy or dominant volunteered that they usually or rarely allowed partners to penetrate them, it is important to note that focus group participants were not asked to describe their own sexual lives. Hence, data from this study cannot confirm or disconfirm the extent to which these 'hard' or 'stone' sexual scripts resonated with the sexual practice of the women in the study.

Illustrating how hard stud sexual scripts were understood by many Black lesbians in the community, two primary reasons were provided by participants for why hard studs would demand that they not be touched during sex. One explanation was that hard studs were not comfortable with the parts of their bodies that defined them as female, mainly their breasts and vaginas. As such, a successful performance of the 'male' role during sex required that the hard stud's female body parts not be touched. Another reason concerned the meaning of being touched and seduced. That is, participants talked about the importance of maintain- ing the appearance of dominance in the sexual act for hard studs and how being touched sexually or being the 'bottom' took away that sense of dominance and control. The vulner- ability of being sexually aroused and pleasured threatened the image of the dominant sexual partner. The contrast between these two explanations is significant. The first explanation, rejecting femaleness, is similar to the comments made by some transgender people regard- ing discomfort with their biological body parts that dictate mainstream society's current gendering system. However, the second explanation, maintaining dominance, is not about denying one's femaleness as expressed through the body but instead about accepting a view that being sexually pleasured and aroused by another makes a person vulnerable. Being vul- nerable does not fit with the hegemonic masculine image and, hence, does not fit with the image of a true stud.

This study was designed to examine sexual discourses – essentially, how Black lesbi- ans discussed sex and what cultural-level sexual scripts were recognized in the community. While examining conflicts between cultural-level norms and individual behaviour was not the aim of the current study, some participants noted that there is some evidence of trans- gressions. Participants in two focus groups (FG1 and FG9) discussed studs they knew who had recently had vaginal sex with men and had children, behaviours that did not fit into the masculine lesbian gender identity role. It is quite likely that many studs and many ultra femmes engaged in sexual behaviour that transgressed expected community norms (beyond the mainstream norms they already transgress through sexual orientation and gen- der presentation), as was found in a study of the level of congruence between butch global presentation and actual self-presentation in sexual settings within a predominantly White sample (Rosenzweig and Lebow 1992).

Feminine expression

Within the masculine/feminine dichotomy that was discussed by participants, there were also the pillow princesses and ultra femmes at the other end of the lesbian gender spectrum. Similar to the hard stud category, these extreme femme labels have clear sexual behaviour roles. In this study 'ultra femme' was a label given to women who expressed themselves in high-fashion feminine ways, usually including heels, make-up and contouring or revealing clothing. Relevant to the current study, 'pillow princess' was a special label for the ultra femme that alluded to the sexual context. In particular, this label described a lesbian who prefers to be the receiver of sexual pleasure and acts, such as having oral sex performed on her. She is not expected or likely to perform any sexual acts on her partner. In a sexual encounter, the expectation is that ultra femmes are the ones that will be vaginally penetrated with sex toys or fingers. While not all participants spoke of the relationship between sexual penetration and femme identities, one group agreed that a requirement to being labelled femme was that an individual liked penetration (FG1). It is notable that outside of acknowledging that this role may be a little selfish, no pathology related to body image or gender identity was ascribed to the role of pillow princess. In general, it was the role of hard stud that engendered the most resistance, as will be described in the next section.

Debate within the community about lesbian gender

As Burch (1998) has noted, some activists and theorists argue that the adoption of femme and stud roles and labels is an attempt to replicate the gendered sexual norms in which lesbians were raised in the mainstream heterosexual society. Several community leaders and focus group participants thought similarly. For example, in FG7, Wanda talked about the differences between White and Black lesbians that she saw:

> They are, and not just Whites, but [also] other non-African American lesbians see it as we are just two women that love each other. Whereas Blacks say we are two women that love each other; however, we do have roles. You know, and we are trying to in a sense maybe ascribe to a heterosexual way of life, or way of operating, in our relationship.
>
> (FG7)

Similarly, one of the community leaders whose work focused on sexuality and spirituality, Vicki, discussed her own experiences with previously claiming a butch identity. She indicated that letting go of this identity represented seeing it for what it was, a replication of heterosexuality. Kendra, another community leader who works in lesbian and gay health arenas, also reported that she felt that femme and butch labels appear to mimic traditional gender roles. However, she cautioned against the assumption that mimicking traditional gender roles automatically made lesbian gender label expression 'artificial'. That is, many African American lesbians genuinely feel masculine or feminine and are truly attracted to 'opposite' lesbian gendered women. Nonetheless, these same women who identify as butch or femme are sometimes frustrated with the strict rules regarding these labels and identities.

In contrast, one focus group participant, Gail, who identified as femme and as a member of the 'butch–femme community', also conveyed to the group that there was a renaissance in the butch–femme movement that included reconfiguring butch and femme to mean more than a replication of heterosexual gender roles. She felt that contemporary butch–femme communities were more egalitarian than they had been when she was younger, where femmes were no longer placed in a subservient or domestic role. Some scholars have argued that femme and stud labels do not attempt to replicate heterosexist norms, but serve as mechanisms for de-gendering gendered lines by claiming masculinity in women's bodies. The butch lesbian in particular functioned as 'images to contradict the prevailing image of female sexuality as passive or even nonexistent' (Burch 1998: 361). However, this argument suggests that lesbians who adopt lesbian gender labels do so as a political statement. While a masculine identity may operate as a radical rejection of traditional female expectations, no data from this study suggest that the adoption of lesbian gender labels among African American lesbians was intended to be a purposeful and political affront to mainstream gender expectations.

Despite the large role that lesbian gender played in organizing Black lesbian sexual life, every focus group discussion revealed individuals' (within the group or people known by group participants) conscious and purposeful rejection of femme and stud labels/roles. There were several strategies used to reject the femme and stud categories within African American lesbian communities: refusing to label oneself; feeling bothered by labels; feeling hopeful that the cultural scripts will change; and avoiding hanging out with people who like labels. Focus group participants reported that they refused to label themselves in terms of femme or stud. As Sheri from FG4 said in response to a comment from another group participant:

> I agree with that ... don't identify in any of those butch/femme things. It is a mystery to me ... I don't disapprove of it, it just isn't who I am ... the role thing, it makes me a little nervous, but I realize that it's out there. That other folks are, that's who they are. And I understand the politics around those roles. But I don't choose it for myself.
>
> (FG4)

Similarly, a participant in another focus group responded to this issue by saying:

> And I'm like, okay, I'm a girl, you know what I'm saying? I'm, we're both women, and it doesn't matter, you know, I don't care what kind of femme I am ... So I, I still have a problem with it ... but ... this is the way I guess our community just, you know, identifies each ... the studs over here, the femmes over there. So I use labels like in my everyday vocabulary, whatever, but when it comes to me personally in a relationship ... I don't look for, like I said, I like the studs, whatever, but I would rather have a female that knows that she's a woman first. I like the masculine type, but I would rather she knows she's a woman first and not come at me all the time like stud this, and stud that, and stud this. In my personal life, that irritates the hell out of me. I'm sorry to say it like that, but it does. It irritates me. And I would just rather, in my personal relationship don't use those labels like that, because we're both females.
>
> (FG6, Tracey)

As illustrated by these quotes, some participants refused the labels for themselves and also expressed being bothered or irritated with the community trend to adopt labels. However, they also conveyed acceptance or tolerance for those that chose the labels. Further, the comments made by Tracey in FG6 indicate that the choice to refuse labels for oneself is not incongruent with having an attraction to women who possess the characteristics those labels define.

In contrast, other focus group participants expressed rejection or avoidance of femme and stud identified women. As discussed previously, Gail was a participant who had previously avoided Black gay spaces because she had experienced butch–femme culture as oppressive, but then later came to adopt a femme identity. In contrast, the two other participants in her group expressed strong negative judgements of the lesbian gender labels, particularly those expressed by stud or butch women. In particular, Anna evaluated masculine identified women in this way by making racial identity confusion analogous to masculine expression (e.g. scratching your crotch) among women:

> … if I walked around saying, 'I'm White, so please address me as such', I think I'd have a mental problem. If I walk around as a woman … and I'm scratching something I don't have, I also see that as a slight mental deficiency.
>
> (FG8)

Stacey then reported that she would like to see lesbians view themselves differently:

> Because I've seen it, seen it all, heard it all, been through a lot of goody stuff, I mean, geez, I used to have a ball, girl. I miss some of that but, ah, I, I've always prayed that gay women would just be as wholesome and caring as possible and not get caught up in all this heavy butch, heavy femme, heavy stud, Dyke, all this shit. Just be who you are. I think you'll be a hell of a lot happier.
>
> (FG8, Stacey)

Several poets at the open mikes spoke about struggling against expectations to label oneself in terms of lesbian gender. For example, one poet who enrolled into the study so that I could quote her poem speaks of wanting to drop these labels as she professes her attraction to a straight girl:

> … the first time I laid eyes on you
> my heart and soul despised of you
> wondering why I couldn't dine with you spend a little time with you
> share a piece of mine with you
> but that was on a Sunday
> one day I took time
> to clear my mind
> of each and every thought of you
> the fucked up labels that I brought to you …
> like STUD and FEMME,
> DYKE and SHEM.
> Just being me was a crime you see
> cause I'm a FEMME living
> STUD LOVING
> thought you was my woman
> till you said you was my husband?????
> Damn! our lifestyle is complex

that's what leaves the straight ones vexed
thinking we all play roles and can't be role models ...

(V-love)

Another poet who was interviewed as a community leader, Warrior, also expressed frustration and anger at being forced into the label of stud and femme. As soon as I asked her to respond to my preliminary findings suggesting that lesbian gender roles were consistently discussed as a unique feature of African American lesbian sexual culture, she commented that she wanted to resist the evidence that the phenomenon of butch and femme belongs to 'us' (i.e. Black lesbians).

Between the extremes

Despite a consistent description of femme and stud at the extremes of lesbian gender expression, participants also discussed several labels that fell between the ultra femme–hard stud ends of the continuum, such as 'soft stud' and 'aggressive femme'. Labels like these represented lesbians that blended both masculine and feminine ways in their public expression and/or sexual behaviours, but with a purposeful leaning toward more masculine or feminine identity. The use of these terms appears contrary to the reports that there were dominant expectations of highly masculine or highly feminine modes of expression. Yet, the sets of sexual discourses that comprise a group's sexual culture are inherently contradictory and often disjointed from one another (Schifter and Madrigal 2001). There was a collective acknowledgement that dominant sexual discourses in Black lesbian communities emphasized an expectation for choosing identities representing opposite sides of a single feminine–masculine continuum. Yet, this expectation did not prevent the existence of informal, less dominant sexual scripts that created room for blending characteristics along both masculine and feminine continua.

One of the community leader interviewees, Kendra, suggested that the mere presence of these alternative labels was evidence of a loosening of the hold that the traditional conceptualization of lesbian gender had on African American lesbians in Chicago. She asserted that the creation of new labels is one form of resistance to the strict dichotomy of stud and femme that arose out of the 'old school' African American lesbian sexual culture and provides more freedom for people to act in various ways and date different types of people. In this way, the development and adoption of more labels, and thus more roles and conceptualizations, could represent a quasi-organized movement toward changing the current gendered sexual discourse among Black lesbians.

Another core feature of sexual discourses, particularly those that are more formal (i.e. explicit) and dominant, is that they engender resistance (Schifter and Madrigal 2001). It was in the theme of lesbian gender that forms of resistance were most evident. As noted previously, resistance strategies ranged from individual choices to not identify with femme or stud roles, to open rejection of other lesbians who chose those identities. Additionally, some Black lesbians discussed the adoption of labels that represented a blend of feminine and masculine traits which simultaneously embraced preferences for gendered ways of relating sexually and romantically and rejected strict rules for lesbian gender roles. Most of the resistance discussed centred on disagreements with the concepts of prescribed roles in romantic and sexual relationships. In cases where the frustration was directed specifically at those who identified with the labels, the discontent was with masculine women, not the femmes. This theme has been observed in other work documenting the experiences of Black studs and aggressives (Moore 2006). This is notable because it indicates that resistance against femme–stud lesbian gender expression is not an unqualified rejection of all Black lesbians who express themselves in gendered ways. The Black lesbians in this study who disagreed with lesbian gender roles were not arguing for a movement toward the androgynous images that characterize many White lesbian communities (Taylor and Rupp 1993). Instead, the resistance is centred on the rejection of masculine women, studs, who dare to transgress the mainstream cultural expectations for proper female expression as well as possible mainstream Black women's cultural expectations of women to operate somewhere between gender-blending and feminine expression.

A radical side to lesbian gender sex roles

The butch/stud and femme phenomenon as discussed by study participants also represents a shift from traditional notions of masculine and feminine expressions of sexuality, even though these views were not labelled as forms of resistance by participants. Though many focus group participants, community leaders and poets at the open mikes argued that stud and femme roles were replications of heterosexual male and female sexual relationships, the sexual scripts for hard studs and pillow princesses appear to turn the traditional conceptualization of fe/male sex roles on its head. Heterosexual men may be expected to be the sexual aggressors (as studs were described to be by participants), but they are typically not socialized to view sexual pleasure of their female partner as the primary outcome. For example, in her historical analysis of the invention of the vibrator, Maines (1999) identified three steps of sex within the dominant US cultural script for sexuality: (1) foreplay or preparation for penetration; (2) penile intercourse; and (3) male orgasm. This type of sex is regarded as the 'real thing' in popular US culture. In contrast to this dominant script, masculine identified stud women prioritize the feminine partner's orgasm. Similarly, whereas pillow princesses and other femmes appear to fall in line with heterosexual conceptualizations of sexual roles for women, where the woman's role is the passive and non-assertive partner, they represent radical departures in other respects. In particular, participants indicated that ultra femmes and pillow princesses fully expected that the sexual act ended with their sexual climax. This appears to be a re-conceptualization of the connection between femininity and sexual prowess, deeming the feminine partner as the primary physical beneficiary. In essence, the feminine partner can be viewed as receptive, rather than passive (Burch 1998).

Conclusion

African American lesbians in this study conveyed a set of sexual beliefs, attitudes and behaviours that influenced what types of sex they had, who they dated and their behaviour within romantic relationships. This study highlighted that femme and stud roles were a dominant norm operating within this African American lesbian community, yet there were clearly informal and less dominant sexual discourses, which included an integration of masculine and feminine forms of representation. Participants expressed various reactions to dominant scripts regarding lesbian gender roles, including various forms of resistance.

While the intent of this study was more explicitly focused on sex than Moore's (2006) study of Black lesbians, many of the findings relating to dating and community expectations around partner choices were similarly reported in the two studies. The similarities of these two studies' findings from different cities, as well as several of the personal narratives discussed earlier, suggest that there may be a persistent sexual cultural script shared among Black lesbians. These scripts may be rooted in an interpretation of African American traditions. The ways in which these similarities are a function of the interaction between race, gender, sexuality and urban living is not known and warrants further investigation. Additional research focusing on significant intracultural or intragroup differences will contribute greatly to theory that accurately represents the diversity of experiences and thinking among groups that have traditionally been silenced around sex and sexuality.

Notes

1 I use the term 'same-gender loving' women to refer to women who partner and have sex with women, some of whom may choose not to use terms like lesbian or bisexual. This is a term that has emerged within US African American gay and lesbian communities to represent the range of labels that may describe non-heterosexual peoples and to counter Eurocentric gay and lesbian terminology.
2 Community leaders were selected for their experience in working within Black lesbian communities or because of their work as sexual health educators in ethnically diverse lesbian communities. Due to confidentiality, the individual demographics are not provided; however, they collectively comprise a group of community organizers, artists, religious leaders, public health directors and sex workshop facilitators.

References

Blackman, I. and Perry, K. 1990. Skirting the issue: Lesbian fashion for the 1990s. *Feminist Review* 34: 67–78.
Brown, W.M., Finn, C.J., Cooke, B.M. and Breedlove, S.M. 2002. Differences in finger length ratios between self-identified 'butch' and 'femme' lesbians. *Archives of Sexual Behavior* 31: 123–128.
Burch, B. 1998. Lesbian sexuality/female sexuality: Searching for sexual subjectivity. *Psychoanalytic Review* 85: 349–372.
Chisholm, K. and Stark, E. (Co-Directed/Produced) 2006. *FtF: Female to Femme*. San Francisco, CA: AltCinema Films. Available at: www.altcinema.com/contact.html [Accessed 22 December 2014].
Crawley, S.L. 2001. Are butch and fem working class and antifeminist? *Gender and Society* 15: 175–196.
Davis, A. 1998. *Blues Legacies and Black Feminism: Gertrude 'Ma' Rainey, Bessie Smith, and Billie Holiday*. New York: Pantheon Books.
Feinberg, L. 1993. *Stone Butch Blues*. Ithaca, NY: Firebrand Books.
Garber, E. 1989. A spectacle in color: The lesbian and gay subculture of jazz age Harlem. In: M.B. Duberman, M. Vicinus and G. Chauncey Jr. (eds) *Hidden from History*. New York: NAL Books, 318–331.
Halberstam, J. 1998. *Female Masculinity*. Durham, NC: Duke University Press.
Hammond, E.M. 2002. Black (w)holes and the geometry of black female sexuality. In: C. Mui and J. Murphy (eds) *Gender Struggles: Practical Approaches to Contemporary Feminism*. Lanham, MD: Rowman and Littlefield, 257–275.
Hampton, M. 1981. Mabel Hampton. In: J. Nestle (ed.) *The Persistent Desire: A Femme–Butch Reader*. Boston, MA: Alyson, 43–45.
Herdt, G.H. 1997. *Same Sex, Different Cultures: Gays and Lesbians Across Cultures*. Boulder, CO: Westview Press.
Hiestand, K.R. and Levitt, H.M. 2005. Butch identity development: The formation of an authentic gender. *Feminism and Psychology* 15: 61–85.

Kluwin, T., Morris, C. and Clifford, J. 2004. A rapid ethnography of itinerant teachers of the deaf. *American Annals of the Deaf* 149(1): 62–72.

Lapovsky-Kennedy, E. and Davis, M. 1993. *Boots of Leather, Slippers of Gold: The History of a Lesbian Community*. New York: Routledge.

Levitt, H.M., Gerrish, E.A. and Hiestand, K.R. 2003. The misunderstood gender: A model of modern femme identity. *Sex Roles* 48: 99–113.

Lorde, A. 1983. Tar beach. In: B. Smith (ed.) *Home Girls: A Black Feminist Anthology*. New York: Kitchen Table – Women of Color Press, 145–158.

Maines, R. 1999. *The Technology of Orgasm: 'Hysteria', the Vibrator and Women's Sexual Satisfaction*. Baltimore, MD: Johns Hopkins University Press.

Massey, D. and Denton, N. 1998. *American Apartheid: Segregation and the Making of the Underclass*. Boston, MA: Harvard University Press.

Moore, M.R. 2006. Lipstick or timberlands? Meanings of gender presentation in Black lesbian communities. *Signs: Journal of Women in Culture and Society* 32: 113–139.

Morris, B. 2005. Negotiating lesbian worlds: The festival communities. In: E. Rothblum and P. Sablove (eds) *Lesbian Communities: Festivals, RVs, and the Internet*. Binghamton, NY: Harrington Park Press, 55–62.

Nestle, J. 1984. The fem question. In: C. Vance (ed.) *Pleasure and Danger: Exploring Female Sexuality*. London: Pandora Press, 232–241.

Parker, R. 1991. *Bodies, Pleasures and Passions*. Boston, MA: Beacon Press.

Peddle, D. (Directed) 2005. *The Aggressives*. Los Angeles, CA: Seventh Art Releasing. Available at: www.7thart.com/current/aggressives/index.html [Accessed 22 December 2014].

Pitman, G. 2000. The influence of race, ethnicity, class and sexual politics on lesbians' body image. *Journal of Homosexuality* 40: 49–64.

Rabin, J. and Slater, B. 2005. Lesbian communities across the United States: Pockets of resistance and resilience. In: E. Rothblum and P. Sablove (eds) *Lesbian Communities: Festivals, RVs and the Internet*. Binghamton, NY: Harrington Park Press, 169–182.

Rosenzweig, J.M. and Lebow, W.C. 1992. Femme on the streets, butch in the sheets? Lesbian sex-roles, dyadic adjustment, and sexual satisfaction. *Journal of Homosexuality* 23: 1–20.

Rothblum, E. and Sablove, P. (eds) 2005. *Lesbian Communities: Festivals, RVs and the Internet*. Binghamton, NY: Harrington Park Press.

Rubin, G. 1992. Of catamites and kings: Reflections on butch, gender and boundaries. In: J. Nestle (ed.) *The Persistent Desire: A Femme–Butch Reader*. Boston, MA: Alyson Publications, 466–482.

Schifter, J. and Madrigal, J. 2001. *The Sexual Construction of Latino Youth*. New York: The Haworth Hispanic/Latino Press.

Singh, D., Vidaurri, M., Zambarano, R.J. and Dabbs, J.M. 1999. Lesbian erotic role: Identification – behavioral, morphological, and hormonal correlates. *Journal of Personality and Social Psychology* 76: 1035–1049.

Smith, B. 1992. The dance of masks. In: J. Nestle (ed.) *The Persistent Desire: A Femme–Butch Reader*. Boston, MA: Alyson Publications, 426–430.

Taylor, V. and Rupp, L. 1993. Women's culture and lesbian feminist activism: A reconsideration of cultural feminism. *Signs* 19: 32–61.

Vaughn, S., Schumm, J.S. and Sinagub, J. 1996. *Focus Group Interviews in Education and Psychology*. Thousand Oaks, CA: SAGE.

Walker, L. 2001. *Looking Like What You Are: Sexual Style, Race and Lesbian Identity*. New York: New York University Press.

Wilson, D. (Directed) 2003. *The Butch Mystique*. Harriman, NY: New Day Films.

Wolcott, H. 1994. *Transforming Qualitative Data Description, Analysis and Interpretation*. Thousand Oaks, CA: SAGE.

Section 4

Sex work

All over the world, sex is exchanged for rewards of various kinds, be these financial, physical or emotional in nature, or linked to the provision of food, warmth or some form of security. Only sometimes, however, are these transactions referred to as prostitution or sex work. Together, the three chapters in this section offer insight into the diverse forms that sex work takes, the different social actors involved, and the contexts in which it occurs.

Against the background of often heated debates about the nature of sex work, Vicky Bungay, Michael Halpin, Chris Atchison and Caitlin Johnston explore the contrast between perspectives which portray all sex workers as the victims of injustice and oppression, and those which see sex work as a form of labour entered into as 'voluntarily' as many other forms of employment. Central to these debates are claims about the agency of those involved in the sex trade. Some researchers argue that those involved are the victims of exploitation and structural and interpersonal constraint, whilst others depict them as individuals and workers exercising choice. Drawing on findings from a review of legal and media accounts of the sex trade and qualitative interviews with indoor sex workers in Vancouver, Canada, the authors argue that both of these perspectives by themselves are insufficient. They argue for a more nuanced perspective, which sees sex work through the complex interplay of *both* structure and agency. While structural analyses highlight the numerous ways in which sex workers are controlled and influenced, agency perspectives point to the means that sex workers use in order to exercise control in contexts of disadvantage. The policy and legal implications of this more sophisticated way of understanding sex work are discussed with reference to modern-day Canada.

Internationally, the literature on sex work focuses primarily on women. Yet, men too sell or exchange sex for financial and other forms of reward. In their chapter, Jerry Okal, Stanley Luchters, Scott Geibel, Matthew F. Chersich, Daniel Lango and Marleen Temmerman provide insights into the sexual practices and life experiences of male sex workers in Kenya. While HIV transmission through sex between men in Africa is increasingly acknowledged, HIV prevention remains focused largely on heterosexual and mother-to-child transmission. Using data from in-depth interviews and focus group discussions in Mombasa, the chapter explores the social and behavioural determinants of sexual risk among men who sell sex to men. Findings point to the diversity of men involved, both with respect to age and social class. First male same-sex experiences occur for diverse reasons, including love and pleasure, as part of sexual exploration, and through coercion and economic exchange. Condom use was inconsistent: being influenced by the common belief that condoms interfere with sexual pleasure, and the motivations of clients. The widespread belief that the risk of HIV transmission through anal sex is lower than vaginal sex compounds sexual risk taking. Traditional values, stereotypes of abnormality, gender norms and cultural and religious influences underlie the intense stigma and discrimination men face. Findings from the study hold the potential to guide the development of peer education programmes, and the sensitisation of health providers, to address unmet HIV prevention needs.

The final chapter in this section focuses on Peru, where sex work involving men and male-born *travestis*, transgenders and transsexuals is usually represented as a dangerous street-based practice engaged in by people experiencing economic hardship and social exclusion. In reality, however, little is known about the complexities of such practices, the social meanings they carry for the individuals involved, and the contexts in which sex work actually takes place. In this chapter, César Rodolfo Nureña, Mario Zúñiga, Joseph Zunt, Carolina Mejía, Silvia Montano and Jorge Sánchez present findings from an ethnographic study of the characteristics, patterns and sociocultural aspects of sex work among men and male-born trans women conducted in three Peruvian cities. The study included participant observation in sex work venues and interviews with sex workers and key informants. In contrast to stereotypical images of sex work, the authors found that sex work by male-born *travestis*, transgenders and transsexuals takes many forms, and is practised in different places by people from various socio-economic levels. In many cases, the practice is linked to ideals about social mobility, migratory experiences and other economic activities. In addition, the increasing use of the Internet and mobile phones is rapidly changing patterns of sex work in Peru and other countries.

Chapter 11

Structure and agency
Reflections from an exploratory study of Vancouver indoor sex workers

Vicky Bungay, Michael Halpin, Chris Atchison and Caitlin Johnston

Introduction

The legality of commercial sex work (remuneration for sexual contact) and the activities of women who work in the sex industry are a source of heated public and academic debate. Assumptions concerning human 'agency' – the freedom to make decisions and enact choices (Sherwin 1998) – sit at the heart of these debates. Scholars and advocacy groups from diverse perspectives seem at an impasse regarding whether sex work is reflective of constraints to women's agency through systemic injustice and violence against women (e.g. Farley 2004; Raphael and Shapiro 2004) or representative of a form of labour in which women have the 'right' to freely choose the nature of their activities (e.g. Betteridge 2005; Jeffrey and MacDonald 2006; Vanwesenbeeck 2001).

Western scholars supporting the abolition of prostitution tend to situate sex workers in a nexus of constraints in which they are subjected to perpetual oppression (e.g. Monroe 2005; Salfati *et al.* 2008). These positions are frequently aligned with assumptions that portray all sex workers as victims of systemic injustice (Weitzer 2005). Farley's (2004) argument that it is impossible to understand sex work as 'work', as it is essentially a form of violence orchestrated by pimps, 'johns' and sex work awareness groups, exemplifies this position.

Proponents of the work perspective situate sex work as a form of labour versus a system of exploitation. Sex workers' decision-making abilities are highlighted to disrupt victimisation assumptions, and many proponents (Bernstein 2007; Jeffrey and MacDonald 2006; Lucas 2005) argue that although sex workers may be constrained by their social conditions, their 'choice' to enter the sex trade represents proof of agency. That is, individuals faced with difficult economic decisions, whether the realities of poverty (Jeffrey and MacDonald 2006) or prosperity-related economic disparities (Bernstein 2007), still choose to enter the sex trade.

An important qualifier of both oppression and work perspectives is the apparent divergence with regards to who the term 'sex worker' represents. Advocates of oppression perspectives tend completely to reject the term sex worker in favour of 'prostituted women' (e.g. Farley 2004) and often point to the most visible examples, particularly those engaged in street-based 'survival sex'. Alternatively, those who favour labour perspectives often frame the identity of individuals engaged in the sex trade as sex workers to reflect their belief that not all who sell sex are severely disadvantaged and emphasise that the majority of sex workers practise their trade within the confines of escort agencies, brothels and the Internet (e.g. Bernstein 2007).

As others have noted (Agustín 2006; Vanwesenbeeck 2001; Weitzer 2005), many current debates appear based on over-generalisations and academic constructions that seem to have been designed to suit particular political ends and as such overlook the benefits of counterpoint assertions. The experiences of sex workers are often more nuanced than debates have led us to believe, particularly when such arguments fail to offer sex workers' own perspectives. There is a growing interest in academia to examine agency within the context of women and sex work in a manner more sensitive to the subtle nuances of structural factors and human agency beyond victimisation or labour perspectives (Agustín 2006). To date, much of this work has been situated within the realm of women's health and the strategies they employ to protect their health (e.g. Choi and Holroyd 2007) or to govern the terms of their labour (e.g. McVerry and Lindop 2005). Our work strives to contribute to this expanding field of research. Aided by the structure–agency theory of Habermas (1984a, 1984b), our aim in this exploratory study was to critically examine the social structures surrounding sex workers (e.g. law and media) in order to compare and contrast societal accounts of sex worker agency with the experiences of sex workers from the Metro Vancouver Region of British Columbia, Canada.

Structure–agency

To support a more nuanced analysis of structure and agency in relation to sex work and the lives of sex workers, our entire analysis drew upon Habermas' theory of structure–agency. For Habermas (1984a), structure–agency rests upon tension between the 'lifeworld' and 'systems'. The lifeworld is the everyday, taken-for-granted domain of individual experience derived from both local knowledge and face-to-face interactions. The possibility for meaningful engagement with others is dependent on our ability to express our lifeworld perspective. The lifeworld, however, is increasingly colonised by social systems (e.g. law, government) that, although essential to our society, can supplant the lifeworld by replacing reciprocal interaction with money, power and bureaucratic practices. Colonisation occurs when lifeworld perspectives are subsumed and silenced by these materialistic concerns (Habermas 1984b). Those who dominate the official economy or administrative state make important social decisions that support the maintenance of the colonising social systems.

Habermas does not privilege structure or agency, but emphasises the complex interplay between structure and agency. His theory is particularly advantageous as he perceives value in analysing social systems and phenomenological accounts (e.g. interviews) in order to better understand the subtle nuances of structure–agency, thereby supporting an analysis of women's experiences as situated within a network of constraints.

Methods

This study was part of a larger community-based project aimed at developing an STI/HIV intervention with employees and clients of massage parlours, the full details of which are under development and reported elsewhere (see Remple *et al.* 2007). Our research focuses on indoor sex markets as it is estimated that 80 per cent of Canadian female sex workers work indoors and are often overlooked by health-care providers and researchers (Hanger 2006; Shaver 2006). While we recognise that women are not the sole proprietors of commercial sex, for the purposes of this exploration we restrict our discussion to women–men exchanges of sex for money.

To explore influential social structures we collected data from two public sources: (1) municipal and federal legislation and related research and (2) regional news media reports (newspapers, news websites) on the sex trade between 1 January 2006 and 31 December 2007. The decision to analyse legal and media texts was guided by Habermas' (1984b) description of the media and legal apparatus as critical institutions in relation to lifeworld and colonisation and the prominence of the legal apparatus in particular in previous sex work reports (e.g. Benoit and Millar 2001; Lowman 2005). Working as a team, we selected and reviewed relevant legislation, related research and media texts to critically examine whether or not these social systems considered or silenced the lifeworld of sex workers. We sought to determine the dominant interests served within the law and media and the extent to which these social systems perpetuated a colonising aim (Habermas 1984a). We also undertook semi-structured interviews with women who identified as working in the indoor sex market. Based on our relationships with 173 women in 39 different indoor settings who were taking part in the larger study, we purposefully selected participants for information they could provide. We purposefully sampled to ensure diversity concerning work venues (e.g. location and structure of venue), length of time in sex work and citizenship and migration status. While we sought diversity, our community partner, which facilitated recruitment, is an AIDS service organisation that specifically targeted Asian women and, as such, our sample reflected the target population of this organisation.[1] All interviews began with describing the project's aim to better understand the experiences of women working indoors, and women were encouraged to describe the nuances of their daily experiences. Interviews were recorded and transcribed verbatim and were reviewed independently by members of the investigative team to identify dominant themes. Results of transcript reviews were discussed in team meetings and we created a coding scheme that reflected the structures relevant in the lives of the participants. Ethical approval was obtained through affiliated universities' behavioural research ethics councils.

Results

Systems and colonisation of the lifeworld

Federal and municipal laws

Canadian federal law concerning the sale of sexual services among adults is paradoxical (see PIVOT Legal Society 2004). For instance, while the sale and purchase of sexual services among adults is not prohibited, a number of activities around selling and buying sexual services are. Section 210(1)(2) of the Criminal Code (Parliament of Canada 1985) prohibits working in, operating or owning a common bawdy house,[2] which renders these venues illegal and encourages sex workers to operate in isolation, thereby increasing the risks associated with the sale of sex (Hanger 2006). Section 213(1) similarly encourages the isolation of sex workers by also deeming public communication for the selling or buying of sex illegal.

Vancouver's municipal bylaws are similarly paradoxical. There are hundreds of massage parlours, escort agencies and dating services operating as legitimate businesses while simultaneously operating as commercial sex venues (Remple et al. 2007). Yet, municipal bylaws prohibit businesses from offering services including nude encounters and out-call body massages (Council of the City of Vancouver [CCV] 1969). Prostitution is explicitly prohibited, with the exception of the activities permitted within body rub parlours defined as the 'manipulating, touching or stimulating by any means, of a person's body' (CCV 1969). Coincidentally, while the annual licence fee for a massage parlour is CAD$172.00, the licence for a body rub parlour is just under CAD$8,000, making the body rub licence the region's third most expensive (Lowman 2000). Additionally, while federal laws encourage isolation, municipal bylaws contribute to increased surveillance of women. Dating and escort services are required to maintain written records of all employees, with the former being required to submit a description of all employees including their addresses to licensing offices (see CCV 1969).

A reading of the municipal and federal laws reveals their lack of responsiveness to the lifeworld of sex workers. Not only are the laws contradictory, but they also place sex workers in situations of risk, rather than safety (Lowman 2005; Shannon *et al.* 2008). The laws do not take an overt stance towards decriminalisation, but appear to provide benefits for municipal coffers.

Law enforcement

As the Canadian Criminal Code needs to be understood within the context of municipal bylaws, the laws must be understood within the context of law enforcement practices. Though proponents of criminalisation argue that many prostitution laws are justified on the basis of protecting sex workers, numerous researchers (Bungay 2008; Lowman 2000; Shannon *et al.* 2008) and legal activist groups (Betteridge 2005; PIVOT Legal Society 2006) have reported that current law enforcement practices disadvantage sex workers. Although heavily weighted towards the experiences of street-based women, several reports indicate that sex workers believe they are more likely to be targeted by authorities than clients (Benoit and Millar 2001; Jeffrey and MacDonald 2006; Lowman 2000; PIVOT Legal Society 2004, 2006). Within the indoor setting, police tend to focus raids on arresting illegal immigrants versus male clients (Remple *et al.* 2007), evidenced when federal and local police raided several indoor venues, arresting more than 100 migrant women (Bolan and Ward 2006).

Sex workers are reluctant to report abuse to police (Benoit and Millar 2001), and those who do frequently meet additional forms of resistance. Specifically, local police often practise non-response, limiting their intervention to criminal acts committed against sex workers (Bungay 2008; Lowman 2000). It has been further suggested that this lack of police engagement increases the chances of violence being used to resolve conflicts between sex workers and their clients, as there is a decreased fear of legal consequences for such actions (Lowman and Atchison 2006; Maher 1997).

As with the laws themselves, law enforcement practices show little sensitivity to the lifeworld of sex workers. Although sex workers encounter exploitation and violence, the police offer little protection. Dismissal and harassment from law enforcement officers place sex workers in positions of disadvantage and vulnerability.

News media

The lifeworlds of sex workers were similarly neglected within media accounts of the sex trade, which is particularly evident by omission of their perspectives in favour of other interests (e.g. police and politicians). This abbreviation is evident in our analysis of local news media reports for the study period. Only 7 of 72 articles from this period cited a sex worker as a source and it was the same individual in every instance. Each of the retrieved articles, with five exceptions, discussed the lives of sex workers as they related to two institutions: law enforcement and law making. Women's lives were reduced to narratives of crime and legal policy.

Of the 72 articles, 41 discussed sex work in relation to crime. These stories included reports of murders[3] (e.g. Altmayer 2007), brothel raids (e.g. Ramsey 2006) and the trafficking of women (CTV News 2006). Articles commonly depicted sex workers in objectified terms. For instance, one quoted a federal police officer as stating that massage parlour workers lived in 'virtual slavery' (CTV News 2006). In another article, the neighbour of a murder victim stated, 'I'm obviously glad that it [the murder] was not random', after it had been revealed the victim was a sex worker (Altmayer 2007). Neither of these reports interviewed sex workers, instead relying on law enforcement officers as key sources. Only one of these articles contained an interview with a sex worker.

The remaining articles discussed larger legal issues related to sex work, the majority of which appeared in three newspapers, *The Vancouver Sun*, *The Province* and *24hours*. These reports focused on the alteration of sex trade laws, such as the potential abolition of prostitution or its legalisation, primarily in the form of a legal brothel (e.g. Loy 2007; Smysnuik 2007). In contrast to the articles on crime, five of these articles included perspectives from one sex worker. However, her statements were bracketed by those from social workers, politicians, police officers and a former journalist who were portrayed as the 'experts' on prostitution. The latter perspectives were given a disproportionate amount of coverage in comparison to those of the sex worker (e.g. Lee 2007: A1–A2).

The media, similar to the laws and law enforcement practices, eliminated the lifeworld perspective of sex workers, who were portrayed as 'victims' and 'slaves'. In contrast, social system representatives (e.g. police) were positioned as possessing a benevolent understanding of the lives of sex workers who did not fully comprehend the totality of their oppression.

Lifeworld perspective: participants' accounts of structure and agency

Twenty-nine interviews were conducted with 21 women (mean age 30; range 19–50). Of these, 15 were Asian migrants to Canada, 11 spoke no or limited English and required translation, 19 worked in massage parlours, and 12 worked in more than one sex venue. Women's length of time in sex work ranged from less than one year to 15 years.

Our analysis of the women's experiences illustrates that the constraints they face and their associated agency in response to these constraints are markedly different than those described by the social systems of law and media. To best illustrate these differences we discuss these interrelationships under the thematic categories of structure and agency.

Although interpersonal relationships were a significant aspect of women's experiences, they also spoke of the difficulties they encountered from larger social structures, particularly in relation to the economic conditions of their work, local law enforcement practices and the quasi-legal nature of prostitution. While each of these social systems were influential, they were not experienced uniformly. Where appropriate, we highlight these differences.

Economy

System views present sex workers as enslaved by pimps, traffickers and addictions (e.g. Bolan and Ward 2006; Lee 2007). These views omit larger economic constraints placed upon women within Canadian culture, which is apparent through participants' accounts of their entrance into the sex market. Entrance narratives focused on the accumulation of economic pressures, familial responsibilities and lack of choices, rather than stories of pimps and addictions. One respondent (Harriet, aged 39) noted, 'I just had no choices after a while and that's what happened.' Another (Ashlee, aged 32) stated:

> The money's really good and I am a single mum … to support my kids and the things they need. The [non-sex work] jobs that I applied for before; they're all minimum wage. I don't really have a lot of education to go work for a big company. I used to be a resident care attendant, but I got really burnt out. I can't do that kind of job any more.

Economic pressures also influenced women's actions within parlours. They described an escalation of sexual acts they performed in relation to time spent employed in these 'legitimate businesses' and their movement between establishments. For instance, in some agencies women are encouraged to perform 'whatever the customer wants'. As a result, the progression into sex for money was not immediate and was often connected to receiving increased 'tips' from clients. Women quickly learned that those providing the most services received more clients and greater income:

> For the first half a month, I only do hand job. The boss gave all the customers who are not doing full service to me. As time gradually passed by, I saw all the other girls are making a lot of money by providing full service. I gradually accepted to do full service.
>
> (Tia, aged 25)

Of additional importance to the economic realities influencing women's work lives was English language proficiency. For many, English proficiency affected their income by influencing clients' decision-making. Participants described how clients preferred women who spoke English: 'If there's two pretty girls, they're going to pick one that they can communicate with' (Emilia, aged 29). Immigrant women who did not speak English also faced unique challenges; for example, being left out of conversations between clients and managers in which services and payment were negotiated. Katherine provided a detailed account of how she was manipulated by both her client and manager as a result of her lack of English skills and, despite knowing she was being cheated, was unable to defend her interests:

> I walked out of the room and talked to the manager. The manager said, 'You didn't do anything for the customer, just return the whole hundred.' I did 25 minutes. She [the manager] said I can keep the 40 dollars and give the customer back 60 dollars. And the customer and the boss were talking and I didn't know what kind of things they were talking about. The manager asked me, 'Give all the money back.' … I returned all money … They were talking in English, so I could not get involved and get my money back. I cannot talk on behalf of myself.
>
> (Katherine, aged 34)

The influence of managers and customers in constraining women's actions and economic gain was not limited to English proficiency. Many managers treated women as third parties in sexual transactions by negotiating fees and receiving payment directly from the client. In these situations, women were often paid a base 'salary' and had little input into the cost of the service, the economic gain or the nature of services performed:

In my parlour the women have no say, the [manager] makes the deal, he takes the money and the woman stays in for as long as the customer wants.

(Alison, aged 29)

The economic control by parlour owners was also evident in the numerous reports of arbitrary fines levied against sex workers:

The door girl keeps your money, that way if you get fined for anything throughout the day, not picking up a towel, not cleaning a sheet, not providing a service the gentleman wanted or so and so, then they fine you ... they fine you $50 for being late ... they will fine you $150 for calling in sick ... I mean what are we going to do? Go to the labour board?

(Judy, aged 36)

While orchestrating the worth of services, managers also increased the services that the women were required to perform:

They [managers] have a way to make them. Like one girl was saying before she got in, she told me she told the guy she was only gonna do the hand job and the other girl said she was only gonna do hand job and blow job. In the end, hand-job girl turned out to be giving him a blow job without a condom. And the second girl, she ended up giving him a blow job without a condom and having sex with a condom.

(Pearl, aged 26)

Despite the women's discomfort, the manager persuaded them to increase their scope of sexual services. Another participant reported a similar act of control, stating that her manager informed her that 'if you're doing more than a hand job then we'd want a portion of the tip' (Julianne, aged 21). This policy had made hand jobs part of the regular service, included with the base client payment. If the woman wanted to make additional money, she must perform more than a hand job. Additionally, the tips that workers received from these additional, potentially 'riskier' services were cut into by the employer. This dynamic ensured the consistent performance of sexual services and the immediate reduction of value of the riskier services, such as oral and vaginal sex. The sex worker is placed into an environment of constant sexualisation and economic disadvantage that established both the sex act and the body of the sex worker as a commodity of the manager, access to which is negotiated with clients.

Legal factors

Absent from system perspectives were the ways that law enforcement and lawmakers constrained sex workers; however, participants' lives were significantly influenced by police surveillance and communication laws. Several women were afraid of being arrested, and these fears intersected with the potential media-related ramifications: 'I am afraid a lot of customer [if] they are a police man ... If I was caught by a police and my face will be on TV ... nobody knows I am working at the massage centre' (Daphne, aged 35). This fear of being arrested was often related to difficulty in distinguishing between police officers and clients:

> We have to be really careful about not soliciting, like verbally soliciting. So the client has to want extras and he has to state clearly what [he wants]. You couldn't offer a blow job ... that [entrapment] is a bit of a fallacy. They can still touch you and charge you ... it wasn't so much if he touched you, it was only about the verbal.
>
> (Julianne, aged 21)

The uncertainty of whether clients were undercover officers, combined with the realities of committing a criminal act, exacerbated economic constraints. Women reported that clients frequently took advantage of the 'illegal' context of their relationships for economic gain. In instances where women negotiated payment, they often could not negotiate before providing services due to restrictions imposed by the communicating law. In these situations, the women took significant financial risks and many reported being paid unfairly once services were rendered:

> I take off my clothes, I do the hand job and I do the service for him. He goes '30 dollars'; 'No!' I take my hand off, they say '30', I say 'no'. I returned 10 dollars back to the customer. This is kind of difficult in this business to say to the customer 'more money'. I said, 'Even if you don't want to pay me 60 dollars, at least give me 40.' The customer still insisted to take the 10 dollars back and not return it to me, so I only ended up with 20 dollars.
>
> (Katherine, aged 34)

Women were also under surveillance by municipal personnel, as Emilia (aged 29) notes:

> He comes and does random checkups and stuff like that ... so he comes in and starts saying, ''Cause you're supposed to wear pants that are up to the knees and up to the elbows.' But some of us weren't. We were wearing shorts and tank tops. So he was complaining about that and we were saying, 'We weren't even working yet.' But you know he was just trying to find anything.

Here, she refers to a municipal bylaw that requires employees in body rub parlours to wear 'garments covering his or her body between the neck and the top of the knee, the sleeves of which do not reach below the elbows' (CCV 1969). These actions did not prevent women from engaging in sex work, but instead necessitated greater secrecy and isolation.

Interpersonal factors

The illegal nature of the women's activities and the negation of their agency by managers contributed to women's significant risk of violence. For example, women's refusal to perform services placing them in vulnerable physical positions (e.g. prone) contributed to heated arguments that often escalated into physical violence:

> I was very afraid and I was screaming at him ... And he even grabbed me and tried to pull me on top of him and wouldn't let me go ... I basically pushed him and on the bed and walked out half naked and I know people could hear me. I could hear people walking down the hall and nobody came to see if, you know, knock on the door, 'Is everything OK?'
>
> (Eve, aged 19)

In this situation, Eve was left to handle the argument in isolation without assistance from co-workers or the manager. With clients able to avoid penalties for assaulting sex workers in some establishments, women risked the possibility of financial loss and violence in their interactions. And while every participant emphasised that there were good venues, several were described in vivid detail that illustrated the ways in which women were constantly kept subservient, sexualised and uncomfortable:

> In an escort agency, everything is relaxed. I bring my homework, I bring my things, I feel more at home. In the massage place, in my experience, you have a schedule. Certain hours you have to do cleaning and it's a lot of running around. Even when you eat, they try to control where you eat. Owners in these kinds of places don't care about the health of the women. They are just bodies and can always be replaced.
>
> (Jami, aged 34)

Although structural analysis of social system perspectives details many constraints faced by sex workers, they risk being hyperbolic and inaccurate. As shown, structural accounts that include the perspectives and experiences of actual sex workers create added nuance, while also detailing the constraints most relevant to the individuals. Most importantly, system perspectives emphasise that women's personal flaws and interpersonal exploitation are the greatest constraints to sex workers. However, when we turn to the voices of the sex workers themselves, it is apparent that the most influential constraints are systemic in nature, both in terms of their economic disadvantage and the ease with which individuals may use sex trade laws to exploit and coerce sex workers.

Focusing exclusively on the constraints and disadvantages faced by sex workers presents only a partial picture of the realities of sex work. To offer a more complete description, we also explored the strategies participants enacted to exercise their agency, often in situations of great constraint. Of particular importance were women's agency with regards to 'choosing' their place of employment, avoiding arrest and managing client interactions to maintain safety.

Employer choice

As noted previously, most women engaged in sex work out of economic necessity. Women also recounted horrendous working conditions. Movement between venues was common as women sought improved working conditions and environments that interacted favourably with other aspects of life:

> I chose this company because I live down the street from here. I don't have to spend money on bus fare, I just walk or take the bike … I just came in and said, 'I am going to start work today.' … I know they need young girls that speak English, so I know that they're not going to tell me to leave.
>
> (Emilia, aged 29)

Other women chose their parlour based on its atmosphere. As Daphne (aged 35) stated, 'I feel this is a big family. The feeling is very, very good. Really comfortable.' While the conditions within some parlours may be exploitative, it is important to note that many participants found their parlour to be safe and supporting. Interestingly, the majority of these parlours were operated by former sex workers, which further emphasises the abilities of sex workers to enact beneficial decisions.

Avoiding arrest

While the legal environment directly impacted the activities of sex workers, women enacted several strategies to avoid arrest. Determining which individuals were law enforcement officers was a priority. Many women described how they relied on clients' non-verbal cues to determine whether they were an undercover officer, and that the ability to read these cues was dependent on their experiences as sex workers:

> This is the key to distinguish policemen from customers. A customer usually will send the signal for a special service. On a particular day, a client requested a 'soft massage' and turned around and touched me. I said, 'Today you want special?' He said, 'Yeah, how much? 40?' Then I just continued negotiating the price with the customer.
>
> (Katherine, aged 34)

Others engaged in more overt behaviours, drawing from their knowledge of how clients 'normally' interacted:

> If it's a policeman, if I touch him, make some body contact with the policeman, some maybe private place, the policeman hand will be 'wait' and try to avoid the touch of the body ... Some policeman will also not take off their clothes, they don't want to expose their whole body and [they] also look into your eyes, very sharp ... because of their demeanour I did not ask [for] something.
>
> (Hue, aged 30)

Managing interactions

Contrary to system perspectives, the relationship between clients and sex workers was not based solely on violence and exploitation. Several women commented that they sympathised with clients: 'I think some of them are just really lonely guys and they get really attached to some of these girls' (Judy, aged 36). Others discussed being indifferent to clients and simply viewed them as a means to an end:

> At first, I was trying to judge, like if he's nice or if I like him. But the more I work in this industry I realise that's not important. It's still money and if he's nice, I don't care if I like him or not because I realise it's just business. I'm not looking for a boyfriend.
>
> (Jami, aged 34)

Participants also detailed their control of client interactions. Many women refused to perform certain acts or have sex in compromising positions that left them physically vulnerable or unable to enforce condom usage. For similar reasons, as well as physical discomfort, many respondents did not perform anal sex; however, clients often encouraged women to try it and asserted that it could be enjoyable. Women noted that the best strategy for refusal was to say that they had previously performed anal sex and did not enjoy it. If the client was dissatisfied by these service options, women also had strategies to appeal to their managers and avoid client confrontations:

> If he did complain I would say he stunk or was hairy or whatever. So I found ways of getting myself out of trouble I guess ... for the most part I pretty much control the situation ... I do what I do and they don't really have anything to say about it. I mean sometimes there's confrontation, but for the most part they do what they're told.
>
> (Eve, aged 19)

Although the women are paid to perform a service, this does not necessitate the disengagement of their ingenuity and ability to make choices, which was most evident in their consistent assertion of condom usage. No participant stated that they performed sexual acts with a client without a condom, regardless of the money offered:

> That's [condom use] a must and that's the woman. That's the masseuse. I mean there's many times where the customer will go, 'Oh, but I'm clean, I'm clean you know, it's OK, you don't have to use a condom.' And you know, I myself would say, 'No way. You know I don't want to catch a disease and what if I have one? I don't want to give it to you, so there's no way that I would go without a condom no matter how much you pay me.'
>
> (Emilia, aged 29)

While sex workers were constrained by their economic position during client interactions, the use of condoms was an area where their choice was consistently maintained. Participants were willing to openly confront clients who did not want to use condoms:

> They say, 'But I don't want to use one.' I'll say, 'OK, if you don't then just get out.' And some cases I'll keep the money and sometimes I'll say, 'Take your money and go. Get the fuck out'; don't trust anybody that way. That's my life and they're [not] going to risk getting me sick.
>
> (Harriett, aged 39)

Women often took physical control of this process; as Eve (aged 19) stated: 'I put the condom on myself. Always, always, always.' Women's emphasis on condom usage signified a general philosophy on sexual health and understanding of the interconnected nature of sex work:

> We kind of educate them: 'We are doing these things for money, many people every day, so kind of safe for you only and also you can go home and be with your wife without a condom. But here you have to have a condom, it's very safe for you.'
>
> (Hue, aged 30)

This sex worker acted as an educator, informing her client about sexual safety while contextualising their interactions within a larger sexual network. The condom keeps the sex worker, the client and the client's partner from being at risk. This view of sexual networks contained both the nuance and structure that was omitted in system perspectives of sex work and sexual health.

Conclusion

Discussions of agency among women in sex work continue to represent significant conflict and diversity of positions among academics, advocacy groups, health-care providers, legal policymakers and law officials (Shaver 2006; Vanwesenbeeck 2001). The positions that underlie the creation of policy and legislation pertaining to prostitution in Canada have important consequences for sex workers, specifically in terms of the relative legality of their actions and their actual everyday experiences in relation to their 'work'. Although our exploratory study was limited to a specific and small subgroup of sex workers within a finite locale, we were able to critically position the discussion within the realm of inter-relationships between structure and agency and to highlight the importance of lifeworld perspectives for these discussions. We suggest that heterogeneity of analytical perspectives is critical to consider the multiplicities of structure–agency.

Additionally, we examined these issues among a subgroup of indoor sex workers who have remained largely invisible within Canadian sex work research. By highlighting the experiences of indoor sex workers, we have added to the growing number of voices that challenge a homogeneous representation of 'prostituted women' or 'sex workers' (see Farley 2004; Raphael and Shapiro 2004; Shaver 2006; Vanwesenbeeck 2001). We discovered that significant heterogeneity exists even within indoor sex workers, and that differences among women's experiences are not limited to work location, but intimately connected to other social forces shaping women's lifeworlds, such as migration, job opportunities and employers. Perhaps this is what Shaver (2006) meant when she argued that in sex work research it was important to shift away from studying sex work as 'identity' and examine more 'general' conditions affecting women's lives.

One of the most important contributions of our work pertains to findings illuminating the negative interrelationships between the Canadian Criminal Code, local municipal bylaws and women's agency. Although this finding has been reported in other contexts (Betteridge 2005; Lowman 2000; PIVOT Legal Society 2004, 2006), the specific nuances of the indoor establishments highlight additional areas of concern. The contradictions created by municipal and federal laws allow government officials to position themselves as being against sex work, while simultaneously extracting the benefits created by sex work and workers. Each of the local businesses operates under the guise of legitimacy, offering escort or massage services without advertising or licensing them as commercialised sex venues. These venues generate significant revenue in licensing fees for the city and contribute to a bureaucratic infrastructure of inspectors and employee registers that position the city officials as experts for these venues and increase surveillance of women. Yet women's income was directly connected to engaging in acts that were not part of the 'legitimate' business. Women were not afforded safe working conditions and had no means of recourse when exploitative acts such as 'fines' by managers were committed against them. It would seem that these bylaws are designed for economic benefit for the city and managers, with little concern for employees. As Habermas (1984a) suggests, social institutions, such as the law, cannot claim legitimacy without engaging with the lifeworld of those that they purport to represent. Perhaps current polemics on the status of sex work are reflective of the lack of legitimacy of these laws, which many (e.g. Farley 2004) have argued from both structural and agency perspectives fail to engage meaningfully with the actual experiences of sex workers.

Regardless of one's stance on sex work, it cannot be denied that the current Canadian criminal laws, local municipal bylaws and law enforcement practices are harmful to women who work in these indoor venues. There are significant challenges in determining what solutions would best address these problems. There is some evidence that suggests legalisation of 'brothels' reduces interpersonal violence and financial exploitation of women by regulating payment and creating a more protective environment (e.g. Brents and Hausbeck 2005). Yet, the legalisation of brothels also has been noted to contribute to increased surveillance of sex workers and restrictions on their basic freedom of movement (Brents and Hausbeck 2005). Abolition does not seem realistic in our research context, given the existing state-sanctioned support. Additional criminalisation would likely serve to further victimise women and exacerbate existing basic human rights violations, including the right to personal security (Betteridge 2005). As researchers, we have struggled with these questions and are unable to reach consensus; however, none support further criminalisation of women. We agree that without the lifeworld experiences of women working in the sex industry, there can be no understanding of the ramifications of the laws or ways in which laws and enforcement officials restrict women's agency.

Habermas (1984a, 1984b) directs us to consider how social structures influence individuals and the consequences for the institutions in society. The law both fails to protect sex workers and to represent their interests. Similarly, the media, with simplistic narratives of personal pathology and archetypes of pimps and johns, fails to reflect the lifeworld of sex workers. Omitted within both of these representations of sex work are accounts of how broader social structures influence and constrain sex workers. Neither the media nor the law account for how the economic disadvantages encountered by sex workers affect their decision to enter sex work, although these broader social realities were much more salient to our cohort than were explanations that relied upon interpersonal coercion. Also omitted are the benefits that social institutions derive from sex work, particularly in the form of fines, business licences, tourism and paper sales. As Habermas would suggest, the inability of these institutions to engage with the lifeworlds of sex workers questions their legitimacy. That is, the media and law's current relationship to sex work questions their ability to accurately and equally represent the interests of all citizens in an equitable manner. Here, Habermas would suggest that it is crucial for these institutions to engage in meaningful communication with sex workers to restore their legitimacy, the importance of which has been stressed by both legal advocacy groups (PIVOT Legal Society 2004, 2006) and the academic community (e.g. Lowman 2005; Shannon et al. 2008).

Notes

1 The larger project known as the ORCHID Project is a community-based HIV and STI intervention project. The community partner, the Asian Society for the Intervention Against AIDS, provides outreach primarily to Asian women in the indoor venues, although all women regardless of ethnic origin are welcome to use the services. The nature of this collaboration and the rationale underpinning targeting Asian women are published elsewhere (see Remple et al. 2007) and are beyond the scope of this chapter.

2 Defined as a place that is kept or occupied, or resorted to by one or more persons, for the purpose of prostitution (Section 197(1), Criminal Code).

3 This does not include articles on the trial of Robert Pickton, as these articles greatly surpass all other articles on the sex trade.

References

Agustín, L. 2006. The conundrum of women's agency: Migrations and the sex industry. In: M. O'Neil and R. Campbell (eds) *Sex Work Now*. Cullompton: Willan Publishing, 116–140.

Altmayer, D. 2007. Neighbourhood fears. *Metro*, 31 August, Local News section.

Benoit, C. and Millar, A. 2001. *Dispelling Myths and Understanding Realities: Working Conditions, Health Status and Exiting Experiences of Sex Workers*. Report for Prostitutes Empowerment, Education and Resource Society, Victoria, British Columbia.

Bernstein, E. 2007. Sex work for the middle classes. *Sexualities* 10(4): 473–488.

Betteridge, G. 2005. *Sex, Work, Rights: Reforming Canadian Criminal Laws on Prostitution*. Canadian HIV/AIDS Legal Network. Toronto, ON: Canadian HIV/AIDS Legal Network.

Bolan, K. and Ward, D. 2006. Massage parlours keep operating. *The Vancouver Sun*, 13 December, p. B5.

Brents, B. and Hausbeck, K. 2005. Violence and legalized brothel prostitution in Nevada. *Journal of Interpersonal Violence* 20(3): 270–295.

Bungay, V. 2008. *Health experiences of women who are street-involved and use crack cocaine: Inequality, oppression and relations of power in Vancouver's downtown eastside*. PhD dissertation, University of British Columbia.

Choi, S. and Holroyd, E. 2007. The influence of power, poverty and agency in the negotiation of condom use for female sex workers in mainland China. *Culture, Health & Sexuality* 9(5): 489–503.

Council of the City of Vancouver (CCV). 1969. *License By-law No. 4450*. City of Vancouver, Municipal Government, British Columbia, Canada.

CTV News. 2006. *108 Arrested in B.C. Massage Parlour Raids*. 8 December.

Farley, M. 2004. Bad for the body, bad for the heart: Prostitution harms women even if legalized or decriminalized. *Violence Against Women* 10(10): 1087–1125.

Habermas, J. 1984a. *The Theory of Communicative Action: Reason and Rationalization of Society*. Boston, MA: Beacon Press.

Habermas, J. 1984b. *The Theory of Communicative Action: Lifeworld and System*. Boston, MA: Beacon Press.

Hanger, M.P. 2006. *The Challenge of Change: A Study of Canada's Criminal Prostitution. Report of the Standing Committee on Justice and Human Rights*. Parliament of Canada. Available at: www.parl. gc.ca [Accessed 8 September 2012].

Jeffrey, L.A. and MacDonald, G. 2006. *Sex Workers in the Maritimes Talk Back*. Vancouver, BC: UBC Press.

Lee, J. 2007. Coalition pushes for legal brothel. *The Vancouver Sun*, 12 November, p. A1.

Lowman, J. 2000. Violence and the outlaw status of (street) prostitution. *Violence Against Women* 6(9): 987–1011.

Lowman, J. 2005. *Submission to the Subcommittee on Solicitation Laws of the Standing Committee on Justice, Human Rights, Public Safety and Emergency Preparedness*. Ottawa, Canada.

Lowman, J. and Atchison, C. 2006. Men who buy sex: A survey in the Greater Vancouver Regional District. *Canadian Review of Sociology and Anthropology* 43(3): 281–296.

Loy, I. 2007. Brothel offered as solution. *24hours*, 23 June, News section.

Lucas, M. 2005. The work of sex work: Elite prostitutes' vocational orientations and experiences. *Deviant Behavior* 26(6): 513–546.

Maher, L. 1997. *Sexed Work: Gender, Race and Resistance in a Brooklyn Drug Market*. Oxford: Clarendon Press.

McVerry, S. and Lindop, E. 2005. Negotiating risk: How women working in massage parlours preserve their sexual and psychological health. *Health Care for Women International* 26(2): 108–117.

Monroe, J. 2005. Women in street prostitution: The result of poverty and the brunt of inequity. *Journal of Poverty* 9(3): 69–88.

Parliament of Canada. 1985. *Criminal Code*. Parliament of Canada.

PIVOT Legal Society. 2004. *Voices for Dignity: A Call to End the Harms Caused by Canada's Sex Trade Laws*. Vancouver: PIVOT Legal Society.

PIVOT Legal Society. 2006. *Beyond Decriminalization: Sex Work, Human Rights and a New Framework for Law Reform*. Vancouver: PIVOT Legal Society.

Ramsey, R. 2006. Police suspect women are victims of human trafficking. *The Province*, 10 December, p. A11.

Raphael, J. and Shapiro, D. 2004. Violence in indoor and outdoor prostitution venues. *Violence Against Women* 10: 126–139.

Remple, V., Johnston, C., Patrick, D., Tyndall, M. and Jolly, A. 2007. Conducting HIV/AIDS research with indoor commercial sex workers: Reaching a hidden population. *Progress in Community Health Partnerships: Research, Education, and Action* 1(2): 161–168.

Salfati, C., James, R. and Ferguson, L. 2008. Prostitute homicides: A descriptive study. *Journal of Interpersonal Violence* 23(4): 505–543.

Shannon, K., Kerr, T., Allinott, S., Chettiar, J., Shoveller, J. and Tyndall, M. 2008. Social and structural violence and power relations in mitigating HIV risk of drug-using women in survival sex work. *Social Science & Medicine* 66(4): 911–921.

Shaver, F. 2006. *Recommendations for Sex Work Policy: An Integrated Approach*. Report to the House of Commons Subcommittee on Solicitation Laws, Ottawa, Canada.

Sherwin, S. 1998. A relational approach to autonomy in health care. In: S. Sherwin (ed.) *The Politics of Women's Health: Exploring Agency and Autonomy*. Philadelphia, PA: Templeton University Press, 19–47.

Smysnuik, S. 2007. The oldest profession. *The Georgia Straight*, 30 August, Letters section.

Vanwesenbeeck, I. 2001. Another decade of social scientific work on sex work: A review of research 1990–2000. *Annual Review of Sex Research* 12: 242–289.

Weitzer, R. 2005. New directions in prostitution research. *Crime, Law and Social Change* 43(4–5): 211–235.

Chapter 12

Social context, sexual risk perceptions and stigma

HIV vulnerability among male sex workers in Mombasa, Kenya

Jerry Okal, Stanley Luchters, Scott Geibel, Matthew F. Chersich, Daniel Lango and Marleen Temmerman

Introduction

Sex between men occurs in all cultures and societies, although its recognition and public visibility vary markedly (Murray and Roscoe 1998). In many parts of Africa, there is evidence showing that same-sex relationships have been an unspoken part of these societies for many years (Evans-Pritchard 1929; Werner 1987; Kiama 1999; Niang *et al.* 2003; Allman *et al.* 2007). Within the African context, male–male sexuality is, however, popularly associated with European or Western influence (McKenna 1996; Murray and Roscoe 1998; Niang *et al.* 2003) and there is widespread denial that it has roots in traditional African society. Sex between men is thought to account for between 5 and 10 per cent of HIV infections globally (UNAIDS 2006) and was estimated to contribute 5 per cent of new HIV infections in Kenya in 2005 (Gouws *et al.* 2006).

In Kenya and Senegal, where overall HIV prevalence is 7 and 1 per cent, respectively (UNAIDS 2008), HIV prevalence among men who have sex with men has been estimated at 38 and 22 per cent, respectively (Wade *et al.* 2005; Sanders *et al.* 2007). Such levels of infection are attributed to a combination of biological, behavioural and sociocultural factors, which together create considerable risk of acquiring and transmitting HIV (Allman *et al.* 2007; Geibel *et al.* 2008; UNAIDS 2008). Several, mainly Western, studies reveal high biological vulnerability to HIV; this is due mainly to highly efficient transmission via unprotected anal sex and extensive sexual partner networks (Roehr *et al.* 2001; Shallock and Moore 2003).

Limited available evidence suggests that sex between men in African settings is commonly unprotected and partner numbers are high (Niang *et al.* 2003; Onyango-Ouma *et al.* 2005; Lane *et al.* 2006; Sanders *et al.* 2007). These studies also showed that men who have sex with men in this setting also frequently have sex with women (Niang *et al.* 2003; Geibel *et al.* 2008).

The law in Kenya criminalises same-sex sexual activity (Government of Kenya 2008), making it difficult for HIV prevention programmes to fully address male sex work. Section 162 of the Penal Code states that 'any person who has carnal knowledge of any person against the order of nature; or … permits a male person to have carnal knowledge of him … is guilty of a felony and is liable to imprisonment of 14 years'. Additionally, Section 165 specifies that any 'male person who … procures another male person to commit any act of gross indecency with him or attempts to procure the commission of any such act by any male person … is guilty of a felony …'.

Other former British colonies in Africa such as Malawi, Nigeria, Uganda and Zambia also criminalise consensual male–male sexual activity, often for 'unnatural offences'. Legislation in these countries reflects UK domestic law-making from the Victorian period

(Baudh 2008). Besides the legal implications, men have to contend with several layers of stigma stemming from sex work and same-sex activities. In the public view, male-to-male sex is often conceived as undermining and challenging powerful assumptions about masculine behaviour and what it means to be a 'real' man (Costigan and Foreman 2002/2003).

Adding to this is the fact that political, civil and religious leaders frequently make public statements claiming that same-sex behaviour is incompatible with traditional 'African' culture (Murray and Roscoe 1998; Kiama 1999; Allman *et al.* 2007). In Kenya, the issue of homosexuality evokes much debate and is emotionally charged. Two former Kenyan presidents are on record disputing the existence and practice of homosexuality, stating that it was 'un-African' and 'even in religion, it is considered a great sin' (Kiama 1998). Leaders across sectors 'close ranks' on this issue, condemning same-sex relationships and invoking religious and cultural reasons to justify their opposition.

Prejudice against men having sex with men, oftentimes expressed as homophobia, limits opportunities for learning about risks of HIV infection and may lead to alienation from HIV prevention and care programmes (Onyango-Ouma *et al.* 2005). In most of Kenya there are no health services that adequately address the diagnosis and treatment of sexually transmitted infections (STIs) for members of this population group. Furthermore, effects of this neglect are exacerbated by socio-economic vulnerability in these settings (UNAIDS 2006).

In Kenya, there has been a near exclusive focus on preventing HIV transmission through vaginal sex or from a mother to her child. There is a long history of providing outreach services to sex workers in many parts of Kenya, including peer-mediated interventions, HIV prevention and control and poverty alleviation strategies (Ngugi *et al.* 1988; Moses *et al.* 1991; Luchters *et al.* 2008). However, male sex workers are seldom targeted in these projects. This chapter aims to enhance understanding of the dynamics of male-to-male sexual activities within the context of commercial sex in Kenya and to guide configuration of targeted HIV prevention services.

Methods

Study setting

Mombasa district, in Kenya's Coast Province, is the site of this study, which took place from October to December 2006. The district has a population of about one million and is a major regional economic centre, with important tourism, port, rail and industrial enterprises. Evidence suggests that the number of men having sex with men in Kenya's coastal region is large (Murray and Roscoe 1998; Geibel *et al.* 2007) and that both Kenyan and foreign tourism are linked with transactional sex in Mombasa and nearby areas (Kiama 1999; Kibicho 2003). This evidence prompted this study, which was conducted in consultation with the Coast Provincial Medical Office and the Kenya National AIDS Control Council. The study is also a response to the National HIV/AIDS Strategic Plan, which stipulates that men having sex with men be included in behaviour change communication for most-at-risk groups (National AIDS Control Council 2005).

Recruitment and initial contact

The study followed a capture–recapture exercise consisting of a mapping and two enumerations one week apart, which located 65 meeting points and estimated 739 male sex workers selling sex to men in May 2006 in Mombasa and its environs (Geibel *et al.* 2007). Initial contact was made through 12 peer mobilisers familiar with male sex work in Mombasa. Potential participants were approached in bars, nightclubs, private brothels, beach areas and other community settings. To be eligible for participation, men had to be 16 years or older and active in Mombasa district. For study purposes, a male sex worker was defined as any man who 'recently sold and/or is currently willing to sell sex to other men in exchange for money or goods'.

Phase I

Structured interviews with 425 men provide background demographic and behavioural data for this study, described in detail elsewhere (Geibel *et al.* 2008). Men were a median 26 years old (interquartile range (IQR) = 22–31), almost all were Kenyan citizens (98.4 per cent; 418/425) and the majority had completed primary school or higher levels of education (68.5 per cent; 291/425). A substantial number (41.6 per cent; 177/425) reported sex work as their sole income source, and more than half the sample uses their income for supporting their family or friends (56.7 per cent; 241/425). During last anal sex with clients, more men reported insertive sexual roles than receptive ones (57.6 per cent; 242/420 versus 34.8 per cent; 146/420), with only a few combining insertive and receptive roles (7.6 per cent; 32/420). In the past 7 days, participants had had a median of two male partners (IQR = 1–3; range = 0–10). Over 80 per cent stated that their last male client was Kenyan. Most respondents (67.1 per cent) had ever had sex with a woman, and one-quarter (25.4 per cent) reported having sex with a non-paying female partner in the past 30 days. Over 12 per cent (51/425) had experienced physical abuse in the past year, while 9.9 per cent had been sexually assaulted or raped over the same period (42/425). Only one-third reported consistent condom use in the past month for insertive or receptive anal sex with male clients (36.0 per cent; 153/425), a figure not surprising given that only 35.3 per cent of those interviewed knew HIV could be transmitted through anal sex.

Phase II

Data presented here describe the experiences of 36 men who reported exchanging sex for money, drawing on three focus group discussions (FGDs) and ten in-depth interviews (IDIs). Study staff identified candidates for either group or individual discussions from among those participating in the Phase I survey. In this process (non-random purposeful selection), staff made a subjective assessment of the likelihood that participants would share their experiences openly.

Men were identified for predetermined IDI subgroups (men who have sex with both men and women; men who have sex with men only; men living with a male partner; younger sex workers [16–24 years]; men older than 25 years; men who sell sex to Kenyans only; men who sell sex to international tourists; men tested for HIV; men seeking clients in multiple venues; and men in high socio-economic strata). While IDIs sought detailed insights on topics at the individual level, FGDs were conducted to elicit debate or consensus on the same topics from preselected subgroups (men who engage in primarily receptive anal sex, men who engage in primarily insertive anal sex, and a third group inclusive of both). The age range of participants was 17–45 years, with 8–10 men per focus group. For both the IDIs and FGDs, identification and definition of these subgroups was based on formative consultations with male sex workers conducted prior to implementation of this study.

A standardised interview guide was developed with open-ended questions followed by probes. The guide was customised for both individual and group participants. Interview instruments specifically sought to establish: the context of first sexual experiences; processes of obtaining clients and negotiations (sexual geography); sexual practices and roles; condom use and risk of HIV infection; partner relations; sexual identity; stigma and discrimination; and access to health services. Trained researchers facilitated the interviews in Kiswahili. The interviews were tape-recorded, transcribed verbatim, translated into English and analysed using QSR NVivo 7 software.

Ethical aspects

The Kenyatta National Hospital Ethics and Review Committee in Kenya and the Institutional Review Board of the Population Council reviewed and approved the study. Written informed consent to interviewing and audio recording of responses was obtained from all interviewees. Participants received 300 Kenya Shillings (US$4.50) for transport reimbursement.

Condom promotion and provision occurred during the quantitative and qualitative phases of the study. Participants also received printed materials on STI, including HIV and referral for HIV testing and counselling. To further promote the health of participants, the interview team was trained to identify respondents who could benefit from free STI treatment or referral and linked participants with such services, where applicable.

Concerns about participant confidentiality and safety made it preferable to have interviews at central venues. For similar reasons participants were asked to provide a nickname during FGDs, which they were encouraged to use when referring to other participants. Pseudonyms are used in presentation of study findings and other participant identifiers are avoided.

Results

Several broad themes were noted in analysis of male sex workers' experiences. These are grouped as follows: first sexual experience; meeting points for obtaining clients; stigma and discrimination; and condom use and perceptions of risk of HIV infection.

Context of first sexual encounter and entry into sex work

Respondents' first sexual experience with men occurred in quite varied circumstances. In general, these experiences can be dichotomised as either being clearly consensual or coerced, and as occurring either with people well known to them or with complete strangers. Men interpreted their first experiences in terms that included love, sexual exploration, coercion and, predominantly, financial incentives. Initial contact with sexual partners was often made in familiar social spaces such as workplaces, schools, public parks, beach areas and other communal settings. In the descriptions of first sex with people well known to them, sexual behaviour often progressed gradually over successive meetings, from physical attraction and appreciative looks to touching, kissing and cuddling, ultimately becoming more intimate and culminating in penetrative anal sex.

For men whose first sexual encounter was at a young age, initiation into homosexual relationships was described as gradual and 'easy', and generally involved people they knew and were comfortable with. In a one-on-one interview, Sam (19 years) explained:

> I have always liked men ... we used to touch one another and joke about our sexuality ... then one day at the beach we decided with my friends to try to have sex and see what happens. That was the first time; we then continued to have sex at home and in school toilets.

Men's narratives often mentioned love and affection and were congruent with accounts of romantic attraction to other men or experiencing pleasure and having sex with other men as part of sexual development. In a deeply personal way, John (18 years) told us of his first sexual experience and how he began selling sex:

> This began when I was in school in class six [about 11 years] and I was first penetrated by my school mate. I was not doing it for money at that time because I did not know what it was all about. All I know is that I loved him ... after I finished class 8, I began commercial sex. This was due to financial problems we have in the family. My parents could not provide clothing and other things that I wanted, and here was money I could make.

Conversely, some men reported entering into a sexual transaction involving anal sex the same day they met with strangers. These decisions were unplanned and influenced largely by an envisaged immediate financial or material gain. This tended to occur among men at an older age and was strongly linked with livelihood opportunities, even as an easy means of survival as well as of acquiring accessories such as phones, shoes and clothing. Minimal probing showed that unemployment and poverty were the overriding drivers. During an IDI, Ken (28 years) explained the circumstances in which he first had sex with another man, demonstrating the key role of poverty in sex work:

> When I first came to Mombasa, I used to visit a local car park. A man came in a car, he called me and talked to me. At first I did not understand. He promised to pay me if I did what he wanted. Since I did not have money I agreed.

For his part, Tim (45 years) described how, upon becoming unemployed, he had no other means of providing for his family. One day when he happened to be in a place where sex work negotiations commonly took place, he was offered money for sex. Tim said that he would stop sex work if he found another way to support his wife and children.

In some cases, initial penetrative sex and subsequent acts were the result of sexual exploitation by friends, relatives or other people trusted and well known to the individuals. This was made evident in the comment of Musa (21 years), who noted:

> My father's friend was very close to me ... when my father died he took care of me and one of my brothers. He used to have sex with us. My brother was about 12 and I was 14. He paid school fees for both of us for 2 years before he also died. When he died I had to take care of things and therefore I got into this business [sex work].

Though no informants reported that their first sexual act was physically forced, cases of cross-generational luring and/or financial coercion had occurred. Often, reports suggested that both subtle and overt coercive strategies were employed by older men. For example, Moha, now 35 years old, explained:

> I was employed as house help. One day my employer asked me if I wanted to have sex with him. He told me that he would add my salary. I agreed and that is how I started.

In these circumstances, considerable power imbalances between partners meant that safe sex was only feasible if the perpetrator opted for protection, which none of our informants mentioned had occurred. For some men, the practice of unsafe sex with their initial partners appeared to extend to sex with subsequent partners, a pattern common to reports of women who have experienced sexual violence (World Health Organization 2005).

Overall, men's first sexual experiences were often recounted with distinct ambivalence. Regardless of whether initial sexual activity was consensual or coerced, a striking commonality in the narratives is the role played by the promise of material or financial reward. Perhaps no other respondent made this linkage clearer than Kim (age unknown), who explained:

> I would say selling sex began with him [first man he had sex with in school] because sometimes after we had sex, he used to ask me what I wanted, and he gave me.

Sexual geography

Examination of solicitation practices provides us with an overview of the different contexts in which clients were acquired and the negotiation of sexual exchange that took place. The stigmatisation and criminalisation of same-sex relationships overwhelmingly shaped where the pursuit of clients occurs. Meeting points were predominantly clandestine, known only to sex workers and their client networks. These locales appeared to shift rapidly between day and night for fear of arrest and from the need to evade public hostility.

Meeting locations were diverse and often aligned with an individual's socio-economic class and age. The demographic characteristics and behaviours of clients (and male sex workers) were thus somewhat specific to a location. Participants in higher social or economic groups reported contacting clients via mobile phones or visiting 'stylish' and secluded locations, such as beach hotels or more exclusive upmarket nightclubs. More experienced and older informants operated from multiple locations outside of Mombasa. Others mentioned having a network of foreign clients and making occasional visits abroad.

Conversely, participants in lower socio-economic groups – more often younger sex workers – mentioned soliciting clients within their local neighbourhood. Favourite meeting spots for members of this group include community nightclubs, video halls, beach areas, public parks and backstreet or mainstreet locations known to them and which offer anonymity and/or secrecy. Once contact has been made, negotiation occurs about the type of sexual activity, price and place. Sex workers based in nightclubs described how agreements are reached while drinking with a client. Both street- and club-based sex workers noted that discussion around condom use only formed a minor component of negotiation, if mentioned at all. Additionally, some street-based venues intrinsically hinder safer sex practices as prevention commodities like condoms or lubricants are not readily available.

According to informants in poorer locations, identifying and successfully concluding speedy negotiations with clients were critical, particularly in the potentially dangerous terrain of public meeting points. Securing clients was achieved using well-rehearsed, non-verbal methods. Men thus positioned themselves to 'assess' and 'signal' to potential sexual partners. Long discussions about safer sex were seemingly out of the question and negotiations mostly covered type of sexual activity. One of the focus group respondents observed:

> When I am on the road [streets] at night, I dress differently, I walk and behave differently. A person who is interested will know that you are on the market [selling sex]. Even on the beaches they will know you from your dress and behaviour.

By and large, success in male sex work was dependent on level of experience, a network of contacts and knowledge of where clients can be obtained. Usually, contact between clients and sex workers occurred without sex-work intermediaries like pimps. However, some informants reported a degree of reliance on informants, friends or newly acquired clients of friends. Bar waiters and other staff in drinking and entertainment venues were especially useful links. Kelly had this view:

> If one of my colleagues has got one [client] already and I have not yet 'fished' one, I will have to wait or use the client my friend has got to link me with other clients, and sometimes we use waiters. We usually give them a tip … there is a lot of coordination you know … waiters play a very big role.

Several men described the use of alcohol and drugs, especially *miraa* (*catha edulis*), as a common pastime. Jim, a middle-aged married man who led two lives – as a husband and father during the day and as a sex worker at night – said he often chewed *miraa* or, 'depending on money in [his] pocket', drank alcohol while awaiting clients.

Most sexual encounters involved selling receptive or insertive anal sex, or occasionally both, but masturbation and oral sex were also practised. When asked, none of the men in the group or individual discussions reported ever having had group sex. Some sexual transactions might occur over a period of hours in lodges or private homes, but some sexual activity also took place 'quickly' in public parks, beach areas, unused buildings or similar places.

In summary, the criminalisation and stigmatisation of male-to-male sex limited negotiation processes; power imbalances in safer sex negotiation and alcohol or drug use portend risky sexual acts for men. Moreover, as Bloor *et al.* (1993) have observed, communication during transactional sex is replete with ambiguity, which includes whether or not safer sex will be practised.

Stigma, discrimination and violence

We aimed to thoroughly explore the types and sources of stigma and discrimination faced by participants. Several respondents cited instances of police harassment, arbitrary arrests for loitering and extortion for money or sexual services. Clients were also reported to inflict abuse upon men through verbal or physical harassment, by not paying after sex or by abandoning them in remote locations. Often, the general public were reported to verbally or physically abuse the street-based sex workers. Many accepted this violence as 'normal' or as 'part of the job'. For some, feminine appearance, behaviour or clothing invited ridicule. To attest to these experiences, one respondent mentioned being called *dume jike* ('man-woman') because of his effeminate looks. Others reported being ostracised by close family members or friends. Another focus group participant reiterated this point:

> I have been discriminated against, where people feel that I am a person of no value. My sisters feel I am useless. They ask why I ... do things that a woman should do.

It was clear that many sex workers lived with secrecy and fear. Men living with their parents or having formal employment mentioned the 'high cost' of being exposed. For them this signalled a loss of vital proximal and distal networks of family and friends and employment. During a one-on-one interview, Jami, age 18, aptly demonstrated this point:

> My parents don't like it, they hate it [sex with other men], they suspect I am doing it and I pretend I don't, so I normally hide my male partner relations or else I can't get anything from them [parents].

Evictions by landlords are commonly reported by African men who have sex with men in other settings (Niang *et al.* 2003; Onyango-Ouma *et al.* 2005), and this was also reported by the Mombasa sex workers. IDI participant Joe (age 45) described how suspicion by neighbours led to his eviction from a rented house:

> According to me it is highly secret [anal sex], but people can detect ... when people [neighbours] came to know that I do this, I was told to vacate a house I was renting. I had to move before getting another house. My belongings were thrown out, and in the course of this, I lost some of my belongings.

After the incident he said:

> These days I don't stay in one place for more than 6 months, I keep on moving from one place to another.

According to Cáceres *et al.* (2008) stigma may lead to self-segregation or forced migration among vulnerable populations. Jamal (IDI participant, age 28), who engaged in insertive anal sex only, describes how this process of separation can take place:

> ... these days I don't talk much ... a very close friend of mine used to see me interact with different people [men]; one day he asked me why I was talking to people some of whom looked like homosexuals. He later talked ill things against me ... even colleagues at my work came to know about this. I almost lost my job.

Most participants spoke of having to make difficult decisions when they became ill, as they feared prejudice in both public and private health facilities. Few health facilities or staff were responsive to their needs, particularly when seeking treatment for rectal infections. This situation led many to seek care from unqualified health professionals or even to self-medicate. Ali (age 26) summed this up as follows:

Services in government hospitals are not good. You will be looked down upon, they can even send you away … or ask you insensitive questions; you see we really need a lot of confidentiality.

Participants in Ali's focus group agreed with these views and expressed a reluctance to visit public health facilities. Another discussant averred:

… when I met the doctor I did not tell him exactly what I was suffering from [rectal infection], I changed what I had to tell him, and only said that I was suffering from a headache.

These participants' narratives powerfully evince the burden of stigma faced from family, friends and society. Like other groups of men involved in same-sex practices in Kenya, most respondents mitigated this by attempting to evade scrutiny, adopting tactics like self-segregation, hiding their sexual identity or seeking social acceptance through marriage or having girlfriends. Most men practising receptive or insertive roles said that they attempt to pass as heterosexual in a strongly heteronormative society. During an IDI, Kasim (age 34) described the steps he took to conform to social expectations:

… I am expected to marry, so I have a wife with two children. We love each other … but I would like to tell you that my feelings for men is much stronger than that for women, that's why I have intimate relationships with men.

In all, only a few men like Brown (age 27), who had a relatively high socio-economic status, felt confident in dealing with stigma. He achieved this by 'carefully selecting' the clients he had sex with and staying away from *mtaa* (housing estates) where he was likely to be stigmatised. He stated:

… I have not experienced that [stigma] because I don't engage in sex with just anybody. It is also because I go to private hospitals when sick … there was some stigma in the *mtaa* and I moved to another *mtaa* the moment I felt it … I select married men because they have families, careers, image, etc., which they would not want to risk.

Interestingly, it appears married men formed a common client group for our participants, which has been noted in other studies (Estep *et al.* 1992; Morse *et al.* 1992).

Condom use and perceptions of HIV risk

Although a 'causal relationship' between homosexuality, unsafe sex and HIV infection has long been dominant in HIV discourses in the West (Wolitski *et al.* 2001; CDC 2005), there is limited evidence for this in Kenya. To obtain more detailed information, participants were asked about frequency of condom use and factors that influenced this, including perceptions of risk of HIV acquisition.

Of the ten men who participated in IDIs, only two reported insisting on condom use, declining clients unwilling to use a condom. First, Brown reported consistent condom use with clients by choosing men carefully based on criteria of 'career and image'. The other, Karim, provided this explanation:

I insist on condom use because in the long run you can use all the money you get from clients to treat yourself.

Although both men called condoms 'cumbersome' because of the time taken to put them on and because they were seen as reducing pleasure, they considered condoms 'very necessary' to avoid infection with HIV or other STIs. Also, men reporting condom use cited unavailability of water-based lubricants as a 'major problem', opting instead to use oil-based lubricants owing to their higher costs.

Respondents rated unprotected anal sex as more pleasurable than protected intercourse. In a focus group session, Lucky (age 23) expressed the common sentiment that:

We are all aware that when you use a condom you don't get that maximum pleasure … so as to get that maximum pleasure we have sex without a condom.

The idea of not using condoms with clients seemed normative; some sex workers even maintained that condom use was 'rarely' discussed with partners. Those proposing condoms with clients reported 'facing resistance', citing client desire for optimal sexual pleasure. To avoid using them, some clients offer additional money for unprotected sex, highlighting the key role of the financial negotiation and transaction process for sex workers. The self-perception of the sex worker as a 'businessman' was reflected in a quote by Kale (age 27), who maintained that:

This [sex work] is like a shop, what is important is to agree on the price. A shopkeeper does not care who comes into the shop.

Many participants expressed the view that using condoms with regular partners was difficult. It appeared that levels of condom use decreased with degree of intimacy and stability of a relationship. As commonly reported within heterosexual relationships, the suggestion of condom use by a regular partner often signified 'mistrust' or was a reflection of his having been 'unfaithful' or even 'HIV-infected'.

In Kenya, the silence of HIV prevention programmes and lack of media reports on anal sex may reinforce perceptions that anal sex is not a high-risk sexual practice. Some informants held a conviction that they would not acquire HIV, despite having unprotected anal sex with both male and female partners. Some participants believed anal sex was 'safer' than vaginal sex and were more likely to report condom use for vaginal sex. Seif (age 24), a man who has sex with both men and women, expressed this view:

There is AIDS and all these but I have never heard of anybody having a sexually transmitted infection in the anus … mostly I think these diseases are found in the vagina and mouth, but I still can't understand it well.

Phil, a focus group participant, observed:

I don't believe that most men use condoms because with the information I get illness is in the vagina and not the anus … I have never heard of anybody getting illness from the anus, even from our teachers.

As mentioned earlier, alcohol was widely available in many sex work locales. Men seeking clients in nightclubs, beach areas and other community settings frequently mentioned the use of alcohol and drugs. Many observed that this often led to poor decision-making, and even those reporting frequent condom use mentioned the lack of such use when intoxicated. Tabu (age 44) described the effects of being intoxicated as:

> I mostly use condoms to protect myself from STIs including HIV. It is for my safety, but there are times when I am drunk, and then I don't use a condom.

Bright (age 29) put it this way:

> When drunk or high you are unable to think properly. When in this state you can easily get into unprotected sex.

This finding is consistent with findings from studies in other sub-Saharan African contexts where alcohol consumption has been associated with unprotected sexual intercourse (Stall et al. 2001; Chersich et al. 2007; Kalichman et al. 2007; Lane et al. 2008; Parry et al. 2008). Similar to what Diaz and Ayala (1999) and Parry et al. (2008) reported, getting drunk or high on drugs was associated with 'relieving stress', 'passing time' or 'instilling courage' prior to selling sex.

It is evident that the practice of unprotected sex is underlined by a dynamic interplay between sex workers and clients. Similar attitudes and condom practices have previously been documented (Colby et al. 2004; Kalichman et al. 2007; Parry et al. 2008). Key factors are: power relations; notions of trust; sexual pleasure; alcohol and drug use; and the belief that male-to-male sex carries a low risk of HIV transmission. Most importantly perhaps, as noted elsewhere, the practice of unsafe sex often occurs in contexts where clients are in control of the encounter and sex workers are unable to contest that control (Browne and Minichiello 1995).

Conclusion

In seeking to explore more fully the lives of male sex workers, this study documented the dynamics of male–male sexual activity and their implications for vulnerability to HIV and overall well-being and health. Reflecting on our findings, we note that alongside individual risk behaviours of participants there exists a range and variation of specific groups, such as low socio-economic strata, younger, aged and incarcerated men, that even further magnifies these risks (Cáceres et al. 2008). Both phases of the study found that most clients are Kenyan, contrary to occasional public pronouncements that male-to-male sex is a foreign import.

Why then does male-to-male sexual activity take place, and how do such notions apply in this population? According to Plummer (1995), male-to-male sexual experience can be classified within four categories: casual homosexuality, situational homosexuality, personalised homosexuality and homosexuality as a way of life. He explains that schoolboy crushes and masturbation, sexual activity in prisons or military camps, secret homosexual desires, and the open acknowledgement of homosexual preference, respectively, fit these classifications. In Kenya, male-to-male sex of a situational nature has previously been documented among men in closed settings (Kiama 1999; Mathenge 2008). However, it is difficult to apply Plummer's categorisation to our population in simple terms. For many men in this study, male-to-male sex was motivated primarily by financial incentives and not as a way of life per se. This, however, is not to say that male–male sex is limited to economic motives alone in this setting. Sex with other men occurred also due to same-sex desire, socio-economic circumstance or a combination thereof.

The study also provides insight into the relationship between health and place. Although understandings of solicitation practices are complex (Macintyre *et al.* 1993; Flowers *et al.* 2000), this study explains, in part, their nexus with high-risk behaviour. The chances of negotiating or acquiring commodities to make sex safer decreases with the class status of the location, and although social class classification has limitations in measuring health (Naidoo and Wills 2000), it does serve as an important indicator of living conditions and access to services. Also, as previously described (de Wit *et al.* 1997), the numbers of anal sexual partners and acts vary according to the venue in which sex occurs. All this suggests locale-based interventional approaches are required for different sex work settings (Flowers *et al.* 2000).

Beyond this, narratives of public prejudice and family ostracism depict the extent of social exclusion experienced by male sex workers. This link has important implications for sexual behaviour, partner relationships and HIV vulnerability. Perceived societal norms bar many men from openly discussing their same-sex experiences or seeking health services. Social structures and beliefs reinforce stigma and violence against these men. Escoffer (1997) and Cáceres *et al.* (2008) argue that stigma frequently promotes increased mobility and vulnerability for such marginalised population groups. Additionally, considerations of family honour and social standing are associated with maintaining concurrent heterosexual relationships. This has potential implications for the broader HIV epidemic, given that male–male sexual networks are often integrated within the general population.

To reduce HIV and STI transmission in male sex work settings in Mombasa, results from the quantitative and qualitative study were analysed and used to inform the development of health interventions. First, patterns of self-identification, client-seeking and health-care avoidance described by informants indicated that an outreach strategy driven by the men themselves may be most effective in reaching peers. Thus, to help facilitate delivery of health information and referrals for STI services, 40 men were recruited as peer educators and trained in basic HIV prevention, harm reduction (hazardous use of alcohol and drugs) and as HIV testing counsellors. Negative experiences at health-care facilities were described by participants. This showed that local health workers were not trained or familiar with anal STI issues, prevention information specific to male-to-male sex, or the public health importance of sensitivity and confidentiality towards these men. To respond to this concern, 20 health service providers in Mombasa attended a workshop to sensitise them to the health-related needs of male sex workers and on how to recognise anal STI symptoms and to tailor HIV prevention advice. These are key first steps towards addressing the unmet prevention needs of men who have sex with men in Mombasa.

Our study has several limitations. Although selection of participants according to preselected categories enabled the study to capture a range of experiences, the sample may not be representative of the male sex worker population. Interview subgroups and discussion topics were also selected based on formative discussions conducted prior to survey implementation and may not have included important issues that emerged in the first-phase quantitative survey. Some of the reported norms, patterns and behaviours may also be specific to the local sex work context in Mombasa, although there are likely to be broad commonalities between the experiences of members of this group and those of other male sex workers in Kenya and other African countries.

Overall, findings from this study show that the HIV prevention needs of men who have sex with men have been largely overlooked. However, policymakers in Kenya have shown an increased willingness to review the evidence and address the issue. Further acknowledgement by African HIV coordinating bodies, as well as informed public discussion, are important steps forward. Evidence indicates that increased awareness and understanding of same-sex issues may help mitigate HIV vulnerability and result in policy action and improved services (De Graaf *et al.* 1994; Cáceres *et al.* 2006; Baral *et al.* 2007; Saavedra *et al.* 2008). Across Africa, comprehensive HIV strategies that include specifically tailored HIV prevention, STI treatment and condom and lubricant provision for men are urgently needed. To facilitate the delivery of these services, it is important for health-care systems to be sensitised and equipped to serve these men in confidential and non-judgemental environments. In Mombasa, targeted interventions that take into account the diverse motivations, socio-economic backgrounds, solicitation patterns and sexual behaviours of male sex workers are also recommended.

References

Allman, D., Adebayo, S., Myers, T., Odomuye, O. and Ongunsola, S. 2007. Challenges for the sexual health and social acceptance of men who have sex with men in Nigeria. *Culture, Health & Sexuality* 9(2): 153–168.

Baral, S., Sifakis, F., Cleghorn, F. and Beyrer, C. 2007. Elevated risk for HIV infection among men who have sex with men in low- and middle-income countries 2000–2006: A systematic review. *PloS Medicine* 4(12): e339.

Baudh, S. 2008. *Human Rights and the Criminalization of Consensual Same-sex Sexual Acts in the Commonwealth, South and Southeast Asia*. New Delhi, India: South and Southeast Asia Resource Centre on Sexuality.

Bloor, M.J., Barnard, M.A., Finlay, A. and McKeganey, N.P. 1993. HIV-related risk practices among Glasgow male prostitutes: Reframing concepts of risk behavior. *Medical Anthropology Quarterly* 7(2): 152–169.

Browne, J. and Minichiello, V. 1995. The social meanings behind male sex work: Implications for sexual interactions. *British Journal of Sociology* 46(4): 598–622.

Cáceres, C., Konda, K., Pecheny, M., Chatterjee, A. and Lyerla, R. 2006. Estimating the number of men who have sex with men in low- and middle-income countries. *Sexually Transmitted Infections* 82(3): iii3–iii9.

Cáceres, C., Aggleton, P. and Galea, J.T. 2008. Sexual diversity, social inclusion and HIV/AIDS. *AIDS* 2: S45–S55.

CDC. 2005. *HIV/AIDS Surveillance Report*. CDC. Available at: www.cdc.gov/hiv/topics/surveillance/resources/reports/ [Accessed 3 June 2009].

Chersich, M.F., Luchters, S.M.F., Malonza, I.M., Mwarogo, P., King'ola, N. and Temmerman, M. 2007. Heavy episodic drinking among Kenyan female sex workers is associated with unsafe sex, sexual violence and sexually transmitted infections. *International Journal of STD & AIDS* 18: 764–769.

Colby, J.D., Cao, N.H. and Doussantousse, S. 2004. Men who have sex with men in Vietnam: A review. *AIDS Education and Prevention* 16(1): 45–54.

Costigan, A. and Foreman, M. 2002/2003. Kenya: Gender, power and AIDS. *The Social Development Review* 7(1). Available at: www.icsw.org/publications/sdr/2003-march/kenya.htm [Accessed 5 March 2015}.

De Graaf, R., Vanwesenbeeck, I., van Zessen, G., Straver, C.J. and Visser, J.H. 1994. Male prostitutes and safe sex: Different settings, different risks. *Aids Care* 6(3): 277–288.

de Wit, J.B.F., deVroome, E.M.M., Sandfort, T.G.M. and van Grievensven, G.J. 1997. Homosexual encounters in different venues. *International Journal of STD and AIDS* 8: 130–134.

Diaz, R.M. and Ayala, G. 1999. Love, passion and rebellion: Ideologies of HIV risk among Latino gay men in the US. *Culture, Health & Sexuality* 1: 277–293.

Escoffer, J. 1997. The political economy of the closet: Notes towards an economic history of gay and lesbian life before Stonewall. In: A. Gluckman and B. Reed (eds) *Homo-economics: Capitalism, Community and Lesbian and Gay Life*. London and New York: Routledge, 165–184.

Estep, R., Waldorf, D. and Marota, T. 1992. Sexual behaviour of male prostitutes. In: J. Huber and B.E. Schneider (eds) *The Social Context of AIDS*. Newbury Park, CA: SAGE, 95–112.

Evans-Pritchard, E.E. 1929. *Witchcraft (Mangu) among the A-Zande*. Sudan Notes and Records XII: 163–248. Khartoum: McCorquodale.

Flowers, P., Marriot, C. and Hart, G. 2000. The bars, the bogs, and the bushes: The impact of locale on sexual cultures. *Culture, Health & Sexuality* 2(1): 69–86.

Geibel, S., van der Elst, E.M., King'ola, N., Luchters, S., Davies, A., Getambu, E.M.N., Peshu, N., Graham, S.M., McClelland, R.S. and Sanders, E.J. 2007. Are you on the market? A capture–recapture enumeration of men who sell sex to men in and around Mombasa, Kenya. *AIDS* 21(10): 1349–1354.

Geibel, S., Luchters, S., Kingola, N., Esu-Williams, E., Rinyiru, A. and Tun, W. 2008. Factors associated with self-reported unprotected anal sex among male sex workers in Mombasa, Kenya. *Sexually Transmitted Diseases* 35(8): 746–752.

Gouws, E., White, P.J., Stover, J. and Brown, T. 2006. Short-term estimates of adult HIV incidence by mode of transmission: Kenya and Thailand as examples. *Sexually Transmitted Infections* 82(suppl. 3): iii51–iii55.

Government of Kenya. 2008. *Laws of Kenya, Penal Code, Chapter 63, Sections 162–165*. National Council for Law Reporting. Available at: www.kenyalaw.org/kenyalaw/klr_app/view_cap.php?CapID=52 [Accessed 2 May 2009].

Kalichman, S.C., Simbayi, L.C., Cain, D. and Jooste, S. 2007. Alcohol use and sexual risks for HIV/AIDS in sub-Saharan Africa: Systematic review of empirical findings. *Prevention Science* 8: 141–151.

Kiama, W. 1998. *Homosexuality Takes Root in Kenya. Worldwide Gay Life, Sites and Insights*. Available at: www.globalgayz.com/kenya-news.html#article1 [Accessed 3 May 2009].

Kiama, W. 1999. Where are Kenya's homosexuals? *AIDS Analysis Africa* 9: 9–10.

Kibicho, W. 2003. Tourism and the sex trade: Roles male sex workers play in Malindi, Kenya. *Tourism Review International* 7: 129–141.

Lane, T., Pettifor, A., Pascoe, S., Fiamma, A. and Rees, H. 2006. Heterosexual anal intercourse increases risk of HIV infection among young South African men. *AIDS* 20: 123–125.

Lane, T., Shade, S.B., McIntyre, J. and Morin, S.F. 2008. Alcohol and sexual risk behavior among men who have sex with men in South African township communities. *AIDS and Behaviour* 12(1): S78–S85.

Luchters, S., Chersich, M., Rinyiru, A., Barasa, M.S., Kingola, N., Mandaliya, K., Bosire, W., Wambugu, S., Mwarogo, P. and Temmerman, M. 2008. Impact of five years of peer-mediated interventions on sexual behavior and sexually transmitted infections among female sex workers in Mombasa, Kenya. *BMC Public Health* 8: 143.

Macintyre, S., MacIver, S. and Sooman, A. 1993. Area, class and health: Should we be focusing on places or people? *Journal of Social Policy* 22: 213–234.

Mathenge, O. 2008. Homosexuality a major cause of AIDS in Kenya prisons. *Daily Nation*, 24 May.

McKenna, N. 1996. *On the Margins: Men who Have Sex with Men and HIV in the Developing World*. London: Panos Institute.

Morse, E.V., Simon, P.M., Balson, P.M. and Osofsky, H.S. 1992. Sexual behaviour patterns of male street prostitutes. *Archives of Sexual Behaviour* 21(3): 347–357.

Moses, S., Plummer, A.F., Ngugi, E.N., Nagelkerke, N.J.D., Anzala, A.O. and Ndinya-Achola, J.O. 1991. Controlling HIV in Africa: Effectiveness and cost of an intervention in a high-frequency STD transmitter core group. *AIDS* 5: 407–411.

Murray, S. and Roscoe, W. 1998. *Boy-wives and Female-husbands: Studies in African Homosexualities.* New York: Palgrave.

Naidoo, J. and Wills, J. 2000. *Health Promotion: Foundations for Practice.* London: Bailliere Tindall, An Imprint of Elsevier Limited.

National AIDS Control Council. 2005. *Kenya National HIV/AIDS Strategic Plan 2005/6–2009/10: A Call to Action.* Nairobi, Kenya: Office of the President.

Ngugi, E.N., Plummer, F.A., Simonsen, J.N., Cameron, D.W., Bosire, M., Waiyaki, P., Ronald, A.R. and Ndinya-Achola, J.O. 1988. Prevention of transmission of human immunodeficiency virus in Africa: Effectiveness of condom promotion and health education among prostitutes. *Lancet* 332(8616): 887–890.

Niang, C.I., Tapsoba, P., Weiss, E., Diagne, M., Niang, Y., Moreau, A.M., Gomis, D., Wade, A.S., Seck, K. and Castle, C. 2003. 'It's raining stones': Stigma, violence and HIV vulnerability among men who have sex with men in Dakar, Senegal. *Culture, Health & Sexuality* 5(6): 499–512.

Onyango-Ouma, W., Birungi, H. and Geibel, S. 2005. *Understanding the HIV/STI Risks and Prevention Needs of Men who Have Sex with Men in Nairobi, Kenya.* Horizons final report. Washington, DC: Population Council.

Parry, C., Petersen, P., Dewing, S., Carney, T., Needle, R., Kroeger, K. and Treger, L. 2008. *Rapid Assessment of Drug-related HIV Risk Among Men who Have Sex with Men in Three South African Cities.* Richmond, VA: Elsevier.

Plummer, K. 1995. *Telling Sexual Stories: Power, Change and Social Worlds.* London: Routledge.

Roehr, B., Gross, M. and Mayer, K. 2001. *Creating a Research and Development Agenda for Rectal Microbicides that Protect against HIV Infection.* Washington, DC: amfAR, The Foundation for AIDS Research.

Saavedra, J., Antonio Izazola-Licea, J. and Beyrer, C. 2008. Sex between men in the context of HIV: The AIDS 2008 Jonathan Mann Memorial Lecture in health and human rights. *Journal of the International AIDS Society* 11(1): 9.

Sanders, E.J., Graham, S.M., Okuku, H.S., van der Elst, E.M., Muhari, A., Davies, A., Peshu, N., Price, M., McClelland, R.S. and Smith, A.D. 2007. HIV-1 infection in high-risk men who have sex with men in Mombasa, Kenya. *AIDS* 21: 2513–2520.

Shallock, R. and Moore, J. 2003. Inhibiting sexual transmission of HIV-1 infection. *Nature Reviews Microbiology* 1(1): 25–34.

Stall, R., Paul, J.P., Greenwood, G., Pollack, L.M., Bein, E., Grosby, G.M., Mills, T.C., Coates, T.J. and Catania, J.A. 2001. Alcohol use, drug use and alcohol-related problems among men who have sex with men: The urban men's health study. *Addiction* 96(11): 1589–1601.

UNAIDS. 2006. *UNAIDS Policy Brief: HIV and Sex Between Men.* Geneva, Switzerland: UNAIDS.

UNAIDS. 2008. *Report on the Global AIDS Epidemic.* Geneva, Switzerland: UNAIDS. Available at: www.unaids.org/sites/default/files/en/media/unaids/contentassets/dataimport/pub/globalreport/2008/jc1510_2008globalreport_en.pdf [Accessed 3 May 2009].

Wade, A., Kane, C. and Diallo, P. 2005. HIV infection and sexually transmitted infections among men who have sex with men in Senegal. *AIDS* 19: 2133–2140.

Werner, D. 1987. *Human Sexuality Around the World.* Unpublished manuscript of the Human Relations Area Files. Yale University. Available at: www.yale.edu/hraf [Accessed 5 May 2009].

Wolitski, R., Valdiserri, R., Denning, P. and Levine, W.C. 2001. Are we headed for a resurgence of the HIV epidemic among men who have sex with men? *American Journal of Public Health* 91: 883–888.

World Health Organization. 2005. *Violence Against Women and HIV/AIDS: Critical Intersections. Violence Against Sex Workers and HIV Prevention.* Geneva, Switzerland: World Health Organization.

Chapter 13

Diversity of commercial sex among men and male-born trans people in three Peruvian cities

César Rodolfo Nureña, Mario Zúñiga, Joseph Zunt, Carolina Mejía, Silvia Montano and Jorge Sánchez

Introduction

Commercial sex involving men and male-born *travestis* (transvestites), transgenders and transsexuals (henceforward referred to as sex work involving men and trans people) is a subject of continued academic interest. This interest grew in the 1980s after the advent of the HIV epidemic (Aggleton 1999; Bimbi 2007). In a review of social science research on the sex trade, Vanwesenbeeck (2001) has detailed how the first approaches to male prostitution considered the phenomenon a form of social pathology, often described as a dangerous behaviour exposing people to disease, violence, discrimination, criminalisation and exploitation (Kaye 2007; Scott *et al.* 2005). These perspectives are still present today, but more nuanced views have emerged recently, with many scholars suggesting that social and sexual practices, as well as the vulnerability of subjects who provide sexual services, are influenced in complex ways by socio-economic factors, gender ideologies, power relations, social norms and culture (Aggleton 1999; Bimbi 2007; Bimbi and Parsons 2005; Browne and Minichiello 1996; Calhoun 1992; Kaye 2003; Perlongher 1999; Prestage 1994; Scott *et al.* 2005; Van der Poel 1992).

Although not a criminal offence in Peru, sex work involving men and trans women is highly stigmatised. According to popular Peruvian stereotypes, the practice is usually associated with poverty, crime and immorality and perceived to be carried out on the streets by socially marginalised people (Cosme *et al.* 2007). Concern about the spread of HIV and other sexually transmitted infections (STIs) has focused scientific interest upon same-sex practices and different forms of sex work (Bautista *et al.* 2004; Clark *et al.* 2007; Konda *et al.* 2008a, 2008b; Lama *et al.* 2006; Montano *et al.* 2005; Paris *et al.* 2001; Salazar and Silva Santisteban 2009; Sanchez *et al.* 2007; Tabet *et al.* 2002; Valderrama *et al.* 2008). Studies have examined the sociocultural context of compensated sex (Fernandez-Davila *et al.* 2008; Salazar *et al.* 2005, 2006), sex work within the framework of male sexual cultures (Cáceres and Jimenez 1999; Cáceres and Rosasco 1999, 2000) and social vulnerability and violence associated with sex work encounters (Caro 1999). The research objectives of studies are diverse, and sex work is not always their main focus, but some reports offer some clues that allow us to infer that sex work is more complex and varied than usually thought from public policy and popular stereotypes, both by the different sexual identities of those who offer sexual services (Konda *et al.* 2008a), as well as the places and ways in which it is practised (Bayer *et al.* 2010; Cáceres and Jimenez 1999). In any case, the complexities and diversity of sex work have not been described or captured in most previous Peruvian studies on this topic, which generally focus on populations of individuals who offer sexual services in public places and suffer social exclusion (such as poor youth and members of sexual minorities).

This situation has some problematic aspects: on the one hand, a partial view of sex work may limit the efficacy of social and health promotion interventions, which will not be able to reach potentially vulnerable but invisible sex workers; on the other hand, public discourses and images about sex work can reproduce stigmatising views of sex workers, based on scientific information that only presents data on marginalised subjects (Tiby 2003; Van der Poel 1992).

The present study is based on an in-depth approach to men and male-born trans individuals who perform sex work. We obtained their individual stories and examined the economic and sociocultural context in which they live and work. Our objective was to identify, describe and analyse the social and cultural factors related to the practice of various forms of sex work among subjects of different social backgrounds. We intentionally did not focus on any one particular group of sex workers but, rather, examined sex work in its multiple manifestations in different groups and social contexts.

Methods

We conducted an exploratory, ethnographic study. Fieldwork was carried out from January to October 2009 in the cities of Lima, Pucallpa and Iquitos, Peru, which were selected because of the high levels of STI and HIV-risk behaviours previously found in these contexts (Lama *et al.* 2006; Tabet *et al.* 2002).

Study sites

Lima, the capital of Peru, has a population of around 10 million people (about one-third of the country's total population) comprised mostly of the descendants of immigrants and their parents who arrived from throughout the country and settled in the city over the last 60 years. The bulk of Peru's businesses, industrial activity, services and cultural affairs is concentrated in Lima and it additionally receives an important share of the revenue generated by the extraction of natural resources in other parts of the country.

Pucallpa and Iquitos are the capitals of the Amazonian regions of Ucayali and Loreto, respectively, located in the north-eastern region of the country. Native ethnic groups living in these areas speak over 40 languages, but the urban centres have a major presence of Spanish-speaking *mestizos* (population of mixed race). Extraction industries (wood and oil) and trade dominate the regional economies. The city of Pucallpa, with a population of approximately 200,000 habitants, is a meeting point for many migratory flows mainly associated with commerce and logging and, to a lesser extent, agricultural and industrial activities. Iquitos, with approximately 400,000 habitants, is accessible only by air or river and has greater economic diversity than Pucallpa.

Recruitment, participants and procedures

We used ethnographic, observational techniques to analyse public behaviour and the physical and social context in 52 sex work venues identified by a previous mapping of the three cities noted previously. Two experienced Peruvian ethnographers (CRN and MZ) visited these locations, sometimes with the support of health promoters and other key informants who facilitated access. In most places, the research team engaged in informal interactions with sex workers, managers and employees of establishments and other persons familiar with the activities of sex workers, including some clients. In other cases, the ethnographers just observed and took notes, for example in public settings where their presence might have compromised the confidentiality or security of sex workers. After each visit, the ethnographers discussed and compared their observations and fieldwork notes before preparing a report for further analysis.

We also conducted in-depth, semi-structured interviews with 42 study participants who provided sexual services (20 in Lima, 11 in Iquitos and 11 in Pucallpa). They were selected in each city by the researchers either directly during the fieldwork using the snowball technique, with the support of health promoters, or by searching sexual services advertisements in print and electronic media, to obtain a convenience sample of maximum variability. The selection criteria for recruiting interview participants were: being a male or male-born trans; being at least 18 years of age; having a history of offering sexual services to men in exchange for money within the 6 months prior to study participation (the commercial character of the exchange was explicit to both sex workers and clients, with payment made either before or after sexual services were provided); and giving verbal consent to participate in the study. Confidential, anonymous interviews, lasting 60–90 minutes, were conducted in private locations. Subjects were asked to narrate their life stories, highlighting their experiences, attitudes and opinions related to the practice of sex work, and were also questioned about other forms of commercial sex they knew or practised themselves. At the end of the interviews, participants were financially reimbursed for transportation costs.

Sex workers interviewed were between 18 and 45 years of age (mean age 27) and had different characteristics in terms of socio-economic background, sexual identity, time and experience in the sex trade and places and modalities of sex work. Educational level was our primary indicator of socio-economic status (SES) (low, low-middle, middle and upper-middle), but was adjusted for monthly income as compared with the legal minimum salary in Peru (approximately US$200 per month in 2010) and occupation (sex work as an occasional or frequent activity and alternative jobs). In each of the three cities we also conducted open-ended interviews with 25 key informants: managers and employees in entertainment establishments, health promoters, sexual rights activists, health professionals and researchers in sexuality and public health. They were asked to share their knowledge and perspectives on sex work.

Field notes obtained through observation in the sex work venues and audio files of the interviews were transcribed verbatim into word-processing files. Data were coded and organised following a grounded-theory approach (Strauss and Corbin 1998) using Atlas.ti™. The information presented here is based on triangulation and contrasts between our different sources of data (fieldwork observations, interviews with sex workers and key informants). The study protocol was reviewed and approved by the Institutional Review Boards of IMPACTA and the University of Washington.

Results

Places and forms of sex work

Sex work involving men and male-born *travestis*, transgenders and transsexuals in Peru occurs in many different venues. During our fieldwork, in addition to sex work on the streets, we found it was also performed in bars and discos, saunas, sex cinemas and video clubs, lodges (hotels and *hostales*), houses and apartments (of individuals, groups or agencies), night clubs, brothels, prisons, river boats, semi-rural areas around cities, highways and timber and oil industry camps (see Table 13.1). A variety of strategies were used to locate and contact clients: face-to-face methods, intermediaries, various forms of internet-based sex work and through mobile phones and the print media.

The most visible and well-known forms of sex work were those involving *travestis* and *fletes* working on the street. In Lima and Pucallpa, some *travestis* worked also in specific peri-urban areas near roads or highways. In the context of sex work in Peru, the term *travesti* is used to refer to individuals born male but with the appearance, attitudes or identities of women (independently of whether they see themselves as transsexual or transgender). Their clients are mostly men who self-identify as heterosexual. In the streets, contacts are negotiated regarding price, location and other details of sexual services, such as sex roles, time, condom use, etc. Almost all *travestis* described clients asking to be penetrated. Although some *travestis* agreed to do this (charging a higher rate), others strongly rejected it.

Fletes are young men with different sexual identities and social backgrounds. Most assume masculine attitudes in their public behaviour and define themselves as heterosexual or bisexual, but there are also some *fletes* who have more feminine manners and self-identify as gay or homosexual. Unlike *travestis*, *fletes* do not dress in female clothes. *Fleteo* is the systematic exchange of sex for money (Cáceres and Jimenez 1999) and includes negotiations similar to those seen among *travestis*. For some young men, *fleteo* is a regular job, while for others it is a temporary or occasional activity. *Fletes* typically work along specific streets or in public squares, bars, discotheques and the gay porn cinemas of Lima. In some of these places we also found groups of soldiers, or *cachaquitos* as they are known. They are recruited by the Peruvian Army from diverse parts of the country, but in their time off some may frequent gay venues in central Lima where they may participate in sex for money, food, drink or overnight lodging. The clients of *fletes* and *cachaquitos* are mostly gay men, bisexual men and closeted homosexuals of different social classes.

Many *travestis* and *fletes* perform street-based sex work in highly competitive environments (for clients, working areas, power and prestige, etc.) and frequently encounter violence from other sex workers, pimps, street delinquents and even public safety officials. However, in the three cities, we also encountered some *fletes* and *travestis* offering sexual services in places and modalities not necessarily associated with violence.

In Iquitos, *fleteo* was similar to *fleteo* in Lima, with low-income youth seeking clients in squares, tourist areas, clubs and gay bars. The demand for sexual services here was more clearly associated with tourism and the local gay subculture. In Pucallpa, unlike in Lima and Iquitos, it was difficult to identify *fletes* in the streets. In the main square, encounters occurred between men that led to sex for money, tips or invitations to eat or drink liquor, but without the negotiation pattern of *fleteo* seen in Lima and Iquitos. Some young men were familiar with the gay scene and self-identified as *fletes*, but offered their services only in gay clubs and bars, using group strategies to contact clients and offer protection.

In some gay entertainment establishments in the three cities there are also *mozos* (waiters) and *anfitriones* (hosts) who interact with clients and may have sex for money in nearby hotels or even inside the establishments, usually with the agreement of the manager of the establishment.

In Lima, a special type of entertainment venue known as *video porno* combines the characteristics of a discotheque and bar with *cuartos oscuros* (dark rooms) for erotic interaction

Table 13.1 Forms and characteristics of sex work in three cities in Peru

Venues and sex workers	Main characteristics
Parks and streets (Li, Iq, Pu)*	The most visible and known modalities, with high social vulnerability and stigmatisation.
Travestis	Markets highly competitive and differentiated, with presence of pimps.
Fletes	*Fletes* are young men with diverse sex identities. Many *fletes* perform sex work for survival. Others from middle classes have diverse motivations (see also Cáceres and Jimenez 1999).
Mototaxistas (Iq)	Some motorcycle taxi drivers who park around gay venues are occasionally solicited for sexual services (see Paris *et al.* 2001).
Bars/discotheques (Li, Iq, Pu) *Anfitriones, mozos*	Some 'hosts' (*anfitriones*) and bar 'waiters' (*mozos*) provide sex services to clients, under arrangements with the bar's owners.
Fletes, travestis	Some *fletes* look for clients in gay bars and discos. When attending these places, *travestis* can eventually contact clients there.
Highways around cities (Pu) *Travestis*	Working along with female sex workers and pimps. Clients from low and working class.
Porn video clubs (Li) *Anfitriones, mozos* Male/gay escorts	Clients seek entertainment and occasional sex with other clients or sex workers. 'Hosts' and 'waiters' provide clients with company and sex services.
Porn cinemas (Li) *Fletes, travestis*	*Fletes* can contact clients in porno cinemas. Some *travestis* have arrangements with cinema administrators for providing sex services inside the cinemas.
Night clubs (Li/Southern Peru) *Travestis*	*Travestis* work along with female sex workers, offering company and sex services to clients, and share the money with the club.
Brothels (Li/Southern Peru) *Travestis*	*Travestis* work in some brothels along with female sex workers, but there are also a few hotels where the administrators offer the sex services of *travestis* to clients.
Agencies (Li, Iq) *Travestis* Male escorts, 'strippers'	Clients call intermediaries and arrange dates with sex workers, who are mainly middle and upper-middle class. Intermediaries usually recruit strippers in gyms to dance in discotheques and private parties, where they can also be solicited for company or sex services.
Independent, media-based *Fletes, travestis* (Li, Iq, Pu) Escorts, 'strippers' (Li, Iq)	Sex services announced in newspapers, personal cards and on the Internet. Contacts made using mobile phones and chat rooms. Confidentiality is highly important, especially for sex workers from the middle and upper-middle classes.
Gay saunas (Li) Masseurs	Mainly young men from working and middle class. They offer massages and sex services to a sauna's clients.

Continued

Table 13.1 Forms and characteristics of sex work in three cities in Peru, *continued*

Venues and sex workers	Main characteristics
Prisons (Li, Iq) *Travestis*	Some incarcerated *travestis* offer sex services inside the prisons, under the rule of pimps. Others have sex (not always paid) with prisoners on visit days.
Boats (Amazon rivers) Gay travellers	Gay men go in boats by fluvial routes and have sex with merchants and travellers (not always for a charge).
Woodwork/oil camps *Cocineros*	In the Amazon jungle, male cooks live in camps for several months with groups of young men and have sex with them. Many obtain additional money by charging workers a fee for sex services (see also Nureña *et al.* 2009).
Infrastructure projects (Pu) *Travestis*, young gay men	Sex workers visit construction sites on payment days and offer sex services to workers.

Note: * 'Li', 'Iq' and 'Pu' are the abbreviations for Lima, Iquitos and Pucallpa, respectively.

and anonymous sex, television screens showing sexual images, and private *cabinas* or small rooms where it is possible to watch pornographic movies and have sex. Some of these venues also have *anfitriones* or *mozos*, and *fletes* may also visit such places to find clients.

In some porn cinemas in Lima we witnessed *travestis* who roamed the halls to contact their clients (mostly heterosexually identified men) during the screening of heterosexual sex scenes. These *travestis* worked under arrangements with the managers of the cinemas, who provided security and rooms for sex services on the premises.

Other sex venues encountered only in Lima were gay saunas. Masseurs who worked in these establishments provided massage to middle- and upper-middle-class clients. These masseurs were mostly young men self-identified as heterosexual or bisexual and offered massage services which could lead to sexual services performed in the same massage rooms.

Some men and *travestis* in Lima and Iquitos worked for intermediaries or agencies that received telephone requests from clients asking for a male companion or escort. Several of these agencies advertised on the Internet or in 'relaxation' sections of some newspapers and charged the sex workers a percentage of the cost of sexual services. This form of sex work also included strippers and exotic dancers. Many of these dancers, in addition to working in nightclubs offering entertainment and shows at private parties, were available for contact by intermediaries or directly by clients to provide sexual services.

In addition, we encountered dancers, masseurs, escorts and many other young men and *travestis* who used the Internet and newspapers, business cards and personal contacts to work independently of any agency or intermediary. Experienced sex workers reported that in previous decades such contacts were made primarily by escort agencies. However, with growing access to the Internet and mobile phones, independent forms of sex work have become more frequent. In fact, most sex workers interviewed reported using mobile phones or the Internet to contact clients, and many noted this allowed them to charge higher rates, remain anonymous and have a relatively steady client base, thereby avoiding the danger associated with working on the street:

I used to work in the street, but now I post my photos online and receive calls on my cell. It's better …

> (Claudia, 26, *travesti*, low-middle-SES, Iquitos)

I no longer have to return to the streets. There are many raids, fights [between *travestis*] for the spaces in the park … So I prefer to work solely on cell phone.

> (Mariela, 30, *travesti*, middle-SES, Iquitos)

Now some [*fletes*] find clients online. They are not coming any more to the square.

> (Rolando, 45, veteran *flete*, middle-SES, Plaza San Martin, Lima)

He [the intermediary agent] has pictures of the strippers in his cell phone. He shows them to clients and says 'choose'.

> (Marcelo, 25, stripper, middle-SES, Lima)

I have a cell phone and a website. So I am available to clients 24 hours a day, and so I can charge more than on the street.

> (Carolina, 21, *travesti*, private escort, low-middle-SES, Iquitos)

Sex work associated with other economic activities

There are forms of sex work clearly linked to specific economic activities. For example, some *travestis* in Pucallpa reported that they occasionally made agreements with the managers of construction projects to provide sexual services to their workers. In Iquitos and Pucallpa, tourism creates a visible demand for commercial sex. In addition, sexual services are offered by men and women during activities related to trade and transport, typically on river boats travelling on the Amazonian rivers and on roads on the outskirts of Lima.

In the Ucayali region we encountered a very distinct but widespread type of sex trade associated with the logging industry. Thousands of young men, mainly from urban centres like Pucallpa, are hired each year by logging companies and sent deep into the forest in groups of 8 to 30 to work for several months. They live in camps, where there is at least one person hired to prepare meals. This person can be a woman or a young man with a homosexual or feminine identity. Several *cocineros* (cooks) reported providing sexual favours to loggers. Although these sexual exchanges do not necessarily involve payment, many *cocineros* have the opportunity to earn additional income from selling sex. They may maintain notebooks with records of the sexual services provided (as in these isolated camps money is absent), and payments are deferred until the end of the work period, when all accrued wages are paid upon return to the city, with the managers of logging companies deducting the payment demanded by *cocineros* from the salaries of workers – sex services are often listed as 'laundry' in the records (see also Nureña *et al.* 2009).

We encountered similar reports of *cocineros* offering sexual services in some camps of oil companies in the Loreto region, but sexual transactions at these camps tended to be more clandestine or covert due to the more rigid rules imposed by companies.

Reasons for involvement in sex work

The majority of *fletes* offering sexual services in the streets rationalised their involvement in sex work as a consequence of social exclusion and lack of other job opportunities:

> I started [to offer sexual services] for the necessity: I have a little daughter and ... I have no job now. The necessity obliged me to become involved ... I needed money.
>
> (Edgar, 24, *flete*, low-SES, Lima)

> When I go [to sell sex], I do it for the money. I really live with this. I cannot do anything else because there is no other job for me.
>
> (Manuel, 20, *flete*, low-SES, Iquitos)

With respect to the *travestis*, social prejudice and stereotypes restricted many of them to working in jobs such as hairdressing and sex work. For example, one *travesti* from Lima, who had completed a university degree in social communication, turned to sex work after several unsuccessful attempts to find employment in this field. However, while social exclusion could be an important factor leading to involvement of many *travestis* in sex work, charging for sex is well accepted among them and sometimes even encouraged through social pressure:

> In the disco I went with a guy and when I returned, my friends [other *travestis*] asked me, 'How much have you earned?' Imagine, everyone said 'I charge so much', and I would not say 'nothing'. They will say 'you're going to ruin the business' ... I did not need it financially because I was living with my parents. At first I went out with the boys for pleasure, but to avoid losing face with the *chivas* ['goats', i.e. men with feminine manners] I also began to collect money.
>
> (Larissa, 25, *travesti*, low-middle-SES, Iquitos)

In contrast, among sex workers from the middle or upper-middle classes there were different motivations for entering into sex work. For example, some reported they began offering sexual services out of 'curiosity', as a 'hobby' or as a way of finding 'adventure' and sexual pleasure. There were also those who saw sex work as a way to meet people from higher social classes – regardless of their sexual identity and mainly when their opportunities of social mobility were perceived as limited. Others mentioned being influenced by their friends:

> I wanted to live the adventure. A friend [*travesti*] came from Lima and told me everything she had lived there. That attracted me and I went to Lima with her. I did not see prostitution as something bad. It was a pleasure ... I enjoyed it.
>
> (Paloma, 30, *travesti*, low-middle-SES, Pucallpa)

> My friends told me they had sex with gay men. It was then that I wanted to experience it too. It was not for economic necessity [their entry into sex work]. A man wanted to pay me and I couldn't say no.
>
> (Ivan, 24, exotic dancer, middle-SES, Lima)

Motivations for performing sex work may vary over time. Some men began to offer sexual services out of curiosity or for pleasure, but then found this provided a good way to earn a significant income. Others entered the opposite way: from the initial need for money, they then turned to sex work for pleasure or habit. There were also those who saw a sex trade as a means of working independently and managing their own schedule. By comparing this activity with salaried work requiring fixed times and places of work, some participants found sex work preferable to other forms of employment:

The first time I went [to offer sexual services] I just wanted to feel the experience. But later, when I had the experience and the client paid me, I began to like the money … I liked the money! Since that time I no longer wanted to work as a cook.

(Mónica, 28, *travesti*, low-middle-SES, Pucallpa)

The multiple meanings of economic necessity

The need for money was often reported by sex workers as a major reason for engaging in sex work. However, an analysis of respondents' social backgrounds and life histories led us to propose that the concept of 'economic need' is relative and may be subject to multiple interpretations dependent on social position and sociocultural context, in which the 'need for money' is not always the same as economic hardship. This is not to deny that there are people performing sex work as a means of survival, as this was reported by many individuals from low-SES in all three cities. However, for most participants, the desire for money through sex work was often strongly linked to ideals of independence, to aspirations of consumption and the lifestyles of the middle class (as often defined by advertising and mass media), or to the desire to access the environments and symbols of prestige of the upper class.

For example, several escorts, masseurs and strippers of middle- and upper-middle-SES engaged in commercial sex to finance their higher education or to rent apartments in middle-class or upper-middle-class districts. Almost all the sex workers, regardless of their SES, used part of the money obtained in commercial sex to purchase consumer goods such as fine clothes, accessories, appliances, etc. Similarly, respondents with different SES (but especially migrants and those from low-SES backgrounds) frequently mentioned and valued their access to places and people (clients) from the higher social strata:

I get the money … 300 soles for 5 minutes [more than US$100]. I needed money, but not so much. I got into this business because they [clients] will take you to fancy restaurants, good places … I like these things.

(Marcelo, 25, stripper, upper-middle-SES, Lima)

What I like about this [sex work] is having fun and free drinks. I dance, drink … talk to people, I get to meet other 'kinds' of people [educated, distinguished, with money].

(Julio, 23, *cachaquito/flete*, low-SES, Lima)

I do it [sex work] because I have to pay for my [professional] studies … Besides, I use the money to pay for my flat, my food, the gym …

(Roberto, 23, stripper, middle-SES, Iquitos)

Geographical mobility and transitions between modalities of sex work

The life stories of sex workers highlighted the recurrent presence of migratory experiences associated with either debut into sex work or the practice itself. One pattern is that of young men who leave home and begin to offer sexual services due to lack of money, job opportunities or social support in the new environment. This was reported by many *fletes* and *cachaquitos* in Lima.

A different pattern of geographic mobility from that of *fletes* and *cachaquitos* was identified among *travestis*. In our interviews, most *travestis* reported temporary or permanent migration resulting directly from sex work. The most common situation was that of a young *travesti* travelling to other cities seeking new sex work markets. This pattern bore a relationship with the demand characteristics, since some clients preferred 'new' and younger *travestis*, as reported both by key informants and *travestis*.

Mobility also occurred in transitions between different places and forms of sex work. This is another feature common to most sex workers interviewed, who claimed to have offered sexual services in more than one form, using different strategies to contact clients. For example, some searched for clients on the streets at times, but at other times waited to be contacted by mobile phone to work as private escorts. In an extreme case of versatility, a young man worked in Lima in the afternoons as a *flete* and then as a *travesti* at night to earn more money.

Discussion

This study in three cities in Peru reveals that sex work is diverse and multifaceted. Contrary to local stereotypes portraying sex work as an obscure and dangerous practice performed mainly on the streets and in squares by *travestis*, *fletes* or other persons considered socially marginalised or extremely poor, we have shown that male sex work in Peru occurs in many places and in various forms, with transitions between different modalities. Sex work moreover involves people from varying social and economic backgrounds with motivations that go well beyond economic need. It is often associated with migration and specific economic activities and has evolved in recent years with the mass dissemination of new media and communication technologies. In addition, new forms of sex work not previously described in Peru are appearing, especially in the cities of Iquitos and Pucallpa and in the logging areas in the Peruvian Amazon.

In comparative terms, our data are consistent with recent studies in other countries. Some have proposed typologies of sex work based on explorations of the diverse forms of this practice between male and female sex workers (Buzdugan *et al.* 2010; Infante *et al.* 2009). For example, one study identified 25 types of sex work practised in different countries (Harcourt and Donovan 2005). Other studies have described the forms of sex work that take place in sexual entertainment establishments or through the provision of private sexual companions (Aggleton 1999; Zuilhof 1999).

A number of factors identified in this study may help explain the diversity of male and trans sex work in Peru. An important issue concerns the reasons that lead subjects of different sexual identities and socio-economic backgrounds to engage in sex work. Beyond economic necessity and its relative meanings, these include aspirations for consumption, social mobility and participation in elevated social circles. In this study we often encountered stories of subjects who were not ashamed to offer sexual services and even saw this activity as preferable to other forms of work. Our research supports the findings from other work that argues that sex work may be a rational choice in pursuit of new income (Calhoun 1996), pleasure and fun (Weisberg 1985) and as an alternative to other forms of employment (Lukenbill 1985; Uy *et al.* 2004). The diversity and varied patterns of sex work practice encountered in this study are best explained by considering specific contexts and the confluence of individual, social, historical and structural factors (and not by focusing only on discrete 'determinants' or isolated psychological traits).

In Peru, the HIV epidemic has been characterised as concentrated mainly in the urban populations of men who have sex with men, with HIV prevalence among such groups ranging from 15 to 18 per cent and even up to 22 per cent depending on sites, subgroups and methods of measurement (Bautista *et al.* 2004; Lama *et al.* 2006; Montano *et al.* 2005; Sanchez *et al.* 2007; Tabet *et al.* 2002). Data on sexual behaviour in these and other studies also show that exchange of sex for money or goods is relatively common among some groups of men who have sex with men (Cáceres *et al.* 2008; Konda *et al.* 2008b; Valderrama *et al.* 2008) and that HIV occurs more frequently among those with more feminine identities (including *travestis*) and those who assume the passive (receptive) sex role in anal sex (Lama *et al.* 2006; Salazar *et al.* 2006; Tabet *et al.* 2002). Recent research has also detected high levels of HIV and STI in *travestis* receiving care at a clinic in Callao (Konda *et al.* 2008a), in different groups of sex workers in the Amazon (Valderrama *et al.* 2008), and among *fletes* in central Lima (Bayer *et al.* 2014).

While prior studies have reported rates of HIV/STI and data on sexual behaviour in the most visible forms of sex work, the present research points to some of the diverse scenarios in which sex work is practised in Peru. Given this diversity, we suggest that the most visible forms are not necessarily the only ones that require attention as part of HIV/STI prevention activities. Although street-based *fletes* and *travestis* may be at greater risk of acquiring STIs and have higher social vulnerability, there are limited data regarding other newer or less visible modalities of sex work. For instance, the widespread use of the Internet and mobile telephones in Peru now allows many sex workers to offer services outside the traditional public venues. While recent studies in the USA and Europe suggest there are significant differences between web-based and street-based sex work in terms of sexual practices and health risks (Cunningham and Kendall 2010), the implications of the use of new communication technologies for sex work remain unclear in Peru.

Our study shows the relationship between migration and sex work. The Joint United Nations Programme on HIV/AIDS (UNAIDS) has emphasised that migrants often face unique situations, such as separation from family and friends, together with the constraints and social pressures associated with new environments and less accessible health services. In the absence of the social norms of their home environment, some may adopt sexual practices they would not normally perform, thereby increasing the risk of acquiring and transmitting STIs (UNAIDS 2001). Many participants in our study reported similar situations and changes in behaviour. These issues need to be explored more deeply in future research on sex work in Peru.

References

Aggleton, P. (ed.) 1999. *Men Who Sell Sex: International Perspectives on Male Prostitution and HIV/ AIDS*. Philadelphia, PA: Temple University Press.

Bautista, C.T., Sanchez, J.L., Montano, S.M., Laguna-Torres, A., Lama, J., Sanchez, J., Kusunoki, L., Manrique, H., Acosta, J., Montoya, O., Tambare, A., Avila, M., Vinoles, J., Aguayo, N., Olson, J. and Carr, J. 2004. Seroprevalence of and risk factors for HIV-1 infection among South American men who have sex with men. *Sexually Transmitted Infections* 80: 498–504.

Bayer, A., Clark, J., Diaz, D., Sanchez, H., Garcia, P. and Coates, T. 2010. *Ethnographic mapping of commercial sex venues with male sex workers or fletes in Peru*. Poster presented at the XVIII International AIDS Conference, 18–23 July, in Vienna, Austria.

Bayer, A., Garvich, M., Díaz, D.A., Sánchez, H., García, P.J. and Coates, T.J. 2014. 'Just getting by': A cross-sectional study of male sex workers as a key population for HIV/STIs among men who have sex with men in Peru. *Sexually Transmitted Infections* 90: 223–229.

Bimbi, D.S. 2007. Male prostitution: Pathology, paradigms and progress in research. *Journal of Homosexuality* 53: 7–35.

Bimbi, D.S. and Parsons, J.T. 2005. Barebacking among Internet-based male sex workers. *Journal of Gay & Lesbian Psychotherapy* 9: 89–110.

Browne, J. and Minichiello, V. 1996. Research directions in male sex work. *Journal of Homosexuality* 31: 29–56.

Buzdugan, R., Copas, A., Moses, S., Blanchard, J., Isac, S., Ramesh, B.M., Washington, R., Halli, S.S. and Cowan, F.M. 2010. Devising a female sex work typology using data from Karnataka, India. *International Journal of Epidemiology* 39: 439–448.

Cáceres, C.F. and Jimenez, O.G. 1999. *Fletes* in Parque Kennedy: Sexual cultures among young men who sell sex to other men in Lima. In: P. Aggleton (ed.) *Men Who Sell Sex: International Perspectives on Male Prostitution and HIV/AIDS*. Philadelphia, PA: Temple University Press, 179–194.

Cáceres, C.F. and Rosasco, A.M. 1999. The margin has many sides: Diversity among gay and homosexually active men in Lima. *Culture, Health & Sexuality* 1: 261–275.

Cáceres, C.F. and Rosasco, A.M. 2000. *Secreto a Voces: Homoerotismo Masculino en Lima: Culturas, Identidades y Salud Sexual* [*Open Secret: Masculine Homoeroticism in Lima: Cultures, Identities and Sexual Health*]. Lima: Universidad Peruana Cayetano Heredia.

Cáceres, C.F., Konda, K.A., Salazar, X., Leon, S.R., Klausner, J.D., Lescano, A.G., Maiorana, A., Kegeles, S., Jones, F.R. and Coates, T.J. 2008. New populations at high risk of HIV/STIs in low-income, urban coastal Peru. *AIDS and Behavior* 12: 544–551.

Calhoun, T.C. 1992. Male street hustling: Introduction to processes and stigma. *Sociological Spectrum* 12: 35–52.

Calhoun, T.C. 1996. Rational decision-making among male street prostitutes. *Deviant Behavior* 17: 209–227.

Caro, L. 1999. *De Cueros y Puñales: Prostitución Masculina y Violencia Juvenil en una Lima de Fin de Milenio* [*On Leathers and Daggers: Male Prostitution and Juvenile Violence in Lima at the Turn of the Millennium*]. Lima: ArteIdea.

Clark, J.L., Cáceres, C.F., Lescano, A.G., Konda, K.A., Leon, S.R., Jones, F.R., Kegeles, S.M., Klausner, J.D. and Coates, T.J. 2007. Prevalence of same-sex sexual behavior and associated characteristics among low-income urban males in Peru. *PLoS ONE* 2: e778.

Cosme, C., Jaime, M., Merino, A. and Rosales, J.L. 2007. *La Imagen In/decente: Diversidad Sexual, Prejuicio y Discriminación en la Prensa Escrita Peruana* [*The In/decent Image: Sexual Diversity, Prejudice and Discrimination in Peruvian Written Press*]. Lima: Instituto de Estudios Peruanos.

Cunningham, S. and Kendall, T.D. 2010. Risk behaviours among Internet-facilitated sex workers: Evidence from two new datasets. *Sexually Transmitted Infections* 86(Suppl. 3): 100–110.

Fernandez-Davila, P., Salazar, X., Cáceres, C.F., Maiorana, A., Kegeles, S., Coates, T.J. and Martinez, J. 2008. Compensated sex and sexual risks: Sexual, social and economic interactions between homosexually- and heterosexually-identified men of low income in two cities of Peru. *Sexualities* 2: 352–374.

Harcourt, C. and Donovan, B. 2005. The many faces of sex work. *Sexually Transmitted Infections* 81: 201–206.

Infante, C., Sosa-Rubi, S.G. and Cuadra, S.M. 2009. Sex work in Mexico: Vulnerability of male, *travesti*, transgender and transsexual sex workers. *Culture, Health & Sexuality* 11: 125–137.

Kaye, K. 2003. Male prostitution in the twentieth century: Pseudohomosexuals, hoodlum homosexuals and exploited teens. *Journal of Homosexuality* 46: 1–77.

Kaye, K. 2007. Sex and the unspoken in male street prostitution. *Journal of Homosexuality* 53: 37–73.

Konda, K.A., Clark, J.L., Segura, E., Salvatierra, J., Galea, J., Leon, S.R., Hall, E.R., Klausner, J.D., Cáceres, C.F. and Coates, T.J. 2008a. *Male sex workers among men who have sex with men in Lima, Peru*. Poster presented at the XVII International AIDS Conference, 3–8 August, in Mexico City, Mexico.

Konda, K.A., Lescano, A.G., Leontsini, E., Fernandez, P., Klausner, J.D., Coates, T.J. and Cáceres, C.F. 2008b. High rates of sex with men among high-risk, heterosexually-identified men in low-income, coastal Peru. *AIDS and Behavior* 12: 483–491.

Lama, J.R., Lucchetti, A., Suarez, L., Laguna-Torres, V.A., Guanira, J.V., Pun, M., Montano, S.M., Celem, C.L., Carr, J.K., Sanchez, J., Bautista, C.T. and Sanches, J.L. Peruvian HIV Sentinel Surveillance Working Group. 2006. Association of herpes simplex virus type-2 infection and syphilis with human immunodeficiency virus infection among men who have sex with men in Peru. *Journal of Infectious Diseases* 194: 1459–1466.

Lukenbill, D.F. 1985. Entering male prostitution. *Urban Life* 14: 131–153.

Montano, S., Sanchez, J.L., Laguna-Torres, A., Cuchi, P., Avila, M.M., Weissenbacher, M., Serra, M. et al. 2005. Prevalences, genotypes and risk factors for HIV transmission in South America. *Journal of Acquired Immune Deficiency Syndromes* 40: 57–64.

Nureña, C.R., Zúñiga, M., Zunt, J., Montano, S., Ortíz, A. and Sánchez, J.L. 2009. *Intercambios sexuales y potencial para la propagación de ITS en campamentos madereros de la selva de Ucayali, Perú [Sexual exchanges and potential for STI dissemination in logging camps, Ucayali's jungle, Peru]*. Paper presented at the V Foro Latinoamericano y del Caribe en VIH/SIDA e ITS, 21–23 November, in Lima, Peru.

Paris, M., Gotuzzo, E., Goyzueta, G., Aramburu, J., Cáceres, C.F., Crawford, D., Castellano, T., Vermund, S.H. and Hook, E.W. (3rd) 2001. Motorcycle taxi drivers and sexually transmitted infections in a Peruvian Amazon city. *Sexually Transmitted Diseases* 28: 11–13.

Perlongher, N. 1999. *El Negocio del Deseo: La Prostitución Masculina en San Pablo [Desire's Business: Male Prostitution in São Paulo]*. Buenos Aires: Paidós.

Prestage, G. 1994. Male and transsexual prostitution. In: R. Perkins, G. Prestage, R. Sharp and F. Lovejoy (eds) *Sex Work and Sex Workers in Australia*. Sydney: University of New South Wales Press, 174–190.

Salazar, X. and Silva Santisteban, A. 2009. *Informe Final de Mapeo y Encuesta Sociodemográfica del Trabajo Sexual en Cuatro Ciudades del Perú [Final Report of Mapping and Socio-demographic Survey on Sex Work in Four Cities in Peru]*. Lima: IESSDEH, REDTRANS, Miluska Vida y Dignidad, UNFPA.

Salazar, X., Cáceres, C., Rosasco, C.A., Kegeles, S., Maiorana, A., Gárate, M. and Coates, T. 2005. Vulnerability and sexual risks: *Vagos* and *vaguitas* in a low-income town in Peru. *Culture, Health & Sexuality* 7: 375–387.

Salazar, X., Cáceres, C., Maiorana, A., Rosasco, A.M., Kegeles, S. and Coates, T. 2006. Influencia del Contexto Sociocultural en la Percepción del Riesgo y la Negociación de Protección en Hombres Homosexuales Pobres de la Costa Peruana [Influence of socio-cultural context on risk perception and negotiation of protection among poor homosexual males on the Peruvian coast]. *Cadernos de Saúde Pública* 22: 2097–2104.

Sanchez, J., Lama, J.R., Kusunoki, L., Manrique, H., Goicochea, P., Lucchetti, A., Rouillon, M., Pun, M., Suarez, L., Montano, S., Sanchez, J.L., Tabet, S., Hughes, J.P. and Celum, C. 2007. HIV-1, sexually transmitted infections and sexual behavior trends among men who have sex with men in Lima, Peru. *Journal of Acquired Immune Deficiency Syndromes* 44: 578–585.

Scott, J., Minichiello, V., Marino, R., Harvey, G.P., Jamieson, M. and Browne, J. 2005. Understanding the new context of the male sex work industry. *Journal of Interpersonal Violence* 20: 320–342.

Strauss, A.L. and Corbin, J. 1998. *Basics of Qualitative Research: Grounded Theory Procedures and Techniques*. 2nd ed. Thousand Oaks, CA: SAGE.

Tabet, S., Sanchez, J., Lama, J., Goicochea, P., Campos, P., Rouillon, M., Cairo, J.I. et al. 2002. HIV, syphilis and heterosexual bridging among Peruvian men who have sex with men. *AIDS* 16: 1271–1277.

Tiby, T.P. 2003. The production and reproduction of prostitution. *Journal of Scandinavian Studies in Criminology and Crime Prevention* 3: 154–172.

UNAIDS. 2001. *Population Mobility and AIDS: UNAIDS Technical Update*. Geneva: UNAIDS.

Uy, J.M., Parsons, J.T., Bimbi, D.S., Koken, J.A. and Halkitis, P.N. 2004. Gay and bisexual male escorts who advertise on the Internet: Understanding reasons for and effects of involvement in commercial sex. *International Journal of Men's Health* 3: 11–26.

Valderrama, M., Blas, M., Carcamo, C., García, P., Bernabe, A., Cotrina, A., Chiappe, M. *et al.* 2008. *High HIV and syphilis prevalences among male commercial sex workers from the Peruvian Amazon.* Poster presented at the XVII International AIDS Conference, 3–8 August, in Mexico City, Mexico.

Van der Poel, S. 1992. Professional male prostitution: A neglected phenomenon. *Crime, Law and Social Change* 18: 259–275.

Vanwesenbeeck, I. 2001. Another decade of social scientific work on sex work: A review of research 1990–2000. *Annual Review of Sex Research* 12: 242–289.

Weisberg, K.D. 1985. *Children of the Night: A Study of Adolescent Prostitution.* Lexington, MA: Lexington Books.

Zuilhof, W. 1999. Sex for money between men and boys in the Netherlands: Implications for HIV prevention. In: P. Aggleton (ed.) *Men Who Sell Sex: International Perspectives on Male Prostitution and HIV/AIDS.* Philadelphia, PA: Temple University Press, 23–39.

Section 5

Sexual violence

While sexual violence is known to take place across all social groups, research has identified displaced and refugee communities as particularly vulnerable to sexual and gender-based violence. However, the majority of work to date has focused on experiences within the country of origin. Ines Keygnaert, Nicole Vettenburg and Marleen Temmerman's chapter therefore provides an important insight into the prevalence of sexual and gender-based violence amongst refugees, asylum seekers and undocumented migrants once they are living within Europe. Drawing on qualitative research undertaken in Belgium and the Netherlands, the authors describe a disturbingly high level and variety of physical and emotional violence experienced amongst study participants. Whilst this was found to be most commonly experienced by young women, the authors show that men and boys also suffer from higher rates of sexual violence than is globally expected. While the perpetrator of the violence was in most cases the current or former partner of the victim, in one-fifth of cases, violence amongst refugees, asylum seekers and undocumented migrants was reported to be perpetrated by professional service providers. Importantly, the chapter identifies how such experiences differ from the sexual- and gender-based violence reported amongst Belgian and Dutch nationals, enabling key risk factors to be recognised and appropriate responses to be identified.

Lesbian, gay, bisexual and transgender (LGBT) young people are known to be vulnerable to high levels of sexual violence despite widening acceptance of gender and sexual diversity across much of the Western world during the past decade. In the second chapter in this section, Elizabeth McDermott, Katrina Roen and Jonathan Scourfield provide key insights into the ways that LGBT young people experience this violence. Importantly, they demonstrate clear connections between non-normative sexual and gender identity, and feelings of distress and self-destructive behaviours such as cutting and suicide. The authors argue that such behaviours act as individualistic shame-avoidance strategies, which close down possibilities or expectations for action or support at wider levels. While recent attempts to mainstream sexual diversity offer a strong step in the right direction, it is clear that more can be done to tackle health inequalities for LGBT people, and that further research is needed to understand how the heteronormative frameworks within which societies operate impact on the mental and physical health of LGBT people.

Over the past 30 years, the physical and psychological impacts of sexual violence have been intensified by concerns relating to HIV infection. While significant advances have been made in expanding access to HIV-related medications, concerns over HIV infection through rape remain very real in many parts of the world. The final chapter in this section relates to post-exposure prophylaxis (PEP) completion after rape in South Africa, where rates of both sexual violence and HIV remain startlingly high. While the past decade has seen a significant increase in the provision of PEP services following sexual assault, Naeemah Abrahams and Rachel Jewkes highlight the significant gaps that remain in health care and the low rates at which women experiencing sexual violence adhere to PEP. Importantly, one key factor influencing access to PEP services relates to the way in which the women themselves interpret incidents of sexual violence against them, with some women either not recognising that they have experienced rape, or not wanting to be associated with the stigma and social repercussions often linked to rape accusations. Abrahams and Jewkes stress that while PEP treatment availability has improved, a number of barriers to PEP adherence remain. These include adverse side effects, self-blame, rape- and treatment-related stigma, family and community perceptions of the incident, understandings of what the medications are for, and the complicated treatment regimens that need to be followed. The need for PEP to be implemented so soon after the emotional trauma associated with the rape is also highlighted as a key issue. Further research is needed not only to support the development of more effective PEP interventions, but also to address the ongoing circumstances in which rape and sexual violence persist.

Chapter 14

Hidden violence is silent rape

Sexual and gender-based violence in refugees, asylum seekers and undocumented migrants in Belgium and the Netherlands

Ines Keygnaert, Nicole Vettenburg and Marleen Temmerman

Introduction

Sexual and gender-based violence (SGBV) is a major public health issue worldwide, a violation of human rights and in some cases a crime against humanity. It comprises sexual violence, emotional-psychological violence, physical violence, harmful cultural practices and socio-economic violence (Basile and Saltzman 2002; UNHCR 2003). In addition to important negative effects on the victim's well-being and participation in society, SGBV may have significant consequences on sexual, reproductive, physical and psychological health (Hynes and Lopes 2000; Norredam *et al.* 2005a; Tavara 2006).

Considered to be vulnerable to SGBV are: first, women – especially the impoverished and those living in shelters, in remote areas or in detention (Wenzel *et al.* 2004); second, adolescent girls and boys, particularly if they live alone or with only one parent and are of low socio-economic status (Holmes and Slap 1998; Tavara 2006); and, third, displaced and refugee communities (Hynes and Lopes 2000; UNHCR 2003; Ward and Vann 2002). People with heightened risk perception and those who were personally victimised or witnessed SGBV during childhood are prone to subsequent victimisation or perpetration of SGBV themselves (Borowsky *et al.* 1997; Brown *et al.* 2005). Research has demonstrated that perpetrators of SGBV are most often known to the victim (Tavara 2006). However, refugees, homeless or impoverished people and young men are often victimised by strangers, persons in authority and those assigned to their protection (Holmes and Slap 1998; Hynes and Lopes 2000; Norredam *et al.* 2005a).

Several determinants in SGBV are thus known. Yet there remain considerable gaps in knowledge when it comes to SGBV victimisation of refugees in Europe, the impact of their victimisation on the individual and public health and effective prevention actions. The aim of this chapter is twofold. First, it explores the nature of SGBV that refugees, asylum seekers and undocumented migrants in Belgium and the Netherlands experienced after arriving in the EU. Second, it discusses which perceived risk and preventive factors may be considered decisive determinants for the prevention of SGBV in this population.

Methods

These research findings encourage the use of an interpretive, feminist, communitarian and dialogical research perspective (Anderson and Doherty 2008; de Laine 2000). Applying a socio-ecological framework (Bronfenbrenner 1979) to the determinants of sexual health and violence, we first identified the potential SGBV determinants in our study population, shown in Table 14.1.

Table 14.1 SGBV determinants, socio-ecologically clustered

Individual determinants

Biology and genes

Gender and sexual orientation

Behaviour

Mental health

Information, knowledge and experience

Individual socio-economic position

Internalised cultural norms

Individual legal status

Interpersonal determinants

Gender

Multiple sexual partners

Social network and support

Information and knowledge exchange

Organisational determinants

Community resilience

Cultural practices

Community gender norms

Community socio-economic position

Service provision

Physical environment

Organisational SGBV prevention and response policy

Societal determinants

Structural gender inequality

Economic hardship

Structural inequity

Asylum and migration policies

Law/justice

Accessibility of services

Societal SGBV prevention policy

We added the concept of Desirable Prevention to this framework. Whereas general prevention can be conceived of in terms of those initiatives that anticipate risk factors in a targeted and systematic way, Desirable Prevention can be defined as 'initiatives which anticipate risk factors even earlier in a targeted and systematic way, are maximally "offensive", have an integral approach, work in a participatory way and have a democratic nature, while aiming at the enhancement or protection of the target group's health and wellbeing' (Vettenburg *et al.* 2003: 20).

Starting from this conceptual framework, we adopted a qualitative and collaborative approach organised around the notion of Community-Based Participatory Research. Community-Based Participatory Research focuses on inequalities and aims to improve the health and well-being of community members by integrating knowledge in action, including social and policy change (Israel *et al.* 2001; Viswanathan *et al.* 2004).

We mobilised a large group of stakeholders: refugee and asylum-seeking communities, policymakers, intermediary organisations, civil society and researchers. We considered the first of these groups to be the project's main beneficiaries and identified a number of inclusion criteria. The first of these was to be a refugee, asylum seeker or undocumented migrant aged between 15 and 49 years old. Second, respondents had to be living in East Flanders in Belgium or the Randstad region in the Netherlands. The application of these criteria resulted in a sample that included participants from Iranian, Iraqi, Roma, Kurdish, Somali, Afghan and former Soviet Union backgrounds.

A total of 14 women and ten men meeting the criteria completed 30 hours of training as Community Researchers (CRs). Topics addressed in their training included sexual and reproductive health, SGBV, gender, psychosocial education, the study conceptual framework and conducting in-depth interviews in an empathic and ethically sound way. Two male CRs dropped out after training because of time constraints. CRs collaborated in every phase of the project, building rapport, capacity and mutual ownership. Other stakeholders participated in a Community Advisory Board (CAB) that met at key moments throughout the duration of the project.

Each CR was asked to conduct 10–12 interviews with respondents meeting the inclusion criteria and of the same gender as themselves. Between January and May 2007, 250 respondents were chain sampled through services and organisations that were members of the CAB, the Red Cross asylum reception centres in East Flanders, and through CRs' networks. Once identified, respondents were informed about the project's objectives, the interview goals, the potential risks and measures taken to protect them from those risks, and modes of participation. Respondents could withdraw from the study at any point during the interview but still participate in later phases of the project. The respondent or his/her nominee signed an informed consent before the interview, and consent was renegotiated during later phases of participation.

The questionnaire comprised four parts: sociodemographic data (closed questions), sexual health, personal or close peer SGBV experiences since arriving in Europe and prevention of SGBV (all open questions). The questionnaire was developed jointly with the CRs and the CAB: first, to enhance the beneficial outcomes of the participatory research approach; second, to maximise the match between 'inner speech' and the language used (Moran *et al.* 2006); and, third, to optimise validity and reliability (Gagnon *et al.* 2004). It was translated into the languages of the respondents by the Belgian CRs and back translated by the Dutch CRs before being pilot-tested and finalised for use in the mother tongue of both the CRs and the respondents. The study protocol applied the World Health Organization (WHO) (Ellsberg and Heise 2005) and the United Nations High Commissioner for Refugees (UNHCR) (UNHCR 2003) ethical and safety guidelines in researching violence and received ethical approval from the Ghent University Hospital Ethical Committee.

Analysis

Interviews were only considered valid when informed consent had been given and when the taped interview matched the notes that were taken by the CR on the interview guide. Excluded from analysis were double interviews, double SGBV cases and cases that were not personal or from a close peer. For the qualitative element of the study, we used framework analysis to sort, code and compare the answers. Thus, we first applied an emic approach to code the data into analytical categories conceived as meaningful to the communities using the respondents' definitions and wordings. We later applied the socio-ecological framework and the concept of Desirable Prevention to interpret the content and context of the findings. Finally, we used SPSS to check the volume of, and diversity within, the qualitative data (Safman and Sobal 2004). Quantitative sociodemographic data were also analysed using SPSS.

Results

Sociodemographic characteristics

In total, 223 of the 250 interviews were considered valid: 132 in Belgium and 91 in the Netherlands. The respondents were 88 men and 135 women, including two transsexuals in Belgium who asked to be included in the analysis as women.

Table 14.2 reveals the main sociodemographic characteristics of respondents. Their general profile was one of highly educated women and men of reproductive age who reported experiencing a major setback in their socio-economic position:

> You are not allowed to work, only to breathe.
>
> (Parvaneh, 37, Iranian asylum seeker)

> You cannot do anything, because you are not a human being.
>
> (Bohan, 20, Kurdish asylum seeker)

In addition, respondents described having poor social networks to rely and build on, and being hampered in participating actively in society impeded their social functioning:

> I have no hope for the future. I live in a reception centre without any contact with other people. I have no money, no work and no contact with girls.
>
> (Zoran, 23, Kurdish asylum seeker)

Subsequently, many indicated suffering from the psychosocial burden of low subjective and socio-economic status:

> My father is a highly educated, intelligent man and held a high position in Iran. When we received our asylum status here he wanted to work, not to live on support. For eight years now he's working as a welder. His hands cannot hold a cup of tea any more and his eyes grow blind. His Dutch colleagues treat him as an idiot. He lost his self-esteem and now stutters.
>
> (Bahareh, 22, Iranian refugee)

Finally, several respondents perceived their asylum situation as a form of violence:

> This family had no right to work, to social support, to rent a house, to have an own account and after four years in the asylum centre they had to leave Belgium. Where are those human rights then here? Nowhere. That's violence too!
>
> (Hawar, 19, Kurdish asylum seeker)

Table 14.2 Sociodemographic profile of respondents

	n = 223	%
Gender		
Female	133	59.6
Male	88	39.5
Transsexual	2	0.9
Age (years)		
< 18	15	6.7
19–29	102	45.7
30–49	106	47.5
Country of origin		
Afghanistan	24	10.8
Former USSR	39	17.5
Iraq	43	19.3
Iran	67	30.0
Slovakia and Czech Republic	36	16.1
Somalia	14	6.3
Residence status		
Asylum seeker	92	41.3
Refugee	103	46.2
Undocumented	28	12.5
Relational status		
No steady partner	119	53.4
Steady partner	104	46.6
Children in care		
0	107	48.0
1	34	15.3
2/> 2	82	36.8
Accompaniment		
Persons > 18 years		
0	65	29.1
1	72	32.3
2/> 2	86	38.6
Persons < 18 years		
0	98	43.9
1	51	22.9
2/> 2	74	33.2

Continued

Table 14.2 Sociodemographic profile of respondents, *continued*

	n = 223	%
Religion		
None	45	20.2
Christian	68	30.5
Muslim	96	43.0
Other	14	6.3
Educational level		
Higher/university	45	20.2
Higher/non-university	46	20.6
Secondary education	99	44.4
Primary education	25	11.2
Not educated	4	1.8
Other	4	1.8
Daily activities		
Country of origin		
Paid at work	101	45.3
At job market	12	5.4
Student	88	39.5
Other	22	9.8
Host country		
Paid at work	50	22.4
At job market	43	19.3
Not allowed to work	45	20.2
Student	51	22.9
Other	34	15.2

> We've got the right to live. Making a difference between asylum seeking and other children is a form of violence!
>
> (Yasemin, 29, Kurdish asylum seeker)

Overview of reported cases of sexual and gender-based violence

A quarter of the respondents did not report violence (57/223). However, 87 respondents had been personally victimised and another 79 respondents knew at least of one close peer – either an (ex-)partner, family member, friend or acquaintance/neighbour – being victimised since arriving in Europe. Together, they described 332 cases consisting of 389 SGBV acts.

All types of violence (except killing and child marriage) were described in both personal as well as peer victimisation, with personal victimisation bearing at least one-third of the proportion within each type of violence. SGBV cases were noted by all CRs in every origin, gender, age and status group interviewed.

Table 14.3 reveals that more than half of the victims were less than 30 years old and female, while perpetrators were predominantly over 30 and male. Nonetheless, one-third of the victims were male and 20 perpetrators were female. Additionally, about half of the perpetrators had acted in a group. The majority of the victims were either refugees or asylum seekers, while one-third of the perpetrators were Belgian or Dutch nationals. The perpetrator was usually the current or former partner of the victim. Yet, in a fifth of the cases, authorities or professionals such as reception centre staff, lawyers, police and security guards were identified as perpetrators.

Table 14.3 Characteristics of victims and perpetrators

	Victim in cases		Perpetrator in cases	
	n = 332	%	n = 332	%
Gender				
Female	230	69.3	20	6.0
Male	95	28.6	241	72.6
Both	5	1.5	5	1.5
Missing	2	0.6	66	19.9
Approximate age				
Youth (< 30)	184	55.4	43	12.9
Adult (> 30)	144	43.4	219	66.0
Missing	4	1.2	70	21.1
Residence status				
Asylum seeker	134	40.4	68	20.5
Refugee	130	39.2	56	16.9
Undocumented migrant	30	9.0	4	1.2
Belgian/Dutch	–	–	113	34.0
Missing	38	11.4	91	27.4
Relationship between	Victim	Respondent	Perpetrator	Victim
Respondent	87	26.2	2	0.6
(Ex-)partner	4	1.2	102	30.7
Family	23	6.9	53	16.0
Friend	71	21.4	12	3.6
Acquaintance/neighbour	147	44.3	49	14.8
Service provider	–	–	77	23.2
Unknown	–	–	37	11.1

Table 14.4 shows the nature of described SGBV experiences. Most cases consisted of multiple forms of violence.

Table 14.4 Nature of SGBV cases

Type of violence	Personal	Close peer	Total (n = 332)	%
Sexual violence	**47**	**141**	**188**	**56.6**
Sexual harassment	32	54	89	26.8
Sexual abuse	8	32	40	12.0
Rape	28	83	111	33.4
• Attempted rape	2	6	8	2.4
• Singular rape	2	19	21	6.3
• Multiple rape	19	45	64	19.3
• Gang rape	4	9	13	3.9
• Forced abortion	1	1	2	0.6
Sexual exploitation	9	31	40	12.0
Emotional/psychological violence	**64**	**142**	**206**	**62**
Verbal abuse	1	4	5	1.5
Humiliation	12	31	43	13.0
Threatening	10	22	32	9.6
Confinement	10	36	46	13.9
Relational	2	18	20	6.0
Asylum procedure related	24	23	47	14.2
Worsening combination	5	7	12	3.6
Physical violence	**40**	**117**	**157**	**47.3**
Singular non-life-threatening	19	54	74	22.9
Multiple non-life-threatening	8	16	24	7.2
Singular life-threatening	3	8	11	3.3
Multiple life-threatening	10	20	30	9.0
Killing	0	18	18	5.4
Socio-economic violence	**44**	**68**	**112**	**33.7**
Discrimination	12	11	23	6.9
Refusal of services	7	18	25	7.5
Refusal of legal assistance	25	39	64	19.3
Harmful cultural practices	**4**	**43**	**47**	**14.2**
Forced marriage	3	3	13	3.9
Child marriage	0	2	2	0.6
Honour-related	1	1	32	9.6

Sexual violence

The bulk of the sexual violence cases consisted of rape, with multiple and gang rape appearing to be common practice. Sexual harassment (no physical contact), sexual abuse (physical contact without penetration) and sexual exploitation were also described. A fifth of all respondents stated being sexually victimised themselves, giving a detailed report of being raped by one or more persons and/or of being sexually exploited on a long-term basis. The victims in the other cases were close peers of the respondents:

> If I wanted an ice cream, I had to lick the head of his soldier first.
>
> (Svetlana, 28, Russian refugee)

> This Dutch guy forced her to have sex to bring money home. He told her that if she didn't sell sex to other men, he'd kill her.
>
> (Muzhdah, 23, Afghan refugee)

> This was awful! That bunch of naked men with burning eyes, they started to fuck me all, it didn't stop.
>
> (Micha, 25, Russian undocumented migrant)

Emotional-psychological violence consisted mostly of humiliation, confinement and emotional-psychological abuse related to the asylum process. Respondents in the Netherlands reported nearly twice as much emotional-psychological violence than in Belgium (68 versus 39 per cent):

> Hitting is better than talking. What he said hurt me more than getting slapped. Sometimes being hit is easier to cope with than psychological torture.
>
> (Esrin, 26, Kurdish asylum seeker)

Physical violence

Physical violence largely took the form of non-life-threatening forms of violence such as beating, punching or kicking. Yet in 58 cases it related to a life-threatening form such as being thrown out of a window, choking, being hit on the head, burning, maiming and killing:

> They were six and hit me so hard on my head that I fell down unconscious and lost a lot of blood.
>
> (Salar, 31, Afghan refugee)

Socio-economic violence

Socio-economic violence consisted most frequently of the denial of legal assistance or obstructive practice related to the asylum procedure, the denial of services such as health care and discrimination/racism. Respondents in the Netherlands reported more than twice as much socio-economic violence cases than those in Belgium (42 versus 19 per cent):

I lived in constant fear and anguish and was not given the prescribed medicine that I needed. I was living in constant pain for days.

(Biixi, 42, Somali refugee)

Harmful cultural practices were mainly honour-related or involved forced marriage or child marriage:

When her father heard that his daughter was raped, he killed her. He couldn't face us fellow citizens any more after this terrible thing.

(Shahrukh, 39, Afghan refugee)

Consequences of victimisation

Respondents indicated that frequently victims had to deal with multiple and long-lasting consequences.

Emotional-psychological consequences

Emotional-psychological consequences occurred in two-thirds of the cases. Respondents described being 'depressed', 'a psychological wreck', 'dispirited' or 'very insecure'. Victims often isolated themselves and no longer trusted anybody. Others dealt with anxiety, sleeping disorders, shame, guilt, anger, frustration and hatred. Many victims did not receive any psychological assistance although they requested this:

Fear, nightmares, we all know it. My children can't bear loud voices or noise. They are very kept to themselves. They have forgotten the meaning of the word 'joy'.

(Parvaneh, 37, Iranian asylum seeker)

Socio-economic consequences

Frequently, violence resulted in a loss of social support. Victims were forcibly separated from their partner or children, were condemned by and expelled from their family or community or had to change reception centres, disrupting their newly built social network. Several victims lost their job, fell behind in their education or could no longer participate actively in society:

The other Afghans soon heard about it … They had a fight, the police investigated the case and her little son was taken from her and put in childcare; she was sent to another asylum reception centre.

(Farozeh, 42, Afghan asylum seeker)

Physical consequences

Physical consequences were described in about half of the cases. They included bruises, bleeding, exhaustion, unconsciousness, heart or gastrointestinal problems, weight loss and other physical complaints. Several victims were permanently injured. Others either died of the immediate consequence of the violence or by committing suicide shortly after:

When I opened my eyes they had thrown me in a park in Ghent. I had to go to a doctor because my anus was as a raw chunk of meat and my penis was blue. After a while I heard I had AIDS, from whom I do not know, the only thing I know is that I'm going to die.

(Micha, 25, Russian undocumented migrant,
died of AIDS shortly after the interview)

Sexual and reproductive consequences

Sexual and reproductive consequences were mentioned in more than a fifth of the cases. In addition to STIs and HIV, these mostly included sexual disorders, unwanted pregnancy, miscarriage due to violence and forced abortion:

He came back and raped me … I became pregnant and I tried to abort the child with alcohol and other means. I lifted heavy things. Nothing worked, so I asked a friend to penetrate my uterus with an awl. I lost a lot of blood and was transferred to a hospital. The doctor told me: after this torture, you cannot get children any more. That is the worst thing that could happen to me.

(Olga, 23, Ukrainian refugee)

Perceived risk factors linked to victimisation

I had no papers and no money, so I only had one option: to be his slave.

(Svetlana, 28, Russian refugee)

In general, respondents identified behavioural factors as the most important risk factor. However, the lack of a social network and economic hardship were also identified as key risk factors. Categorising their answers on individual, interpersonal and societal socio-ecological levels, the following findings emerge.

Individual level

Individual determinants mostly comprised behavioural factors including drug/alcohol use, verbal and non-verbal attitudes and being alone on the streets at night. One-third of the respondents identified lack of knowledge and information as a risk factor. This included 'not knowing the language and culture of the host country' and lack of 'sexual knowledge' and 'self-defence skills'. About the same number of respondents indicated that mental health problems put one at risk of SGBV. They described this as 'being down', having 'no self-confidence', 'being mentally ill' and 'not having a lot of brains'. A quarter of the respondents saw also risk related to gender. They described this as 'being weaker as a woman', 'being too free as a girl' and 'being a beautiful woman'.

Interpersonal level

Half of the respondents identified issues relating to social networks as important risk factors. Examples included 'not having somebody to turn to', 'trusting people too easily' and 'having bad examples as friends or parents'.

Societal level

More than one-third of the respondents mentioned economic hardship as a risk factor, including 'having a bad financial situation', 'poverty' and 'taking risks to earn money'. Having no legal residence permit, having an unprotected status and not having full rights were identified as residence-related risk factors. A bad physical environment was described as 'sharing housing with too many people' and 'living in a deprived area':

> I don't think refugees choose to become victims of violence. They are thrown into it by society itself, inhuman treatment, bad policy and a lack of guidance.
>
> (Arun, 31, Kurdish refugee)

Desired prevention measures

Subsequently we enquired about the respondents' perceptions and suggestions concerning prevention. The following themes emerged.

Individual level

Some respondents indicated that an individual could not do much. However, the majority were convinced that an individual had an important role to play in SGBV prevention. A quarter of respondents stated that an informed individual was less at risk; therefore, one should inform oneself. Mental health factors such as 'being self-confident', 'knowing your own limits', 'having a strong mind' and 'respecting yourself before you respect others' were also seen as preventive. At an individual level, behavioural factors such as 'avoiding risks', 'choosing suitable clothes' and 'avoiding drugs and alcohol' were seen as important.

Interpersonal level

A larger number of behavioural factors were in relation to others. These included 'avoiding relationships with strangers or bad friends', 'choosing your friends carefully' and 'being careful, also in intimate relationships'. The majority of respondents felt that others should react when violence occurs and provide social and parental control and support. Therefore, prevention measures should seek to enhance social networks. Successful strategies included 'making sure that parents and children are good friends', 'enhancing networks among the same age groups' and 'organising meetings in which people can share their experiences and feelings'. Sharing knowledge was also considered preventive, and key strategies here included 'giving general information and education to others', 'sensitisation and advice from parents on risks' and 'making violence debatable'.

Organisational level

Although some respondents stressed that a victim should seek help by 'notifying the police', 'looking for help from knowledgeable people' and 'looking for legal aid', most respondents stated that others should help in accessing services. They identified the need to have services that are safe and trustworthy for refugees, asylum seekers and undocumented migrants, and that offer psychological assistance. Although few respondents pointed to cultural norms and values as protective factors, a quarter believed that prevention measures should address cultural norms and values, including informing the host society about refugee issues.

Societal level

For more than half of the respondents, prevention should seek to enhance knowledge through sensitisation, education on sexual health, risks and SGBV, and training about rights. Others felt that the overall legislative framework should become more preventive. They suggested, for example, that the government should 'assure protection against violence for all', 'enforce laws on violence' and 'enhance general public safety'. Furthermore, the system of residence status should change to enhance the research population's possibilities of enjoying rights and actively participating in host communities. This could be done by 'giving all migrants the right to work', by 'shortening the asylum procedure' and by 'educating asylum seekers on their rights and duties'.

The vast majority of respondents felt that the suggested preventive measures would work for both women and men. However, prevention for young people should be adapted to their own language and culture. Nearly three-quarters of respondents stressed they would like to participate in future SGBV-prevention activities, welcomed the focus of the research and thanked the research team for being genuinely interested in their lives. This is in line with Sikweyiya and Jewkes's (2011) suggestion that risks in SGBV research can remain minimal when protocols are followed and that it can even generate a positive impact.

Discussion

Victimisation

This study explored the nature of SGBV that refugees, asylum seekers and undocumented migrants in Belgium and the Netherlands experienced since arriving in the EU (see Table 14.4). Within the limited scope of our research population, we found a high incidence of combined forms of victimisation, which sometimes resulted in a fatal outcome. Not only the extent to which sexual violence was part of their victimisation, but also its nature (e.g. frequent gang and multiple rape), differs from what is known about SGBV among Belgian and Dutch nationals (MOVISIE 2009; Pieters *et al.* 2010). Furthermore, unlike what is expected in the general population (Tavara 2006), but in line with findings for refugees, people in poverty and adolescent boys (Holmes and Slap 1998; Hynes and Lopes 2000; Norredam *et al.* 2005a), an important number of perpetrators in our study were either persons in authority – including those assigned to their protection – or were unknown to the victim. Our study also confirms the finding that impoverished women and girls and those living in remote areas and shelters may be especially vulnerable (Wenzel *et al.* 2004). Finally, it is interesting to note that the men and young boys in our study appear to be more prone to sexual and other kinds of violence than is globally expected in men (Holmes and Slap 1998; Tavara 2006).

Together, the data highlight the vulnerability of refugees, asylum seekers and undocumented migrants to SGBV in Belgium and the Netherlands. Because research has demonstrated that people with a heightened risk perception and those who have been personally victimised and/or witnessed SGBV during childhood are prone to subsequent victimisation or the perpetration of SGBV themselves (Borowsky *et al.* 1997; Brown *et al.* 2005), there is an urgent need for intervention.

Prevention

With respect to prevention at the individual level, the great majority of our respondents were highly educated, which – according to the available literature – should in principle help to protect them against the onset of ill health (Herd *et al.* 2007). However, respondents also reported a decline in socio-economic position and low subjective social status, linked to their immigration status restricting them from working officially and from participating freely in civil society. Thus, even with a higher education degree and former professional experience, respondents were structurally hampered from investing in the host society by turning their human capital potential into economic and social capital. Both low objective and subjective social status are considered important predictors of ill health (Demakakos *et al.* 2008; Marmot 2001), and low income is associated with the progression of ill health (Herd *et al.* 2007). As a result, it is not unreasonable to assume that SGBV puts our research population at great risk of high morbidity.

At an interpersonal level, respondents identified social networks and social support, information exchange, awareness-raising and community resilience as important prevention factors. However, respondents reported (see Table 14.2 and sociodemographic profile) living alone, being members of truncated networks with restricted opportunities for societal participation and building social capital. Social networks provide social and emotional support, self-esteem, trust, identity, coping, shared purpose and perceptions of control, the absence of which is demonstrated to have negative impacts on health (Bracke *et al.* 2008; Cohen and Wills 1985; Norris *et al.* 2008).

People in truncated networks are at risk of not having a confidant or receiving appropriate instrumental and social support (Cattell 2001; Weyers *et al.* 2008), an issue that is magnified in refugee contexts where the need to belong and the risk of social exclusion are key determinants of healthy sexual development as well as positive resettlement outcomes (McMichael and Gifford 2010). Beyond this, a high degree of social isolation and low quality of relationships with male confidants may lead to inappropriate sexual behaviour in men (Gutierrez-Lobos *et al.* 2001). Evidence also shows that social networks have a significant impact on exposure to health information, on shaping of health-related norms (Rose 2000; Scott and Hofmeyer 2007) and on health-risk perceptions and the adoption of health preventive behaviours (Kohler *et al.* 2007; Viswanath *et al.* 2006). Lack of participation as a citizen, sense of community and attachment to a place can hamper community resilience to stressors, such as SGBV (Norris *et al.* 2008).

Organisational and societal factors, including unhealthy and unsafe housing, unemployment, poverty, restricted access to health care, higher education, participation in civil society and legal protection, all contribute to the ill health that refugees and asylum seekers face on a daily basis (Deaton 2002; Robert and House 2000). These factors connect closely with basic human rights (Beyrer *et al.* 2007; Gruskin *et al.* 2007), but the fulfilment of these rights is far from self-evident when the opportunity to enjoy them is linked to legal residence status. Refugees receive an official residence permit which, in Belgium and the Netherlands, assures access to health-care services and entitles refugees to realise most rights, notwithstanding the multiple barriers they might encounter when trying to do so. Asylum seekers, on the other hand, are in the insecure process of achieving this status or having it denied, and undocumented migrants do not have a status, which implies that their access to health care is often left to the arbitrary decisions of individual health care and other service providers (Norredam *et al.* 2005b).

Conclusion and future research

Specific health-promotion and violence-prevention interventions are urgently needed to correct the unequal health conditions described in this chapter. At an individual level, behavioural change, sensitisation to SGBV and its risk and protective factors, and the enhancement of objective and subjective social status are of major importance. At the interpersonal level, it is paramount to empower our research population to build social networks that improve social capital and enhance the exchange of transferable knowledge skills through social learning, the creation of social support and community resilience. At the organisational level, it is crucial that health care and other services are made accessible to everyone, regardless of residence status. At the societal level, structural changes in asylum policies to enable everyone to enjoy and fulfil their human rights are urgently required.

In all these measures, the participation of the target population is crucial. This accords with research findings suggesting that prevention of SGBV in migrants should be based on culturally competent interventions, empowerment, the enhancement of structural elements (Bhuyan and Senturia 2005) and the adoption of comprehensive prevention approaches in which community resilience is integrated (Krieger *et al.* 2002; Maciak *et al.* 1999; Mosavel *et al.* 2005).

Finally, further research is needed: first, to enquire into the protective role of education in this research population, given the impediment of residence status, and, second, to determine whether (reverse) causation between socio-economic position and health applies and, if so, how much exposure to a setback in socio-economic position suffices to trigger ill health. The long-term evaluation of Desirable Prevention measures and their impact on the health and well-being of this population compared to others would help to clarify the relationship between the different determinants.

Limitations

This study has several practical limitations. Respondents were sampled through criterion and chain sampling, following the networks of the CRs and CAB. Although we excluded (among others) cases that were not personal or from a close peer, we respected the respondents' definition of a close peer. Furthermore, although all CRs were trained alike and the questionnaires were translated thoroughly, it cannot be guaranteed that their epistemological perspective while conducting and translating the interviews did not differ from those of the main researchers. These elements might introduce some biases in the data which we consider not to be generalised. However, we believe the results are transferable to similar populations in comparable settings.

References

Anderson, I. and Doherty, K. 2008. *Accounting for Rape: Psychology, Feminism and Discourse Analysis in the Study of Sexual Violence.* New York: Routledge.

Basile, K. and Saltzman, L.E. 2002. *Sexual Violence Surveillance: Uniform Definitions and Recommended Data Elements.* Atlanta, GA: NCIPC-CDCP.

Beyrer, C., Villar, J.C., Suwanvanichkij, V., Singh, S., Baral, S.D. and Mills, E.J. 2007. Neglected diseases, civil conflicts and the right to health. *Lancet* 370(9587): 619–627.

Bhuyan, R. and Senturia, K. 2005. Understanding domestic violence resource utilization and survivor solutions among immigrant and refugee women. Introduction to the Special Issue. *Journal of Interpersonal Violence* 20(8): 895–901.

Borowsky, I.W., Hogan, M. and Ireland, M. 1997. Adolescent sexual aggression: Risk and protective factors. *Pediatrics* 100(6): E7.

Bracke, P., Christiaens, W. and Verhaeghe, M. 2008. Self-esteem, self-efficacy and the balance of peer support among persons with chronic mental health problems. *Journal of Applied Social Psychology* 38(2): 436–459.

Bronfenbrenner, U. 1979. *The Ecology of Human Development: Experiments by Nature and Design.* Cambridge, MA: Harvard University Press.

Brown, A.L., Messman-Moore, T.L., Miller, A.G. and Stasser, G. 2005. Sexual victimization in relation to perceptions of risk: Mediation, generalization and temporal stability. *Personality & Social Psychology Bulletin* 31(7): 963–976.

Cattell, V. 2001. Poor people, poor places and poor health: The mediating role of social networks and social capital. *Social Sciences & Medicine* 52(10): 1501–1516.

Cohen, S. and Wills, T.A. 1985. Stress, social support and the buffering hypothesis. *Psychological Bulletin* 98(2): 310–357.

Deaton, A. 2002. Policy implications of the gradient of health and wealth. *Health Affairs* 21(2): 13–30.

de Laine, M. 2000. *Fieldwork, Participation and Practice: Ethics and Dilemmas in Qualitative Research.* London: SAGE.

Demakakos, P., Azroo, J.N., Breeze, E. and Marmot, M. 2008. Socioeconomic status and health: The role of subjective social status. *Social Sciences & Medicine* 67(2): 330–340.

Ellsberg, M. and Heise, L. 2005. *Researching Violence Against Women: A Practical Guide for Researchers and Activists.* Washington, DC: World Health Organization and Program for Appropriate Technology in Health (PATH).

Gagnon, A.J., Tuck, J. and Barkun, L. 2004. A systematic review of questionnaires measuring the health of resettling refugee women. *Health Care Women International* 25(2): 111–149.

Gruskin, S., Mills, E.J. and Tarantola, D. 2007. History, principles and practice of health and human rights. *Lancet* 370(9585): 449–455.

Gutierrez-Lobos, K., Eher, R., Grunhut, C., Bankier, B., Schmidl-Mohl, B., Fruhwald, S. and Semler, B. 2001. Violent sex offenders lack male social support. *International Journal of Offender Therapy and Comparative Criminology* 45(1): 70–82.

Herd, P., Goesling, B. and House, J.S. 2007. Socioeconomic position and health: The differential effects of education versus income on the onset versus progression of health problems. *Journal of Health and Social Behavior* 48(3): 223–238.

Holmes, W.C. and Slap, G.B. 1998. Sexual abuse of boys: Definition, prevalence, correlates, sequelae and management. *Journal of the American Medical Association* 280(21): 1855–1862.

Hynes, M. and Lopes, C.B. 2000. Sexual violence against refugee women. *Journal of Women's Health & Gender Based Medicine* 9(8): 819–823.

Israel, B.A., Schulz, A.J., Parker, E.A. and Becker, A.B. 2001. Community-based participatory research: Policy recommendations for promoting a partnership approach in health research. *Education for Health* 14(2): 182–197.

Kohler, H.P., Behrman, J.R. and Watkins, S.C. 2007. Social networks and HIV/AIDS risk perceptions. *Demography* 44(1): 1–33.

Krieger, J., Allen, C., Cheadle, A., Ciske, S., Schier, J.K., Senturia, K. and Sullivan, M. 2002. Using community-based participatory research to address social determinants of health: Lessons learned from Seattle Partners for Healthy Communities. *Health Education & Behavior* 29(3): 361–382.

Maciak, B.J., Guzman, R., Santiago, A., Villalobos, G. and Israel, B.A. 1999. Establishing LA VIDA: A community-based partnership to prevent intimate violence against Latina women. *Health Education & Behavior* 26(6): 821–840.

Marmot, M. 2001. Inequalities in health. *New England Journal of Medicine* 345(2): 134–136.

McMichael, C. and Gifford, S. 2010. Narratives of sexual health risk and protection amongst young people from refugee backgrounds in Melbourne, Australia. *Culture, Health & Sexuality* 12(3): 263–277.

Moran, R., Mohamed, Z. and Lovel, H. 2006. Breaking the silence: Participatory research processes about health with Somali refugee people seeking asylum. In: B. Temple and R. Moran (eds) *Doing Research with Refugees: Issues and Guidelines*. Bristol: Policy Press, 55–74.

Mosavel, M., Simon, C., van Stade, D. and Buchbinder, M. 2005. Community-based participatory research (CBPR) in South Africa: Engaging multiple constituents to shape the research question. *Social Sciences & Medicine* 61(12): 2577–2587.

MOVISIE. 2009. *Seksueel Geweld: Feiten en Cijfers [Sexual Violence: Facts and Figures]*. Utrecht: MOVISIE.

Norredam, M., Crosby, S., Munarriz, R., Piwowarczyk, L. and Grodin, M. 2005a. Urologic complications of sexual trauma among male survivors of torture. *Urology* 65(1): 28–32.

Norredam, M., Mygind, A. and Krasnik, A. 2005b. Ethnic disparities in health: Access to healthcare for asylum seekers in the European Union – a comparative study of country policies. *European Journal of Public Health* 16(3): 285–289.

Norris, F.H., Stevens, S.P., Pfefferbaum, B., Wyche, K.F. and Pfefferbaum, R.L. 2008. Community resilience as a metaphor, theory, set of capacities and strategy for disaster readiness. *American Journal of Community Psychology* 41(1–2): 127–150.

Pieters, J., Italiano, P., Offermans, A. and Hellemans, S. 2010. *Ervaringen van Vrouwen en Mannen met Psychologisch, Fysiek en Seksueel Geweld [Experiences of Women and Men with Psychological, Physical and Sexual Violence]*. Brussels: IGVM.

Robert, S. and House, J. 2000. Socioeconomic inequalities in health: An enduring sociological problem. In: L.E. Bird, P. Conrad and A.M. Fremont (eds) *Handbook of Medical Sociology*. Upper Saddle River, NJ: Prentice-Hall, 79–97.

Rose, R. 2000. How much does social capital add to individual health? A survey study of Russians. *Social Sciences & Medicine* 51(9): 1421–1435.

Safman, R.M. and Sobal, J. 2004. Qualitative sample extensiveness in health education research. *Health, Education & Behaviour* 31(1): 9–21.

Scott, C. and Hofmeyer, A. 2007. Networks and social capital: A relational approach to primary healthcare reform. *Health Research Policy & Systems* 25: 5–9.

Sikweyiya, Y. and Jewkes, R. 2011. Perceptions about safety and risks in gender-based violence research: Implications for the ethics review process. *Culture, Health & Sexuality* 13(9): 1091–1102.

Tavara, L. 2006. Sexual violence. *Best Practice & Research. Clinical Obstetrics & Gynaecology* 20(3): 395–408.

UNHCR. 2003. *Sexual and Gender-based Violence Against Refugees, Returnees and Internally Displaced Persons: Guidelines for Prevention and Response*. New York: UNHCR.

Vettenburg, N., Burssens, D., Melis, B., Goris, P., van Gils, J., Verdonck, D. and Walgrave, L. 2003. *Preventie Gespiegeld: Visie en Instrumenten voor Wenselijke Preventie [Prevention Mirrored: Vision and Instruments for Desirable Prevention]*. Tielt, Belgium: Lannoo Uitgeverij.

Viswanath, K., Randolph, S.W. and Finnegan Jr., J.R. 2006. Social capital and health: Civic engagement, community size and recall of health messages. *American Journal of Public Health* 96(8): 1456–1461.

Viswanathan, M., Ammerman, A., Eng, E., Garlehner, G., Lohr, K.N., Griffith, D., Rhodes, S. et al. 2004. Community-based participatory research: Assessing the evidence. *Evidence Report & Technology Assessment* 99: 1–8.

Ward, J. and Vann, B. 2002. Gender-based violence in refugee settings. *Lancet* 360(Suppl.): 13–14.

Wenzel, S.L., Tucker, J.S., Elliott, M.N., Marshall, G.N. and Williamson, S.L. 2004. Physical violence against impoverished women: A longitudinal analysis of risk and protective factors. *Women's Health Issues* 14(5): 144–154.

Weyers, S., Dragano, N., Mobus, S., Beck, E.M., Stang, A., Mohlenkamp, S., Jockel, K.H., Erbel, R. and Siegrist, J. 2008. Low socio-economic position is associated with poor social networks and social support: Results from the Heinz Nixdorf Recall Study. *International Journal for Equity in Health* 7: 13.

Chapter 15

Avoiding shame

Young LGBT people, homophobia and self-destructive behaviours

Elizabeth McDermott, Katrina Roen and Jonathan Scourfield

Introduction

The intimate life of the Western developed world is going through a process of transformation and transition that is creating the possibility for sexual/gender diversity to flourish (Giddens 1992; Weeks 2007). Recent UK legislation has enshrined in law same-sex relationships (Civil Partnership Act: UK Parliament 2004) and provided protection against discrimination and homophobia (e.g. The Employment Equality [Sexual Orientation] Regulations: UK Parliament 2003; The Equality Act [Sexual Orientation] Regulations: UK Parliament 2007; Criminal Justice and Immigration Act: UK Parliament 2008). The British Social Attitudes survey (Park 2005) shows increasing popular acceptance of same-sex partnerships, especially among younger people. Despite this mainstreaming of sexual diversity, there is ongoing marginalisation of and stigma associated with sexual minorities. This is illustrated in the disproportionately high rate of suicidal thoughts and suicide attempts among young people who are lesbian, gay, bisexual or transgender (LGBT).

Youth suicide has received widespread attention as a subject of research, a focus of health policy and a concern of broader public debates (Cantor 2000; Hawton *et al.* 2006). However, within these discourses, the ways in which young people's sexual identities may influence mental health have been marginalised (Valentine and Skelton 2003). For example, it is only very recently that the National Suicide Prevention Strategy for England has identified sexual identity as a risk factor for suicide (King *et al.* 2008).

There is a substantial international body of evidence that highlights the elevated rates of self-destructive behaviours in LGBT youth (e.g. Fenaughty and Harre 2003; Molloy *et al.* 2003; Savin-Williams and Ream 2003; Wichstrøm and Hegna 2003; D'Augelli *et al.* 2005), as well as the negative effects of homophobia and victimisation on the mental health of young LGBT people (Pilkington and D'Augelli 1995; Rivers 1999, 2000). Existing research on LGBT youth and suicide and self-harm, which is framed by psychological perspectives and quantitative methodologies, has been important for our understanding of the relationship between sexual identity and mental health. There is rather less qualitative research that has sought to access LGBT young people's own views about engaging in self-destructive behaviours (King *et al.* 2008). This chapter outlines findings from an original qualitative research study that aimed to access the perspectives of young LGBT people about how non-normative sexual and gender identities are linked to feelings of extreme distress and self-destructive behaviours including suicidal and self-harming behaviours. The study draws upon literatures across sociology, psychology, geography and cultural studies to frame the investigation. The chapter focuses upon the ways in which young LGBT people must negotiate homophobia in their everyday interactions and manage being positioned as 'deviant'. It suggests that important to that process of negotiation is shame avoidance.

LGBT youth, homophobia and self-destructive behaviours

International research has demonstrated a clear link between experiencing homophobic abuse, suffering negative psychological consequences and engaging in self-destructive behaviours. Recent North American and New Zealand-based studies of large populations reveal that young LGBT people can have rates of suicide attempts at least four times those of their heterosexual counterparts (Bagley and Tremblay 2000). In the UK, Rivers' (1999) work suggests that one out of every three gay, lesbian and bisexual persons is victimised during adolescence because of their actual or perceived sexual orientation.

Rivers (2000) also examined how exposure to violence or harassment may be detrimental for psychological well-being. Across LGB respondents in his study, 19 per cent had attempted self-destructive behaviour once and 8 per cent had attempted self-destructive behaviour more than once due to sexual orientation difficulties. For those who reported having been bullied at school, however, this figure rose dramatically, with 30 per cent having engaged in multiple self-destructive attempts. Valentine et al.'s (2002: 13) research describes self-destructive behaviour as an effect of homophobia:

> [H]omophobia can contribute to young people feeling bad about their own sexuality and developing low self-esteem or even self-loathing. These emotions can trigger self-destructive cycles of behaviour such as drinking, drug-taking, unsafe sexual practices [and] self-harm.

They suggest that homophobia can make it harder to access support, and the ensuing isolation can contribute to young people's self-destructive behaviours. International evidence on suicide risk and young LGBT people has been dominated by psychological perspectives. Fullagar (2003, 2005) argues for more attention to be paid to the social relations that shape young people's emotional distress, and challenges the dominance of normalised discourses about risky individual behaviour in the suicide and self-harm psychological literature:

> Power relations that shape the way that young people are socially positioned and come to feel about themselves are rendered invisible through risk discourses that reify identity and mobilise mental health discourses to explain suicide.
>
> (Fullagar 2005: 37)

In support of Fullagar's argument, our study investigates the social and cultural influences on young people's sexual identities and self-destructive behaviours. In emphasising the heteronormative and homophobic context within which young people negotiate their sexual identities, we hope to avoid the danger of pathologising LGBT mental health as inherently fragile.

Young adulthoods, heterosexuality and mental health

There is some agreement that the journey into adulthood has become more complicated, extended and uncertain (for an overview of debates see MacDonald and Marsh 2005). In addition, some young people find the transition to adulthood particularly difficult and are at increased risk of homelessness, unemployment, social isolation (Coles 1997) and mental health problems (e.g. suicide, self-harm, eating disorders and depression) (Giddens 1991; Furlong and Cartmel 1997; Henderson *et al.* 2007). However, rarely included within these debates are LGBT young people and the particular difficulties they may experience negotiating non-normative sexual identities in the transition to adulthood (Valentine *et al.* 2002; Valentine and Skelton 2003).

For young LGBT people, sexuality may become an additional aspect of uncertainty and stress. In the UK, for example, Valentine and Skelton (2003) have revealed the hazards some young LGBT people encounter in the process of becoming adults. These include: homelessness; homophobic bullying at school disrupting education; family rejection; and difficulties finding safe spaces to form supportive relationships. Similarly, a recent longitudinal biographical investigation into young people's transition to adulthood shows that young LGBT people leave home earlier than their peers due to difficulties of coming out and living as LGBT (Henderson *et al.* 2007).

Young LGBT people must find ways to 'invent and sustain' adult LGBT identities within overwhelming heterosexual norms. Epstein *et al.*'s (2003) work on the reproduction of heterosexuality in education argues that 'normative heterosexuality is promoted, sustained and made to appear totally natural' (2). They state that the reproduction of heterosexuality requires a 'tremendous amount of work that ... young people, regardless of their own sexual identifications, must do in dealing with, resisting, coming to terms with, negotiating or adopting normative versions of heterosexuality' (145).

LGBT young people experience many of the problems common to young people in becoming adults, whatever their sexual identity. But they are confronted with the additional challenges of creating LGBT identities within discourses of 'compulsory' (Rich 1993) heterosexual and gender normative adulthood and the accompanying risk of homophobia, bullying and social isolation.

Homophobia, shame and distress

Shame and pride are powerful emotions (Scheff 1994) that have been historically linked to non-conformist sexual identities (Munt 2000). Cultural and queer theorists have suggested that the pride/shame binary remains strategically essential for LGBT people's negotiation of everyday life (Munt 2000; Probyn 2000; Sedgwick 2003). Sedgwick (2003: 64) states:

> I would say that for at least certain ('queer') people, shame is simply the first, and remains a permanent, structuring fact of identity.

Munt (2000) argues that for the 'homosexual subject' the increasing consciousness of same-sex desire generates feelings of marginality. An individual may be shamed by their feelings or may refute shame through discourses of pride. What is proposed by such theorists is that LGBT identity, however it is formed, is formed through the shame/pride binary. They contend that pride relies on the 'erasure of shame', and shame remains unspoken. Probyn (2000) suggests 'pride operates as a necessity, an ontology of gay life that cannot admit its other' (19–20). There is a complex negotiation of both emotions in the construction of sexual identities.

Shame arising from the transgression of social and cultural norms has also been found to be significant in literature on health and illness; for example: suicide (Cottle 2000; Fullagar 2003); lung cancer (Chapple *et al.* 2004); HIV/AIDS (Duffy 2005); eating disorders (Monro and Huon 2005); and depression (Andrews 1995). Fullagar's (2003, 2005) work on youth suicide demonstrates the centrality of shame in young people's accounts of suicidal experiences and argues that the social dynamics of shame are important to understanding young people's subjectivities. She connects shame to the failed or shamed self and suggests that suicidal thoughts enable young people to escape those pressures which make them feel unworthy or failed. In other words, it allows them to escape from being positioned as shamed. She gives an example of a young woman who is bullied at school for the 'fluidity of her sexual identity' (2003: 297):

> Shame is very much connected to the embodied performance of identity in relation to cultural norms, as it produces feelings of self-hatred, disgust and loathing that are not easily detached from the self as 'cognitions'.
>
> (299)

Although shame is recognised across a range of disciplines (e.g. anthropology, psychology, sociology, cultural studies) as a powerful emotion, it is one that is 'invisible' or 'hidden' in modern Western societies (Lewis 1992; Gilbert 1997; Scheff 2003; Probyn 2005). Scheff (2003) suggests that 'a large part of the cultural defence against shame is linguistic; the English language, particularly, disguises shame' (240). In this study we did not directly set out to investigate shame, nor did our participants often use shame explicitly to name their emotions, but through a discourse analysis of the data it became evident that shame was the unspoken emotion of the young LGBT research participants' accounts.

This chapter considers connections in the data between homophobia and self-destructive behaviours. It then explores the most prominent ways in which the young LGBT participants avoided the shaming of homophobia. The chapter argues that these strategies of shame avoidance might lead young LGBT people to manage homophobia individually, without expectation of support, and as such may make them vulnerable to self-destructive behaviours.

Methods

The research involved 13 interviews and 11 focus groups with young people aged 16 to 25 years, in the North West of England and South Wales, with 69 young people participating. For three of the 11 focus groups we specifically recruited young people who identified as LGBT and for the other groups we did not specify sexual or gender identity. We aimed for diversity in terms of the ethnicity and socio-economic circumstances of participants, as well as collecting data in both rural and urban locations.

The findings presented here draw on a subset of data consisting of interviews and focus groups with specifically LGBT young people (n = 27). We did not aim to recruit young people to the study who had experiences of suicide or self-harm, but participants may have been motivated to take part because of their own experiences. In this subsample, at least half (n = 14) had themselves attempted suicide or self-harmed. The LGBT participants were all white and were recruited via LGBT support groups. The young people may have been referred to a support group through professional networks (social services, education, health) or found the group themselves via the Internet, leaflets or word of mouth. They are, therefore, not a representative sample of all LGBT young people in the regions where we conducted the research.

The research employed ethical practices to ensure young people were not harmed by participating. We paid particular attention to ensuring that the young people were carefully informed and understood the nature of the research. Confidentiality was maintained by anonymising the data and utilising pseudonyms for the name of participants, youth organisations and their location. At each interview or focus group we arranged for a support worker, whom the young people trusted, to be available if necessary. We also provided an information sheet with support contacts. The research proposal was reviewed by the relevant university ethics committee.

This chapter presents data analysed using a Foucauldian discourse analytic approach drawing upon the work of Gavey (1989), Hook (2001) and Willig (2003). Language and discourse are understood as social practices through which meaning, knowledge and beliefs are produced. The authors worked with the texts to: identify key discourses through which self-harm, suicide, homophobia and sexuality are understood; describe the relationship among those discourses; identify points of tension and resistance; and identify silences and contradictions. Following Willig (2003), where key steps in the analytic process are detailed, the discourse analysis was guided by questions about the effects of the discursive constructions, the subject positions that are offered as a result, and the consequences for participants of taking up those subject positions.

In the following section we discuss the connections the LGBT participants made between homophobia and self-destructive behaviours (we use the term 'self-destructive behaviours' to mean suicide, self-harm or other risky practices). Then we present an analysis of the ways in which young LGBT participants attempted to negotiate homophobia through strategies of shame avoidance. We focus upon the three most prevalent strategies: the routinisation and minimising of homophobia; maintaining individual 'adult' responsibility; and constructing 'proud' identities.

Homophobia and self-destructive behaviours

The young LGBT participants in this study drew a strong link between homophobia and self-destructive behaviour. In the following extract, David and John, two young Welsh gay men, talk about the connection between homophobia, suicide and being gay:

> David: I know of a few people who've, well rumours were going round that they were supposed to be gay although they didn't, they hadn't come out if they were or, you know, they could just have been straight but their life was made such a misery that they actually did kill themselves … he was about 18 to 19, so he'd left school but that was when he actually killed himself.
> Researcher: What was it about him that made him kind of not fit in?
> David: Um, yes, eh, he had a feminine voice, eh, and he did look, he did look gay.

John: It's just like the guy from *EastEnders*, the one who used to play I think it was Spencer.
Researcher: Oh yeah.
John: In *EastEnders*, he tried to commit suicide 'cause people said he was gay and like. So some people say you're gay just tell them to piss off.
Researcher: ... he had a feminine voice, what else?
John: People think people are gay just because they've got feminine voices, it's not really true, some people just do.
David: Well the thing is this, this boy he's actually, down here he had quite a few girlfriends as well.

(Focus group: city, South Wales)

David and John connect the labelling of an individual as gay (David's friend and the *EastEnders* actor) with homophobia and suicide. The two important points in this exchange are that, first, they present an implicit understanding that being labelled 'gay' is a term of abuse, which, potentially, can cause an individual considerable distress, which may lead to suicidal behaviour. Second, while people who carry out suicidal acts may be either straight or gay, the significant fact is whether others judge them as gay. They consider this judgement to be based upon visible and/or audible markers of sexuality and gender normativity such as voice tone ('feminine'), appearance ('he did look gay') and the gender of sexual partner ('girlfriends').

Homophobia is discursively constructed by our research participants as punishment for the transgression of heterosexual norms. The punishment was through physical and verbal abuse, rejection or isolation, but this went beyond the immediate hostility of, for example, a physical attack in the street. Homophobia works to punish at a deep individual level to create psychological distress; it shames the self and requires a young person to deal with being positioned, because of their sexual desire, as abnormal, dirty and disgusting. In the previous extract, in response to homophobia, David and John offer two possibilities for action: suicide, which is a result of extreme distress and a shamed-subject position, or defiance ('tell them to piss off'), which involves a subject position that refuses the shaming of homophobia.

Some of the young LGBT participants explained their own self-destructive behaviours as resulting from the emotional distress caused by homophobia. Paul explained:

Just before I left school I got myself in really a bad state ... I got myself really down because I was having a load of trouble with people at school. And I think everybody thought they could take the piss because they got away with it. I was a right mess, I couldn't move some days, I just felt like, argh, and then I started cutting myself on my arm and I was just a mess. I was upset because of the way people were with me because I was gay and it just aggravates me so much.

(16, gay, interview: small town, North West of England)

Cutting is presented as a coping strategy for the distress Paul experiences as a result of homophobia. This method of coping, as distinct from other coping strategies, such as drinking, avoidance, seeking safe space and resistance, which he also describes in his interview, is for when he is very distressed. 'The way people were' with him, ridiculing him because he is gay, 'aggravates' him, and anger is one of the emotions he names when describing self-harming through cutting:

It's [cutting is] weird, it distracts everything going on in your head really; at the time you are doing it you are angry but after you just like, argh, you are thinking why did you do that? You were stupid but … I don't want to punch walls as much any more.

Anger is associated with shame (Gilbert 1997). It is argued that when shame is unacknowledged by individuals they can become withdrawn or angry (Scheff 1994). Lorraine appeared very angry throughout the discussion on homophobia and self-destructive behaviours. She explains her way of coping with homophobic bullying at school:

> … the only reason I didn't kill myself is because when I got bullied I started taking drugs and I was so high off cocaine I just didn't care what people said about me any more.
>
> (19, lesbian, focus group: small town, North of England)

The strong relationship articulated by some of the young LGBT people between homophobia, emotional distress and self-destructive behaviours was not straightforward; not all young people who are subject to homophobia try to take their own life. Our interpretation of the data suggests that an important factor in negotiating homophobia in everyday interactions is avoiding being shamed. In the following section we explore the complicated, contradictory and multiple ways in which young LGBT people negotiate homophobia. We argue that what we are uncovering are possible 'modalities of shame-avoidance' (Munt 2000: 534).

Avoiding homophobic shaming

Our participants' accounts suggest they used various strategies, tactics and manoeuvres when negotiating homophobia. These were influenced by individual personal factors, their own economic and social circumstances, and the setting in which the hostility occurred (e.g. family home, public street, school). Cherie, for example, a 17-year-old lesbian from the North West of England, managed homophobia in diverse ways such as moving schools, avoiding eye contact, and tackling hostility in public spaces through fighting, as well as coping through self-harm in private spaces. In this section we focus upon some of the most prominent ways in which the young people negotiated the shaming-spotlight of homophobia.

Routinisation and minimisation

The participants' accounts indicate that homophobia was both expected, and constructed as ordinary and routine:

> Jane: I got bottled actually in a homophobic attack and, eh, ended up in hospital a few years ago, which is nothing you know really serious, plenty of people get bottled anyway (laughs).
>
> (25, gay, interview: city, South Wales)

> Cherie: I used to get beaten up on the way back and like, are you a boy as well? The usual stuff.
>
> (17, lesbian, interview: small town, North West of England)

Cherie's 'the usual stuff' constructs a routinisation around the verbal and physical abuse she has experienced. She expects the hostility and knows what form it will take. Similarly, Jane's description of her attack as commonplace ('plenty of people get bottled') posits homophobia as a mundane fact of life. Our interpretation proposes that constructing homophobia as routine or mundane reduces the significance of the attack/abuse to an individual level – in Jane's words, 'nothing [...] really serious'. This minimising strategy may enable the young LGBT participants to position themselves as unaffected by the abuse and deflect the shaming effects of homophobia. Clarke *et al*.'s (2004) research on lesbian and gay families also found that parents minimised homophobia that was directed towards their children. The parents were conscious of the negative discourses around same-sex parenting and wanted to avoid feelings of failure and guilt that their sexuality may have a negative impact on their children's well-being. A close examination of Andrew's account of his experience of a violent homophobic incident at university highlights this minimising strategy:

> I was just in my room one night and they came back in and one of the guys was drunk, and he was quite violent anyway and he started grabbing a chair from the kitchen and banging it against my door telling me that he wanted to ... swearing and saying how he wanted to kill me, because, like, 'you gay fucker', um, 'you gays are blah, blah, blah' and I was just like OK, what's your problem here? ... I didn't report it or anything because I was just used to how he was because he was quite a violent person anyway. But that was probably the scariest thing that happened in the first year of university.
>
> (19, bisexual, interview: university, small city, North of England)

Andrew attempts to reduce the severity of the attack by normalising the behaviour of the perpetrator ('he was quite a violent person anyway') and presenting the abuse as mundane ('you gays are blah, blah, blah'). Then he positions himself as virtually unaffected by the incident through his rational and emotionally controlled response ('what's your problem?'), although he does admit it was a frightening experience. Finally, he justifies not reporting the incident by minimising the effect on him ('I was just used to how he was').

The problem with attempts to minimise homophobia by undermining it or constructing it as an unlucky occurrence is that it closes down the opportunities for taking action beyond the individual level. Andrew did not report his homophobic attack to the university. To have done so may have drawn attention to the incident and turned the shaming-spotlight of homophobia towards him.

Our concern is that young LGBT people, in their efforts to minimise homophobia, may be hesitant to seek help. It was clear from the young people that they did not expect support either from education and welfare services or their families (although some received support). Furthermore, it is a shame-avoidance strategy that relies on individual resources and resourcefulness. Andrew had the support of the university LGBT group. He says, 'I had seen how strong they were, reacting, it gave kind of an idea.' Other participants with fewer resources may be less able to undermine the significance of homophobia and avoid the shaming effects. This in turn may make them more vulnerable to self-destructive coping methods.

Adult identities and individual responsibility

> Deborah: I'm not 10 years old any more, I'm 16, I've grown up and I'm leaving home soon, so just get over the fact that I am what I am, that I like girls as well as lads, and just say, tell him, 'fuck off'.
>
> (16, bisexual, focus group: small town, North West of England)

Deborah is describing how she manages her father's hostility to her sexuality. She positions herself as an adult ('I've grown up') as a way of asserting the legitimacy of her bisexual identity. She constructs her emerging adult identity by drawing on both discourses of independence ('leaving home') and maturity (declaring her sexual desire). We suggest that a significant influence on the young LGBT participants' attempts to negotiate homophobia was their desire to position themselves as adults. In the following extract, Jane describes how she manages homophobia:

> I'm quite outwardly gay and ... when people make homophobic comments then I will let them know that I'm actually gay and because I don't think attitudes will ever change unless they're challenged.
>
> (Jane, 24, gay, interview: city, South Wales)

Similarly, Andrew states after his homophobic attack:

> I think I probably made it worse because I think I made a point of being even more open about it ... Because I was like they need to be personally made aware of it.
>
> (Andrew, 19, bisexual, interview: university, small city, North of England)

Jane and Andrew, both university educated, draw upon individualising discourses of the neo-liberal self that demonstrate adult status by being rational, self-reliant and responsible (Rose 1989; Moran and Skeggs 2004). Through managing homophobia in an emotionally controlled and responsible manner, they are able to position themselves as adult. Our analysis suggests that important to the young LGBT people's sense of adult self was an individual responsibility to cope with homophobia. Fullagar's (2003) research on youth suicide found that feeling worried or ashamed about not coping was a key factor in understanding young people's suicide. In the following extract, David describes how homophobia led to a very difficult period in his life:

> David: I can remember lying back on my bed in October thinking oh my life's all sorted out, and the next day I get kicked out of my house so I had to leave college, the course that I loved more than anything ... and then I had to come down to [city] and I was in the YMCA and it was just the people in, in the YMCA weren't very nice people as well, so on top of all that, you know, being kicked out, not speaking to your mother.
> Researcher: When you say kicked out of your house – was that your family home ...?
> David: Yeah. And, and then having people say horrible stuff ... it was really, yeah it was stressful ... I didn't deal with it at the time, I would take it out on my partner at the time ... as well so ... eventually ... me and my partner broke up as well, which got really bad ... and it was a time in my life where I had to like ... you know get up and do

things as well like, em, you couldn't you know lay in bed and get over it that way. I had to ... you know, sort housing out and, em, well, be an adult.

(17, gay, interview: city, South Wales)

David describes the cumulative effects of homophobia. He is thrown out of his family home and as a consequence is unable to pursue his college course and his imagined future. He is therefore made homeless and seeks refuge in an unfamiliar city at the YMCA where he encounters further hostility to his sexuality. The psychological stress eventually causes his relationship to end. David was in temporary hostel accommodation, in a new city, without any obvious forms of support or financial income. Coping with the situation, he states he had to 'be an adult'; he positions himself as individually responsible for managing the emotional distress ('I didn't deal with it'). Later in the interview David describes the physical and psychological effects:

> David: At the time I was ... getting really bad chest, you know like, bad chest pains. It was like as if I was holding my breath and then all of sudden just letting go of it and it would be a sort of rush from my chest. Like a rippling feeling or something ... I didn't have the money to drink a lot but I, I did. Whenever I found it I would drink ... And because of the, because I was in a hostel I wouldn't go to the ... to the canteen to get food, so I wouldn't eat because there was, there was people who might have said things.

Clearly David was finding it difficult to cope, and later in the interview he admits contemplating suicide. Fullagar (2003) argues that the failure of young people to manage their emotional self can induce profound shame. In David's very distressing circumstances and with few resources but his own personal capacities he feels he has failed to cope ('I didn't deal with it').

We would suggest that David's construction of the adult LGBT self as responsible for coping with homophobia, his failure to do so, the ongoing homophobia and his few resources create psychological distress and a shamed self where self-destructive behaviours, in this case alcohol abuse and suicidal thoughts, become a viable option. Our concern again is that young LGBT people like David feel that, as young adults, they must take individual responsibility for negotiating homophobia and they may be reluctant to seek support.

Proud identities

In addition to discourses of adulthood, the young people drew upon discourses of pride in order to position themselves with a positive gay identity. The following short extract is taken from a longer conversation between Cherie and the interviewer about her ways of managing homophobia, and the transphobia directed at a close relative:

> Cherie: I have always been about 10 years ahead in my head than what I actually am.
> Researcher: It sounds like you've had to take responsibility.
> Cherie: Yeah, you learn quickly. It was really strange because my [close relative] was 24 and I was 14 when she died, but she looked up to me rather than me looking up to her and whenever she had a problem she rang me up. So I've always learnt, I look after my friends that way as well, because a lot of my friends are gay. Um, and I've always learnt to stand up for people and I would never tell anybody I wasn't gay or disown her.
>
> (17, gay, interview: small town, North West of England)

Cherie's identity and coping strategy pivots upon the notion that she is mature ('ahead in my head'), responsible (caring for others) and proud (not denying her sexuality). She constructs coping with distress through individualising 'adult' discourses that invoke rhetorics of responsibility, emotional maturity and personal autonomy. As well as positioning herself as mature and responsible, Cherie draws upon gay pride discourses ('I would never tell anybody I wasn't gay') to position herself with a positive gay identity that is unashamed about her sexuality. It is an individual refusal to be shamed by homophobia. Our data suggest that the proud LGBT subject position can be a strategy of resilience in the face of homophobia. In the following extract, the participants are discussing whether a young man who wants to be a ballet dancer is normal and the level of distress he may feel. At the beginning of the extract, Lorraine gives the example of her gay male friend, an arts student, who suffers homophobic abuse, including homophobic graffiti on his home:

> Lorraine: He is completely comfortable with who he is. He's not bothered by what people say. But when they're getting to the stage that they are, doing things to his family home and stuff, it is very distressing for him …
> Researcher: Do you think a young man wouldn't find it distressing?
> Stuart: If a young man actually wan…
> Samuel: I think if they've reached that … themselves they won't find it distressing.
> Lily: They don't find it distressing themselves. The stress comes from external sources from people who are giving them hassle because of it.
> Samuel: Yes, yes.
> Stuart: It's, um, everybody's personal thing, though if they feel normal then they're normal and it doesn't really matter about what everybody else thinks.
> Researcher: Yes, yes.
> Stuart: So even if it is distressing they can still feel themselves.
>   (Focus group: small town, North of England)

Lorraine directly connects a positive gay identity ('comfortable with who he is') and a type of 'immunity' to distress arising from homophobia ('not bothered by what people say'). Sexual identity is constructed by the group as an individual, internal dialogue and personal choice that is unproblematic in terms of causing distress ('if they feel normal … it doesn't really matter about what everybody else thinks'). Distress is constructed as arising when homophobia is 'external' to the self; it is directed at others (e.g. family) by 'other' perpetrators. Queer cultural theorists (Munt 2000; Sedgwick 2003; Probyn 2005) have argued that counter-discourses of gay pride are intrinsic to a community movement dealing with shame. Within these pride counter-discourses, an individual 'in the closet' is hiding their sexual identity and must, therefore, be ashamed. In other words, 'outness' is constructed as the proud subject position, and a 'closeted' sexual identity is the failed, shamed LGBT subject position. Our analysis suggests that the young people drew upon gay pride discourses to position themselves as unashamed sexual subjects and refuse the shaming of homophobia. In the previous extract, the participants are constructing and inventing a proud young LGBT adult as able to cope with homophobia ('even if it is distressing they can still feel themselves').

The proud sexual subject can provide resilience against homophobia. It allows young LGBT people to position themselves positively in regard to their sexual and gender identity. However, some of the focus group participants had talked about their own suicide attempts, self-harm practices and excessive drinking and drug-taking resulting from homophobia. As this suggests, the proud subject position which can inoculate against distress from homophobia is, in reality, more difficult to maintain than perhaps is presented by the young LGBT people.

Our interpretation suggests that, by drawing upon shame–pride discourses, a binary is established that appears to allow for only two subject positions: the successful, proud self who can cope with homophobia, and the failed, ashamed self who is distressed by homophobia. This binary tends not to allow for more nuanced and complex manoeuvring within these discourses to subject positions which may be proud in some spaces, but less so in other situations. Sustaining a proud sexual identity requires resilience, experience, expertise (of the self) and resources that go beyond the individual's capacity to hold their head high.

Conclusion

This research is one of the few UK studies to investigate young LGBT people and self-destructive behaviours. By eliciting the perspectives of young LGBT people, it sought to understand why young people with sexual and gender identities that do not fit with heterosexual and gender norms may consider engaging in self-destructive practices. Our findings indicate a complex relationship between young LGBT people's sexual identities and self-destructive behaviours. The participants connected (although not exclusively) the distress arising from homophobia to suicide attempts, self-harm practices, risky sexual practices and excessive drinking and drug-taking. We acknowledge the potential for research on this topic to pathologise LGBT identities, but to guard against this we have tried to emphasise the context of heteronormative (and homophobic) sexual and gender relations within which this issue needs to be understood. So, for example, recent research findings demonstrate that the difficulties young LGBT people may face can be overcome by the right support (Stonewall 2007).

Our concern about the effects of homophobia on the mental health of young LGBT people is deepened by these findings, which suggest that young LGBT people may employ individualistic shame-avoidance strategies to negotiate homophobia that closes down the opportunities for taking action beyond the individual level. They may reduce the possibility, or expectation, of action or support at community, institutional or national levels. In a wider context, the construction and reproduction of heterosexuality as the most legitimate sexual orientation seems to remain persistent in the face of major transformations associated with advances in acceptance of sexual diversity. For example, Henderson et al.'s (2007: 25) research found that almost all the young people that took part in their study 'imagined' a heterosexual future. They assert that 'what is surprising in this time of change is the power of the normative model and how few young people are pushing against the constraints, and imagining a different future'.

Savin-Williams (2005) argues that LGBT identity may no longer be the risk to young people's mental health it was 20 years ago. Our research is limited by size and scope (the participants were all members of LGBT youth groups) but it suggests that for some young LGBT people who transgress the heavily enforced heterosexual norms, they still, despite evidence of the widening acceptance of different sexual identities (Weeks 2007), must learn to manage homophobia. Some of the participants in our study struggled to find ways to refuse the shaming of homophobia, which might potentially have made them more vulnerable to self-destructive practices. It is only recently that the UK government has begun to take seriously the tackling of health inequalities for LGBT people (Department of Health

2008). More research is required to develop understanding of the mental health consequences, for young LGBT people, of negotiating everyday settings framed by the normative discourses, institutions and structures of heterosexuality.

References

Andrews, B. 1995. Bodily shame as a mediator between abusive experiences and depression. *Journal of Abnormal Psychology* 104: 277–285.

Bagley, C. and Tremblay, P. 2000. Elevated rates of suicidal behaviour in gay, lesbian, and bisexual youth. *Crisis* 21: 111–117.

Cantor, C.H. 2000. Suicide in the Western world. In: K. Hawton and K. van Herringen (eds) *The International Handbook of Suicide and Attempted Suicide*. Chichester: John Wiley, 9–28.

Chapple, A., Ziebland, S. and McPherson, A. 2004. Stigma, shame and blame experienced by patients with lung cancer: Qualitative study. *British Medical Journal* 328: 1470–1473.

Clarke, V., Kitzinger, C. and Potter, J. 2004. 'Kids are just cruel anyway': Lesbian and gay parents' talk about homophobic bullying. *British Journal of Social Psychology* 43: 531–550.

Coles, B. 1997. Vulnerable youth and processes of social exclusion: A theoretical framework, a review of recent research and suggestions for a future research agenda. In: J. Bynner, L. Chisholm and A. Furlong (eds) *Youth Citizenship and Social Change in a European Context*. Aldershot, Hants: Ashgate.

Cottle, T.J. 2000. Mind shadows: A suicide in the family. *Journal of Contemporary Ethnography* 29: 222–255.

D'Augelli, A.R., Grossman, A.H., Salter, N.P., Vasey, J.J., Starks, M.T. and Sinclair, K.O. 2005. Predicting the suicide attempts of lesbian, gay, and bisexual youth. *Suicide and Life-Threatening Behavior* 35: 646–660.

Department of Health. 2008. *Reducing Health Inequalities for Lesbian, Gay, Bisexual and Trans People*. London: Department of Health.

Duffy, L. 2005. Suffering, shame and silence: The stigma of HIV/AIDS. *Journal of the Association of Nurses in AIDS Care* 16: 13–20.

Epstein, D., O'Flynn, S. and Telford, D. 2003. *Silenced Sexualities in Schools and Universities*. Stoke on Trent: Trentham.

Fenaughty, J. and Harre, N. 2003. Life on the seesaw: A qualitative study of suicide resiliency factors for young gay men. *Journal of Homosexuality* 45: 1–22.

Fullagar, S. 2003. Wasted lives. *Journal of Sociology* 39: 291–307.

Fullagar, S. 2005. The paradox of promoting help-seeking: A critical analysis of risk, rurality and youth suicide. *Critical Psychology* 14: 31–51.

Furlong, A. and Cartmel, F. 1997. *Young People and Social Change: Individualization and Risk in Late Modernity*. Buckingham: Open University Press.

Gavey, N. 1989. Feminist poststructuralism and discourse analysis: Contributions to feminist psychology. *Psychology of Women Quarterly* 13: 459–475.

Giddens, A. 1991. *Modernity and Self-identity*. Cambridge: Polity Press.

Giddens, A. 1992. *The Transformation of Intimacy: Sexuality, Love and Eroticism in Modern Societies*. Cambridge: Polity Press.

Gilbert, P. 1997. The evolution of social attractiveness and its role in shame, humiliation, guilt and therapy. *British Journal of Medical Psychology* 70: 113–147.

Hawton, K., Rodham, K. and Evans, E. 2006. *By Their Own Hand: Deliberate Self-harm and Suicidal Ideas in Adolescents*. London: Jessica Kingsley.

Henderson, S., Holland, J., McGrellis, S., Sharpe, S. and Thomson, R. 2007. *Inventing Adulthoods: A Biographical Approach to Youth Transitions*. London: SAGE.

Hook, D. 2001. Discourse, knowledge, materiality, history: Foucault and discourse analysis. *Theory and Psychology* 11: 521–547.

King, M., Semlyen, J., See Tai, S., Killaspy, H., Osborn, D., Popelyuk, D. and Nazareth, I. 2008. *Mental Disorders, Suicide and Deliberate Self-harm in Lesbian, Gay and Bisexual People: A Systematic Review*. London: National Institute for Mental Health England.

Lewis, M. 1992. *Shame: The Exposed Self*. New York: Free Press.

MacDonald, R. and Marsh, J. 2005. *Disconnect Youth? Growing up in Britain's Poor Neighbourhoods*. Basingstoke, Hampshire: Palgrave.

Molloy, M., McLaren, S. and McLachlan, A.J. 2003. Young, gay and suicidal: Who cares? *Australian Journal of Psychology* 55: 198.

Monro, F. and Huon, G. 2005. Media-portrayed idealized images, body shame and appearance anxiety. *International Journal of Eating Disorders* 38: 85–90.

Moran, L. and Skeggs, B. 2004. *Sexuality and the Politics of Violence*. London: Routledge.

Munt, S.R. 2000. Shame/pride dichotomies in Queer As Folk. *Textual Practice* 14: 531–546.

Park, A. 2005. *British Social Attitudes: The 22nd Report*. London: SAGE.

Pilkington, N.W. and D'Augelli, A.R. 1995. Victimization of lesbian, gay and bisexual youth in community settings. *Journal of Community Psychology* 23: 33–56.

Probyn, E. 2000. Sporting bodies: Dynamics of shame and pride. *Body and Society* 6: 13–28.

Probyn, E. 2005. *Blush: Faces of Shame*. Minneapolis, MN: University of Minnesota Press.

Rich, A. 1993. Compulsory heterosexuality and lesbian existence. In: H. Abelove, M. Barale and D. Halperin (eds) *The Lesbian and Gay Studies Reader*. London: Routledge, 227–254.

Rivers, I. 1999. *The psycho-social correlates and long-term implications of bullying at school for lesbians, gay men and bisexual men and women*. PhD thesis, University of Surrey.

Rivers, I. 2000. Long-term consequences of bullying. In: C. Neal and D. Davies (eds) *Issues in Therapy with Lesbian, Gay, Bisexual and Transgender Clients*. Buckingham: Open University Press, 146–159.

Rose, N. 1989. *Governing the Soul: The Shaping of the Private Self*. London: Routledge.

Savin-Williams, R. 2005. *The New Gay Teenager*. Cambridge, MA: Harvard University Press.

Savin-Williams, R.C. and Ream, G.L. 2003. Suicide attempts among sexual-minority male youth. *Journal of Clinical Child & Adolescent Psychology* 32: 509–522.

Scheff, T.J. 1994. Emotions and identity: A theory of ethnic nationalism. In: C. Calhoun (ed.) *Social Theory and the Politics of Identity*. Oxford: Blackwell, 277–303.

Scheff, T.J. 2003. Shame in self and society. *Symbolic Interaction* 26: 239–262.

Sedgwick, E. 2003. *Touching, Feeling: Affect, Pedagogy, Performativity*. Durham, NC: Duke University Press.

Stonewall. 2007. *School Report: The Experiences of Young Gay People in Britain's Schools*. London: Stonewall.

UK Parliament. 2003. *The Employment Equality (Sexual Orientation) Regulations*. London: The Stationery Office.

UK Parliament. 2004. *Civil Partnership Act*. London: The Stationery Office.

UK Parliament. 2007. *The Equality Act (Sexual Orientation) Regulations*. London: The Stationery Office.

UK Parliament. 2008. *Criminal Justice and Immigration Act*. London: The Stationery Office.

Valentine, G. and Skelton, T. 2003. Finding oneself, losing oneself: The lesbian and gay 'scene' as a paradoxical space. *International Journal of Urban and Regional Research* 27: 849–866.

Valentine, G., Skelton, T. and Butler, R. 2002. The vulnerability and marginalisation of lesbian and gay youth: Ways forward. *Youth and Policy* 75: 4–29.

Weeks, J. 2007. *The World We Have Won*. London: Routledge.

Wichstrøm, L. and Hegna, K. 2003. Sexual orientation and suicide attempt: A longitudinal study of the general Norwegian adolescent population. *Journal of Abnormal Psychology* 112: 144–151.

Willig, C. 2003. Discourse analysis. In: J. Smith (ed.) *Qualitative Psychology: A Practical Guide to Methods*. London: SAGE.

Chapter 16

Barriers to post-exposure prophylaxis (PEP) completion after rape

A South African qualitative study

Naeemah Abrahams and Rachel Jewkes

Introduction

In South Africa, being infected with HIV during rape is a great concern for women (Christofides *et al.* 2005). Where it occurs, the assault leaves an indelible and often fatal legacy. In order to prevent this, South Africa's Cabinet approved the provision of post-exposure prophylaxis (PEP) in public health services following sexual assaults in April 2002. Many services were initiated across the country with new models of care, including the use of nurses trained in forensics; the introduction of one-stop centres (Thuthuzela Centres); training initiatives; facilities with dedicated rape rooms; and partnerships with non-governmental organisations (NGOs). This was followed in 2005 by the development of the Sexual Assault Policy and Clinical Management Guidelines (South African Department of Health 2005), which articulated a vision of a holistic, needs-centred health service. In 2007, the provision of PEP after a sexual assault was legislated via the Sexual Offences and Related Matters Amendment Act No 23 (South African Government 2007), and this law ensures services are provided free by the state, in designated facilities, with development of minimum standards and the training of providers. Despite these service developments, huge questions remain about rape care in general and the completion of PEP.

Varied levels of adherence and poor follow-up of patients following initiation of PEP have been reported both internationally (Linden *et al.* 2005; Wiebe *et al.* 2000) and locally (Christofides *et al.* 2005; Vetten and Haffejee 2004). Comparisons between studies are complicated by different samples and methods used to measure adherence, and the few South African studies report adherence levels of between 15 and 57 per cent in the public health services (Carries *et al.* 2007; Christofides *et al.* 2005; Collings *et al.* 2008; Mugabo *et al.* 2005; Vetten and Haffejee 2004). Only one example of much higher completion rates was reported by an NGO, the Thohoyandou Victim Empowerment Programme, in Limpopo province (Vetten and Haffejee 2004). Similar low levels of adherence after occupational exposure have been reported in a Cochrane review (Young *et al.* 2009) and other studies (Gupta *et al.* 2008; Siika *et al.* 2009).

Adherence to medication is complex, and research on this has burgeoned in response to the challenges (and research resources) of the highly active antiretroviral therapy (HAART) era. A systematic review of patient-reported barriers and facilitators to antiretroviral therapy (ART) found barriers to be fairly consistent across countries. The 34 qualitative studies (32 from developed countries) identified patient-related, drug-related and interpersonal relationship-related barriers (Mills *et al.* 2006a: 438). Although not as much research has been done on compliance to PEP after sexual violence and occupational exposure, many similar reasons for non-adherence were reported globally (Jagannathan *et al.* 2007; Loutfy *et al.* 2008; Siika *et al.* 2009; Wiebe *et al.* 2000) and in South Africa (Carries *et al.* 2007; Collings *et al.* 2008; Vetten and Haffejee 2004).

Strategies to support adherence (Adamian *et al.* 2004; Golin *et al.* 2006; Mills *et al.* 2006b; Nachega *et al.* 2006) are viewed as critical aspects of the ART programmes and, although not all are applicable to PEP adherence after a sexual assault, of potential relevance are: providing information; using tools like adherence diaries; supporting disclosure; and having social support structures during the period of pill-taking. Many sexual assault services in South Africa appear to neglect the emotional elements that are barriers to care. The higher levels of adherence of the Thohoyandou Victim Empowerment Programme are reported to be related to the multiple strategies developed by this NGO as part of the support and management of rape survivors. These included the employment of a range of personnel to support survivors; regular face-to-face contact; monitoring of side effects; immediate treatment or referrals for further medical management; and active treatment literacy (Vetten and Haffejee 2004).

Mental health barriers have been identified in studies of adherence to HAART (Ammassari *et al.* 2004; Gonzalez *et al.* 2004; Mills *et al.* 2006a; Safren *et al.* 2003) and in qualitative studies of occupational exposure (Chunqing *et al.* 2008; Roets and Ziady 2008), and this may be particularly pertinent to the situation of most rape victims, who struggle with life disruptions and the emotional trauma of the rape. The acute fear and anxiety that follows rape reduces concentration and creates an overwhelming desire to avoid memories of the traumatic event (Burgess and Holmstrom 1974; Resnick 1993). Furthermore, rather than abating, anxiety levels generally increase in the immediate weeks after rape and this can potentially impact greatly on the 28 days during which PEP should be taken.

While the data are patchy, it seems that most rape survivors are not gaining the highly prized protection from HIV transmission because they are not completing their courses of tablets. This chapter presents the findings of a study undertaken to explore rape experiences and PEP use after rape, including the circumstances that facilitate and obstruct these.

Methods

This qualitative study included 29 women aged 16 to 73 years who were recruited at two public health facilities, the Sinawe Centre in the Eastern Cape Province (16 women) and the Karl Bremer sexual assault service in the Western Cape (13 women). Semi-structured, individual, in-depth interviews were conducted with women who tested negative for HIV after rape and agreed to take PEP.

The Sinawe Centre is located in Mthatha, a town of about 250,000 Xhosa-speaking people in an otherwise rural province. The centre forms part of the Mthatha Hospital complex and is managed by the Forensic Services Department of Walter Sisulu University. The centre is exclusively a sexual assault service, open during the daytime, and its staff include a dedicated police officer and social worker. Psychological support for patients and court preparation is available from the social worker or, if necessary, the hospital psychiatric service. There are no NGOs supporting rape survivors in the town.

The Karl Bremer service is one of five public sexual assault services in the urban Cape Metropole. Located within a secondary hospital complex, it provides a 24-hour service. The hospital generally serves the northern suburbs of Cape Town, and its catchment includes large areas of subeconomic housing and informal settlements. There is a local working class community that lives on the periphery of the hospital, and most patients come from backgrounds characterised by high levels of unemployment, poverty and overcrowding. The service at the centre is exclusively medical, and rape survivors are referred to volunteer counsellors. There is no NGO working on rape in the area.

The services provided PEP according to the South African policy of prescribing combination therapy of Zidovudine and Lamivudine for 28 days, started within 72 hours of the rape in HIV-negative individuals. Dispensing practices depended on the availability of HIV testing and counselling, resources for return visits, and patient readiness to test for HIV. The majority of the women were tested immediately, and only two women at the Cape Town site were given a 3-day starter pack of PEP and asked to return for the test. The assortment of medication prescribed included: PEP medication to be taken twice a day for 28 days, with most women given prescriptions initially for 7, 14 or 28 days, with return visits planned to collect the remaining medication; antibiotics to be taken for 7 days for the treatment of sexually transmitted infections; and emergency contraception (if not pregnant) taken for 2 days and anti-emetics normally prescribed for between 5 and 7 days. In addition, in Mthatha women received the PEP drugs as separate drugs, while in Cape Town the combination drug was dispensed. The women left the service with many different pills and complex instructions on dosage, with great potential for side effects.

Interviews were conducted in 2005–2006, first in Cape Town and then Mthatha. In Cape Town, between one and three interviews were conducted with each woman. All 13 women had one interview during the time of taking PEP, 9 women had a second interview at the end of taking the course and one woman had a third interview (total of 23 interviews). In the Eastern Cape site, for logistical reasons, one interview was conducted with each woman (16 interviews) within a week after the expected completed date of the PEP. The majority of the interviews took place at participants' homes, and a few interviews took place in the researcher's car if privacy in the home could not be ensured.

Permission to access the sites was granted by the relevant health authorities. Information sheets were left at the centres, and the nursing staff approached HIV-negative women aged 16 years or over who accepted PEP medication to ask them to give consent to be contacted by a researcher. The details of those agreeing were forwarded to the researcher. The researcher contacted the women, explained about the study, and made arrangements to meet, at which point the final agreement to participate was sought and a consent form signed.

The scope of enquiry for the interviews included experiences of the rape, health service use, support received, responses from others, disclosing to others, coping after the rape, and experiences of taking PEP, including motivations and barriers to its use. We assessed adherence by self-disclosure and probed whether participants returned to collect follow-up medication and if any tablets were missed. If possible, we asked to see the tablet containers and had a discussion around medication that was not used. The interviews were conducted in the respondent's preferred language, Xhosa, English or Afrikaans. They were recorded and transcribed verbatim before being translated into English. The data were analysed inductively, with analysis commenced during data collection and, where there were multiple interviews, the first interviews were analysed before the follow-up interviews. This assisted in planning the follow-up interviews. The interviews were initially coded into categories that drew on the main themes of the scope of enquiry and with subcoding stages driven by ideas emerging from the data. The data were analysed by both authors.

The Medical Research Council's Ethics Committee gave ethical approval for the study, but ethical issues that arose included women requiring further psychosocial support and the removal of leftover medication. As part of the study plan, provision was made to refer women who demonstrated mental health problems to relevant services.

Results

Sample

The women's ages ranged from 16 to 73 years, with only two from Mthatha below the age of 18 years. The mean age of women from Mthatha was 32.2 years, and 26.6 years for Cape Town. The majority of participants based in Cape Town were single and urban, while 9 of the 16 women from Mthatha lived in rural settings. Only 9 completed their PEP medication: 4 from Mthatha and 5 from Cape Town.

Incident of rape

The interviews commenced with accounts of the rapes that demonstrated their diversity. In Mthatha, rapists were generally known to the women as young men of the village and, if their name was not known, others in the community could often recognise them. In Cape Town, in contrast, perpetrators were often strangers attacking women walking alone. Some were intimate partners, and in all of these cases the women were in the process of leaving their husbands after long periods of abuse.

Two sisters were raped by two men on the eve of a family funeral. They were instructed by them to hand over their phones and the men demanded the money that was paid by the funeral scheme (*umbutho*) for the funeral at gun point. Some women were tricked. In Mthatha, a woman had opened the door at night because the perpetrator pretended to be her brother. A Cape Town woman was raped accompanying a man purporting to offer a room to rent. Another was escorted home by an acquaintance from a tavern and dragged into an empty school ground. Other rapes were by men who had propositioned them, been rejected and then raped them. Such violence in the face of outright rejection of a proposition has been discussed by researchers (Wood *et al.* 2008).

Another common pattern described in Mthatha was rape occurring when sharing a room with friends or acquaintances after a night drinking together. A common practice in this region was for people to share sleeping space in a room at the *shebeen* (tavern) or at the nearest homestead rather than risking a dangerous walk home. Vatiswa, a 29-year-old woman from Mthatha, explained:

> We were drinking alcohol because there was a party and we went to sleep like we used to in the sitting room. When I woke up around 12 o'clock in the middle of the night a boy that was sleeping in the same room was on top of me.

Barriers experienced

All participants reported experiencing one or more barriers that could potentially have influenced the taking of medication, and although the side effects of the drugs was the dominant experience reported by 18 participants, it was not necessarily a barrier to taking the medication, as discussed later. The second most common factor that appeared to have influenced adherence was being blamed or fear of being blamed for the rape (reported by

11 women), followed by poor knowledge (9 women) and poor social support (9 women). However, most women experienced multiple barriers, and a supportive social environment and knowledge of the role of the PEP appeared to have mediated other barriers such as fear of HIV, which was less common and reported by 5 participants from the rural site and 2 from Cape Town. Also more common in Mthatha was the role of poverty, such as not having transport money, which was mentioned by only one woman in Cape Town.

Pathways to care

Most women received assistance from the police, often having had help from family members and neighbours. In the process the meanings of events evolved. Two women were told by police that their experience included rape when they reported physical assault by their partners to the police. A woman explained she had not realised a husband could rape his wife:

> I was assaulted. So first it was just an assault case. He didn't really force himself on me ... I didn't put up any resistance – and I didn't say no either. I just lay down. I just waited for him to finish and to go ... It was probably for 10 minutes, but I felt nothing. I was so angry ... But my case wasn't really as bad, I am not worried as much about the rape itself. It was more about the beating that has been happening for many years.
>
> (Norma, from Cape Town, aged 44 years)

A 16-year-old was taken to the police by her mother, but she believed her experience was not rape. She explained:

> I went to East London with this man, we slept in a hotel, he told me he wanted to sleep with me and I did not want to. He forced me ... I believe when I went to East London ... it was my choice, it was not rape to me but my mother believed it was rape and the police told me that it was not good for an old man to sleep with me. So they want me to call it a rape.
>
> (Bongwekazi, from Mthatha, aged 16 years)

Rape stigma also played a role in accessing care and was clearly demonstrated by Busi, a young woman (aged 22 years) who, despite being encouraged by her boyfriend to report the rape to the police, initially refused to do so because she 'did not want to be associated with rape'. For other women, not being believed or expecting to be blamed were often the reasons why they did not tell others about the rape.

Accounts of help-seeking demonstrated that, even after rape, women often had multiple priorities. A woman who was a street vendor was raped in the early morning and was only able to go to the local hospital after she had set up her business and found someone to watch her products. Through this she missed a day's work, and explained that she decided not to attend further appointments to collect medication because without help she would lose earnings and perhaps her business.

In the rural area, women were transported back to their homes by the police. This did not happen as often in the urban site where family or friends assisted with transport. Many women spoke about spending time at home before returning to work or school. One young woman from Mthatha was very distressed and stayed home for a month after the rape.

Assigning blame and receiving support

Fear of being blamed for the rape often influenced help-seeking. Some young women blamed themselves when they were raped while drinking alcohol, visiting *shebeens* or walking around at night. More than one woman concealed the rape from her parents because of self-blame. Another told her parents but they preferred to believe that she was lying and the perpetrator was a boyfriend. Victim-blaming was also seen when a schoolgirl raped by a fellow learner was ridiculed by the community for reporting the rape to police, leading to the consequent arrest of the perpetrator.

Silence and non-communication from others about the rape incident were also perceived as signs of being blamed for the rape. A woman who had serious self-esteem problems because of feelings of guilt and shame said that, although she lived with her mother and saw her daily, she never asked about the rape, the progress of the police investigations or about the outcome of the HIV tests.

Responses from family members were not all negative, but were influenced by the victim's age and a notion of 'deserving victimhood'. Older women were often considered more credible, even if they had been drinking, and self-blame and shame were less evident in their experiences. They were also more likely to be supported by community members in the identification and arrest of the perpetrators. Assistance and support were more forthcoming if the perpetrator was a known troublemaker. In contrast, if a community feared a perpetrator, they were not as willing to assist.

Although community members were more willing to assist in the rural setting, some reluctance to get involved and judgement about worthiness for support was also visible. Two women, both married, and raped in similar circumstances while walking home at night, called for help. One, whose husband was out of town, received no further support, while the other, who was older and who was raped by a nephew, was accompanied home and her husband was told what had happened. With the former, the perpetrator's explanation that 'nothing happened' was accepted despite there being witnesses to her calls for help. This created much distress and she feared being blamed by her husband. After 2 days, a friend accompanied her to the rape centre, at which time her primary motivation was to avoid pregnancy and being accused by her husband of bringing HIV into the relationship.

In the rural Eastern Cape, village Headmen were often the first source of assistance. Usually, the rape and its perpetrator(s) were reported to them and they were asked to facilitate transport to the police. This assistance was not always provided. One woman aged 60 was not helped because the young perpetrator was related to the Headman, while another woman was evicted by the local Headman from the village after she reported her uncle to the police after many years of rape.

A few women were assisted by family, colleagues, neighbours and friends with transport money to return to the clinic. Carol, a 25-year-old woman from Cape Town, explained how caring her husband became, 'paying much more attention to me. He is caring. He would phone me during the day to hear how I am doing.' At the same time she was distrustful as he was also 'withdrawn' at times and she felt that 'later I know he's going to throw it back to my face'. The way in which rape affected relationships was further illustrated by a woman who had initial support from her boyfriend, who later moved out saying he was 'very angry, he wanted to beat them [the rapists] … he decided that he cannot stay here and went to build that shack …' (Donna, a 43-year-old woman from Cape Town).

Women's position in their social milieu also determined their support from others and their worthiness of sympathy. A woman did not bother to seek assistance from others because she said she was already isolated in the community because of her alcohol drinking and absence of family, whereas the sisters raped at the family funeral received immediate help with the identification of the perpetrators and their banishment from the community.

Gossip was also feared, and prevented many women from telling others about the rape. Ann, a 39-year-old woman from Cape Town, said she considered 'suicide rather than to face people' because 'everyone has something bad to say about me'. She felt that her family was 'rejoicing' as they had been jealous of her rich husband. The additional layer of racist slurs was added when she was called a '*kaffir meid*', a racist label given to Coloured[1] or White women who have relationships with African men.

Women who spoke of fear of being stigmatised for the rape were often already marginalised in the communities, had little social support, and often had had other traumas in their lives, including previous sexual assault. Busi, a 22-year-old woman who was living with a friend while attending school, explained that 'I was scared of stigma' as the reason why she did not want to report the rape. Very distressed, she had stayed away from school for a month. Vatiswa (29 years old) withdrew her case because of the community's responses in blaming her; she later explained that she had been raped before by her brother, and her family didn't do anything, and she said, 'I realise that they don't care.'

Taking of PEP, and side effects

While grappling with these complex aspects of the context of rape, women found they also had to negotiate the taking of medication.

> The first packet I used to take three times a day, the other one two times a day and the last one in a bottle two times a day also. But there [in the clinic] they gave me four, I think they were four, and they said I must swallow them all together. Four tablets and then the other ones were also four and then two.
>
> (Lebo, from Mthatha, aged 44 years)

The previous extract shows how enormously complex the taking of tablets after rape is and how it may require considerable concentration and determination.

Nausea was a common side effect, and most women were given anti-emetics and found they could cope well. Some said they did not have any side effects, explaining, 'I didn't feel anything.' And yet, when this was further probed, we learned they had experienced nausea and vomiting, but their expression of not experiencing the side effects rather meant they could cope, as the following extract from an older woman who lived in Mthatha shows:

> Participant: No, I did not notice anything … What I noticed was a discharge …
> Interviewer: OK, otherwise you did not notice anything like nausea?
> Participant: Yes I used to have nausea, I would tell the others … if I was still able to reproduce I would say I am pregnant … [laugh].
>
> (Chumisa, from Mthatha, aged 49 years)

Other side effects described by women included diarrhoea, itchy rash (which may actually have been ringworm), headaches, dizziness and 'becoming blind', described as a side effect compounded by hunger. One woman who adhered attributed her emotional state to the taking of the tablets and their side effects:

> ... one minute I'd be the happiest person under the sun, I'll be so healthy ... and the next I'll be so down and feeling so awful. Some mornings I just won't get up you know, and it makes me so nauseous. Sometimes it makes me like I can't eat or anything.
>
> (Debbie, from Cape Town, aged 23 years)

Not coping with side effects

There was a group of women who spoke of not being able to cope with their side effects and explained this to be a contributing factor to the stopping of the medication. A notable feature of this group of women from Mthatha was that they were all distressed by the notion of taking antiretroviral (ARV) medication because 'ARVs are only given to people that are HIV-positive'.

A woman who explained she had been given 'ARVs to clean the virus' became tormented by the fear of taking 'HIV tablets'. In the next extract she emphasised the problem with nausea in a way that contradicted the earlier part of her interview, and this suggested that the combination of feeling ill from the medication and the association of the drugs with the AIDS illness created immense distress and was a barrier to taking PEP:

> I took the tablets and when I got home it was like they said I was HIV-positive. For 2 weeks taking the tablets became more and more difficult knowing that I am taking HIV tablets ... I think maybe if I did not know that they were for HIV maybe I would have taken the tablets with more enthusiasm ... It's like, I'm going to live like this, to take the tablets and feel nauseous, and you think, oh my God if I am HIV-positive I will vomit up until I die and becoming sick every day ... I promise you the time you take the tablets it's difficult to take them even to swallow and you feel like not up to it ... it's a sentence, sentence for being raped.
>
> (Busi, from Mthatha, aged 22 years)

This same individual responded to the fear by taking the pills once a day instead of twice. The taking of medication reminded both Busi and Ntombekhaya of the rape and created much distress. This was despite having tested HIV-negative and having been told that the tablets were for HIV prevention:

> Participant: I tried to take the tablets several times but I vomited and I decided to stop taking it. I did not go back to Sinawe because I did not want to cheat.
> Interviewer: How many days did you take the tablets?
> Participant: Once, after taking the tablets in the morning I vomited, then I tried to take another tablet during the day but still I was vomiting and at night I took the tablets but I could not sleep. I realised that what would be troubling me was to know why I was taking these tablets ... I decided to stop.
>
> (Ntombekhaya, from Mthatha, aged 23 years)

Information management

In general, rape services provided patients with a lot of information and most of the women interviewed had a very good basic understanding of the tests that were done at the clinic, the different tablets, how to take them and follow-up appointments. This was quite impressive as the treatment was complex and, without printed information, patients were required to recall what they were told or refer to notes jotted down for them. However, there was one group of participants who seemed to have focused knowledge gaps around HIV-related matters. While this may indicate a lack of explanation about HIV by service providers, the data suggest that this may not be the explanation and could be another manifestation of the fear of HIV. The knowledge gaps seem to have been deployed by the rape survivors as a way of enabling them to comply with treatment, which they would have found more difficult if they had made themselves face up to the HIV implications of this.

Knowledge had a complex relationship with adherence. One of the two women who completed all their pills was notably ill-informed. Another had a great deal of uncomplicated faith in her treatment; she said she had never thought of not completing the course because she was told by the policeman that he would take her to the clinic where she will receive 'good stuff'. While other women who took their medication demonstrated very clear understanding of its purpose, very often they had no more understanding than others who did not adhere. One explained:

> I believe that I should not take the pills as people who are HIV-positive take them to keep them healthy. I was not HIV-positive so that is why I stopped taking the tablets because I was negative.
>
> (Bongwekazi, from Mthatha, aged 16 years)

Some of the women struggled to organise their pill-taking schedule. Such forgetfulness and trying to fit the pill-taking into daily routines have been reported as common barriers among patients taking ART (Mills *et al.* 2006a: 438). In the study, it was not clear whether women were told what to do if they missed doses, but those who were more motivated to complete the pills developed strategies to try and complete the medication. These included taking the pills as soon as they remembered, doubling the dose the next time or just continuing with the schedule and completing in much more than 28 days.

Social support, poverty and adherence

Several of the research participants described receiving support in taking their medication, which they identified as helpful. Women were reminded by employers, mothers, aunts and school friends. One girl explained, 'I was taking them every day, even my friends at school used to remind me.' However, others, conspicuously, were not supported. Two women who complained to the sister and boyfriend about the PEP medication and clinic visits were advised just to stop them.

Poverty was a particular barrier in Mthatha as the site drew clients from a broad catchment area and transport costs were high and the local population generally poorer. The clinic practice provided pills for 2 weeks and then required a further visit to collect the final 14-days' tablets. A few women had not returned, citing lack of money, although it was unclear whether this was the only reason or seemed a more acceptable explanation. One research participant who did not take her pills did so because she did not have enough food. Other participants said they were working, travelling or attending a funeral on the day of their appointment so did not return. These women who did not return did not speak about concerns about the threat of HIV infection either.

Impact of psychological responses to rape and adherence

When the project was conceptualised we had envisaged hearing many accounts of the way in which psychological reactions to rape impacted on treatment adherence. With the exception of blame and the pills serving as a reminder of the rape, the interviews were more notable for the infrequency with which general psychological responses were discussed. One notable exception was a woman from Cape Town, who was suffering severely from memory impairment and demonstrated avoidance behaviours, both of which are recognised symptoms of post-traumatic stress. She took almost none of her tablets because they reminded her of the rape. She explained:

> One moment I remember ... and then I can't ... One moment I want to remember everything – and the next moment I want to wipe it all out ... I should have been taking more than I have done ... but I really can't ... it's like a reminder of something bad. Often I don't take the tablets on time – especially if I want to just be myself – then the tablets really are in my way. Now, there are days when I take it and there are days when I don't ... [The participant also described how she had attempted to commit suicide.]
> (Ann, from Cape Town, aged 39 years)

There was one other woman whose immediate reactions to rape (described as being 'stressed') seemed to have influenced her adherence. She left the clinic and went to a friend's place and got drunk there. It was not clear whether she actually had a substance abuse problem or had just medicated her initial response to the rape with alcohol, but having not started the tablets as directed because she was drinking, she then never took them. She was one of the women who had a severe problem with HIV stigma associated with ARVs.

Discussion

Adherence to ART in the period after rape is a challenging process; only one-in-three informants completed their PEP regimen, and only two women seemed not to have missed any doses. While medical advice on adherence very strongly emphasises the importance of trying to achieve high levels of overall adherence to the 28-day course, as well as striving to keep doses 12 hours apart, many complex factors coalesce to prevent this happening. Taking the many tablets and following intricate dosage instructions in the first week after the sexual assault was a particularly complex process and it was notable that, despite side effects and other barriers, many of the women tried hard to take the prescribed pills.

On the face of it, factors influencing adherence were similar to those identified for patients on HAART (Mills *et al.* 2006a: 438). These were individual barriers such as self-blame; emotional upheaval created by the trauma of the rape; social support factors including fear of disclosure and being blamed for the rape; factors related to beliefs about the medication, such as complicated regimens and having knowledge gaps about the medication; and not being able to fit medication into a daily schedule. Findings reveal that perceptions of the rape also impacted on adherence. If rape was contested by either the women or those in their social environment, any risk of HIV infection became of secondary importance. Similarly, some women who had knowledge gaps and who were not very conscious of the threat of HIV transmission from rape seemed easily distracted by other priorities. Social support was extremely helpful, but if those in the social networks blamed the victims, or did not believe them, support was not forthcoming. Who the victims and the perpetrators were, the circumstances of the rape, family cohesion and the community perceptions of sexual violence all influenced the women's credibility and offers of support. Blame had a profound psychosocial impact on the women and was notably disempowering and, through this, impacted on adherence.

Fear of HIV had an important impact on adherence to the HIV prevention medication for those from Mthatha. This was mediated by the emotional vulnerability created by the rape experience. Many studies have documented the devastating mental health impact following rape, including depression (Foa and Riggs 1993; Jewkes and Abrahams 2002; Resnick 1993), and although this dimension of the rape was not hugely visible, it appeared that the additional burden of fear of HIV illness played a debilitating role, preventing women from taking the medication. Although the role of HIV stigma has been discussed extensively as a huge impediment for the successful implementation of HIV treatment (Malcolm *et al.* 1998), in contrast, the fear of HIV infection has been discussed as a facilitator in the preventive management of HIV, while for a few women in this study it acted as a barrier. This fear emerged in particular when combined with drug-induced nausea, which created immense distress when they brought to mind ideas about developing HIV-related illnesses. The physical effects of the drugs clearly exacerbated the fear of HIV infection, and the associated illness and sexual assault services should be aware of this as a potential barrier to PEP adherence.

Adherence to PEP medication was also related to having knowledge of the prevention mechanism of the drugs, good relations with health workers and support from important others, which mediated the psychological impact of the rape. Even some women with very shaky knowledge were able to adhere if they had good relationships with the health service and good social support. In contrast, HIV fear and the absence of support interfered with adherence in those who had good knowledge.

The failure of the health services to adequately support PEP course completion was evident in the study. Most women were not actively followed up by the services and, indeed, without this research the services might not have known how low completion rates were. Women were offered no psychological support beyond containment in the immediate post-rape visit and there was no support for adherence either. This was, however, a small qualitative study. We used multiple contacts and interviews with many of the women to try to enhance rapport and understand how barriers to adherence might evolve throughout the first month after the rape. Nonetheless, the findings cannot be generalised outside the study population. The main strengths of the study lie in the ability of the methods to allow unexpected influences on adherence to become visible. In particular, we had not previously expected to see a strong influence of HIV fear on PEP adherence. The extent to which this is a feature more broadly among rape survivors needs to be further explored.

Conclusion

The study has important implications for the understanding and assistance of rape survivors in the period of taking PEP. The medication regimen after rape is complicated for women and often entails navigating drug side effects and the important role of support and transfer of knowledge during this period. The study found fear of rape stigma to be a compelling factor that causes distress, and this should be recognised as a critical aspect in mental health support in the period after rape. These findings are important since PEP adherence following a sexual assault has been relatively resistant to interventions to improve it, and recent intervention research, for example using a leaflet, pill diary and telephonic adherence motivation, was unable to secure any substantial improvement (Abrahams *et al.* 2010). The findings from this qualitative research suggest that the reasons for poor PEP adherence are complex. Fear of being blamed, fear of HIV infection, and poor support have not adequately been taken into account in developing post-rape services, and this clearly points to the need for further research to support the development of programmes that take into account the many complexities involved.

Note

1 During the apartheid era, South Africans were classified by race into Black, Coloured, White and Indian. In using these terms here we do not endorse these distinctions but do continue to reflect a social reality that was created at this time through the segregation of all aspects of daily life.

References

Abrahams, N., Jewkes, R., Lombard, L., Mathews, S., Campbell, J.C. and Meel, B. 2010. Impact of telephonic psycho-social support on adherence to post-exposure prophylaxis (PEP) after rape: A randomised control trial. *AIDS Care* 22(10): 1173–1181.

Adamian, M.S., Golin, C.E., Shain, L.S. and DeVellis, B. 2004. Brief motivational interviewing to improve adherence to antiretroviral therapy: Development and qualitative pilot assessment of an intervention. *AIDS Patient Care and STDs* 18(4): 229–238.

Ammassari, A., Antinori, A., Aloisi, M.S., Trotta, M.P., Murri, R., Bartoli, L., Monforte, A.D., Wu, A.W. and Starace, F. 2004. Depressive symptoms, neurocognitive impairment and adherence to highly active antiretroviral therapy among HIV-infected persons. *Psychosomatics* 45(5): 394–402.

Burgess, A.W. and Holmstrom, L.L. 1974. Rape trauma syndrome. *American Journal of Psychiatry* 131(9): 981–986.

Carries, S., Muller, F., Muller, F.J., Morroni, C. and Wilson, D. 2007. Characteristics, treatment and antiretroviral prophylaxis adherence of South African rape survivors. *Journal of Acquired Immune Deficiency Syndrome* 46(1): 68–71.

Christofides, N.J., Jewkes, R.K., Webster, N., Penn-Kekana, L., Abrahams, N. and Martin, L.J. 2005. 'Other patients are really in need of medical attention': The quality of health services for rape survivors in South Africa. *Bulletin of World Health Organization* 83(7): 495–502.

Chunqing, L., Li, L., Zunyou, W., Sheng, W. and Manhong, J. 2008. Occupational exposure to HIV among healthcare providers: A qualitative study in Yunnan, China. *Journal of the International Association of Physicians in AIDS Care* 7(1): 35–41.

Collings, S.J., Bugwandeen, S.R. and Wiles, W.A. 2008. HIV post-exposure prophylaxis for child rape survivors in KwaZulu-Natal, South Africa: Who qualifies and who complies? *Child Abuse and Neglect* 32(4): 477–483.

Foa, E.B. and Riggs, D.S. 1993. Posttraumatic stress disorder and rape. In: J.M. Oldham and A. Tasman (eds) *Review of Psychiatry*. Washington, DC: American Psychiatric Press, 273–303.

Golin, C., Earp, J., Tien, H.C., Stewart, P., Porter, C. and Howie, L. 2006. A 2-arm, randomized, controlled trial of a motivational interviewing-based intervention to improve adherence to antiretroviral therapy (ART) among patients failing or initiating ART. *Journal of Acquired Immune Deficiency Syndrome* 42(1): 42–51.

Gonzalez, J.S., Penedo, F.J., Antoni, M.H., Duran, R.E., Pherson-Baker, S., Ironson, G., Isabel, F.M., Klimas, N.G., Fletcher, M.A. and Schneiderman, N. 2004. Social support, positive states of mind and HIV treatment adherence in men and women living with HIV/AIDS. *Health Psychology* 23(4): 413–418.

Gupta, A., Anand, S., Sastry, J., Krisagar, A., Basavaraj, A., Bhat, S.M., Gupte, N., Bollinger, R.C. and Kakrani, A.L. 2008. High risk for occupational exposure to HIV and utilization of post-exposure prophylaxis in a teaching hospital in Pune, India. *BMC Infectious Diseases* 8: 142.

Jagannathan, P., Landovitz, R. and Roland, M.E. 2007. Post-exposure prophylaxis after sexual exposure to HIV. *Future HIV Therapy* 1(1): 35–47.

Jewkes, R. and Abrahams, N. 2002. The epidemiology of rape and sexual coercion in South Africa: An overview. *Social Science and Medicine* 55(7): 1231–1244.

Linden, J.A., Oldeg, P., Mehta, S.D., McCabe, K.K. and LaBelle, C. 2005. HIV post-exposure prophylaxis in sexual assault: Current practice and patient adherence to treatment recommendations in a large urban teaching hospital. *Academic Emergency Medicine* 12(7): 640–646.

Loutfy, M.R., Macdonald, S., Myhr, T., Husson, H., Du, M.J., Balla, S., Antoniou, T. and Rachlis, A. 2008. Prospective cohort study of HIV post-exposure prophylaxis for sexual assault survivors. *Antiviral Therapy* 13(1): 87–95.

Malcolm, A., Aggleton, P., Bronfman, M., Galvão, J., Mane, P. and Verrall, J. 1998. HIV-related stigmatization and discrimination: Its forms and contexts. *Critical Public Health* 8(4): 347–370.

Mills, E.J., Nachega, J.B., Bangsberg, D.R., Singh, S., Rachlis, B., Wu, P., Wilson, K., Buchan, I., Gill, C.J. and Cooper, C. 2006a. Adherence to HAART: A systematic review of developed and developing nation patient-reported barriers and facilitators. *PLoS Medicine* 3(11): e438.

Mills, E.J., Nachega, J.B., Buchan, I., Orbinski, J., Attaran, A., Singh, S., Rachlis, B., Wu, P., Cooper, C., Thabane, L., Wilson, K., Guyatt, G.H. and Bangsberg, D.R. 2006b. Adherence to antiretroviral therapy in sub-Saharan Africa and North America: A meta-analysis. *Journal of the American Medical Association* 296(6): 679–690.

Mugabo, P., Shabodien, A., Mahlobo, H., Phillips, A., Makiti, S., Africa, D. and Mbalo, M. 2005. *Management of HIV infection in rape survivors in the Cape Metropole*. Paper presented at South African Gender Based Violence and Health Conference, 16–18 October, in Stellenbosch, South Africa.

Nachega, J.B., Knowlton, A.R., Deluca, A., Schoeman, J.H., Watkinson, L., Efron, A., Chaisson, R.E. and Maartens, G. 2006. Treatment support to improve adherence to antiretroviral therapy in HIV-infected South African adults: A qualitative study. *Journal of Acquired Immune Deficiency Syndromes* 43(Suppl. 1): S127–133.

Resnick, P.A. 1993. The psychological impact of rape. *Journal of Interpersonal Violence* 8(2): 223–255.

Roets, L. and Ziady, L.E. 2008. The nurses' experience of possible HIV infection after injury and/or exposure on duty. *Curationis* 31: 13–23.

Safren, S.A., Gershuny, B.S. and Hendriksen, E. 2003. Symptoms of posttraumatic stress and death anxiety in persons with HIV and medication adherence difficulties. *AIDS Patient Care and STDs* 17(12): 657–664.

Siika, A.M., Nyandiko, W.M., Mwangi, A., Waxman, M., Sidle, J.E., Kimaiyo, S.N. and Wools-Kaloustian, K. 2009. The structure and outcomes of a HIV postexposure prophylaxis program in a high HIV prevalence setup in western Kenya. *Journal of Acquired Immune Deficiency Syndromes* 51(1): 47–53.

South African Department of Health. 2005. *National Sexual Assault Policy*. Pretoria: South African Department of Health.

South African Government. 2007. *Sexual Offences and Related Matters, Amendment Act No 23*. Pretoria: South African Government.

Vetten, L. and Haffejee, S. 2004. *Factors Affecting Adherence to Post-exposure Prophylaxis in the Aftermath of Sexual Assault*. Johannesburg: Centre for the Study of Violence.

Wiebe, E.R., Comay, S.E., McGregor, M. and Ducceschi, S. 2000. Offering HIV prophylaxis to people who have been sexually assaulted: 16 months' experience in a sexual assault service. *Canadian Medical Association Journal* 162(5): 641–645.

Wood, K., Lambert, H. and Jewkes, R. 2008. 'Injuries are beyond love': Physical violence in young South Africans' sexual relationships. *Medical Anthropology* 27(1): 43–69.

Young, T.N., Arens, F.J., Kennedy, G.E., Laurie, J.W. and Rutherford, G. 2009. Antiretroviral post-exposure prophylaxis (PEP) for occupational HIV exposure. *Cochrane Database Systematic Review* 1: CD002835.

Section 6

Mobility and migration

A considerable literature exists which seeks to examine the intersections between health, sexuality, migration and mobility. The three chapters in this section provide excellent insights into some of the key themes that have emerged within these fields in recent years, and reflect the diverse population groups and geographical contexts in which such important research has taken place.

Published at a time when HIV prevalence was rising and evangelical and Pentecostal Christian churches were rapidly expanding their influence across much of West Africa, Daniel Jordan Smith's chapter examines the ways in which religious moral frameworks influence perceptions of HIV-related risk amongst young rural–urban migrants in Nigeria. Central to this chapter is recognition of the role of the church in providing an important community for young Igbo people who have moved away from kinship groups to pursue their ambitions in urban areas. While many churches were found to provide positive support for people affected by HIV, a more prevalent discourse of immorality was found to contribute to the ongoing stigmatisation of the disease. Smith explores the ways that young migrants use these kinds of religious discourses to make sense of the HIV epidemic and, importantly, how they then conceptualise their own sense of risk in relation to their sexual behaviour as 'born again' Christians. His findings suggest that popular religious interpretations of HIV led many young migrants to believe themselves to be at little or no risk of HIV, and to contribute to inconsistent protective practices. At the same time, however, the potentially important role of the church is acknowledged in delaying sexual debut and partner reduction amongst young rural–urban migrants. There is a need to move away from simplistic one-dimensional intervention strategies, to more holistic approaches that recognise the intersections between religion, health, sexuality and morality.

The importance of transcending too narrowly defined forms of health intervention is also the focus of the second chapter in this section. Here, Elanah Uretsky argues that it is necessary to look beyond traditional target groups for HIV prevention, to also include other populations that are known to engage in 'high risk' sexual behaviour. Implicit within this argument is the need to respond to the local sociocultural and politico-economic context in which sexual activity takes place. In this chapter, Uretsky examines the potential for high-risk sexual behaviour amongst wealthy, mobile businessmen and government officials in urban China, where HIV prevalence has risen sharply in recent years. While political and social status has precluded these men from being engaged with as part of HIV prevention, it is increasingly recognised that the unofficial aspects of their work that are required to build and maintain successful business relationships, i.e. through entertainment which involves sex with female entertainers and 'minor' wives, expose them and their partners to the risk of sexually transmitted infections, including HIV. As Uretsky reminds us, work within the field of public health and human rights has helped to define sex work primarily as work undertaken by women. Yet as this chapter makes clear, it is important to also recognise the contexts in which the soliciting of sexual services is defined as an inherent and expected component of men's work, and to understand how the increasingly mobile nature of many professions can exacerbate risky sexual behaviour.

Over the past two decades, research has demonstrated the increasingly disparate health and well-being experiences reported by migrants from different sociocultural and economic backgrounds. Very often, such research has shown how migrants from economically developed countries and those classed as highly skilled are able to access and make productive use of key health services both within the host country and beyond, whilst those from less advantaged backgrounds struggle to access health care and support. In the third chapter in this section, Pardis Mahdavi examines how migrants from different countries working in the United Arab Emirates' sex industry are both racialised and spatialised. Emerging alongside Dubai's development as a key global city over the past two decades, the sex industry now includes women from the Middle East, Eastern Europe, East Asia and Africa. Through in-depth qualitative research undertaken over several years, Mahdavi explores the ways in which certain monetary and moral values are placed on these women's bodies through forms of localised racism, which are in turn reinforced through what Mahdavi argues are misinformed Western assumptions relating to victimhood and agency. Such thinking, she argues, makes overly simplistic assumptions which construct those relegated to the lower end of the sex industry by virtue of their perceived 'race' as innocent victims of 'trafficking', whilst simultaneously stereotyping those at the higher end of the industry as guilty and undeserving of support. These responses not only overlook the agency of those at the lower end by creating an artificial dichotomy of force and choice, but also deny support to those working at the higher end, even when they may require protection.

Chapter 17

Youth, sin and sex in Nigeria

Christianity and HIV/AIDS-related beliefs and behaviour among rural–urban migrants

Daniel Jordan Smith

Introduction

In Nigeria, as in much of sub-Saharan Africa, young people are embracing evangelical and Pentecostal Christianity in rapidly growing numbers. While the reasons for the popularity of what Nigerians call 'new breed' or 'born again' churches are multiple and complex, these churches provide systems of meaning that are appealing to young people and especially to those who have migrated from their rural communities of origin to urban areas in search of further education, employment or business opportunities. These churches provide powerful symbolic interpretations of contemporary Nigerian society, aiding people in navigating a social world in which ambitions are expanding but poverty and inequality remain profound. Church teachings explain social injustices in terms of morality and promise prosperity to those who have faith and live righteously. To some extent, church congregations also create new communities, building social networks that replace, or at least augment, the kinship groups from which young migrants can be somewhat removed because of their mobility and alienated from because of their ambitions and frustrations. For young Nigerians who are 'born again', and indeed for many others who do not belong to these 'new breed' churches, but are heavily influenced by increasingly dominant public discourses about the connections between individual religious morality and the prospects for prosperity, a Christian world view strongly influences the understanding of social problems.

By the end of 2001, the HIV prevalence rate among adults (aged 15–49) in Nigeria was estimated to be 5.8 per cent (UNAIDS 2002), with a total of approximately 3.5 million people infected. A widely publicized US intelligence report called *The Next Wave of HIV/AIDS* suggested that Nigeria's adult prevalence rate would increase to 18–26 per cent by 2010, and that the number of infected individuals would increase to 10–15 million (National Intelligence Council 2002). While numbers and estimates regarding HIV/AIDS in Nigeria must be interpreted with caution and have wide margins of error, nothing of this magnitude has come to pass. More recent estimates are that Nigeria's HIV prevalence among people aged 15–49 is 3.1 per cent (UNAIDS 2014). Nonetheless, Nigeria has the third largest absolute number of people living with HIV/AIDS in the world, after only South Africa and India.

To a significant extent, Nigerians view HIV/AIDS as a social problem that is the result of immorality, emblematic of a widely shared sense that most of the country's worst problems – poverty, inequality, corruption, crime and now HIV/AIDS – are the result of immoral behaviour. The sense of moral decline in Nigeria long precedes HIV/AIDS, and is related to complex political economic issues such as the disappointments of development and democracy (Achebe 1983; Orewa 1997; Nwankwo 1999), the decline in economic well-being following the collapse of Nigeria's oil boom in the 1970s (Watts 1992), and tensions between kin that emerge with urbanization and exacerbated inequality (Bastian 1993). Christianity is by no means the only idiom through which these discontents are expressed. The older generation wields notions of tradition and custom to criticize the young, and young people mobilize ideas about modernity to disparage the constraints of village life (Geschiere 1997; Renne 2003). But in the era of AIDS, the 'born again' Christian perspective is a primary lens through which many young Nigerians, especially young migrants, interpret the disease, assess their risk, and negotiate their sexual relationships.

In this chapter, the intersection of HIV/AIDS and Christianity in Nigeria is examined, focusing on understanding the social processes whereby HIV risk is equated with religious immorality. Drawing on a 2-year study of young rural–urban migrants in two cities in Nigeria, I describe and analyse how young Nigerians use a Christian moral framework to make sense of the epidemic, but also how they conceptualize their own sense of risk in relation to their sexual behaviour. The connections between religion, morality and sexuality for young migrants are complex. For some, religious views serve as a reason for abstinence; for others, religion provides a justification for the morality of certain sexual relationships (and, therefore, the lack of risk in those relationships); and for still others, such views are a source of ambivalence and denial, when sexual behaviour cannot legitimately fit into a Christian framework, but people are nonetheless affected by powerful moral sanctions.

Methods

The study reported here was undertaken between 2001 and 2003, and looked at HIV/AIDS-related beliefs and behaviour among Igbo-speaking adolescent and young adult rural–urban migrants in two Nigerian cities, Aba and Kano.[1] The primary research methods included sample surveys of 863 young migrants in the two cities, in-depth life history interviews with 20 young migrants in each city, several months of participant observation by the author, and 18 months of continuous participant observation conducted by a young migrant who was hired as a research assistant. Criteria for inclusion in the survey were that respondents were between the ages of 15 and 24, had migrated to the city after age 12, had lived in the city for at least 3 months, were of Igbo ethnicity, and had never married. Respondents were selected randomly, using a grid to divide the study areas into zones from which interviewers identified eligible migrants. Approximately 50 per cent of the sample was female. Igbo-speaking undergraduates, graduate students and young faculty members from local universities were trained to conduct the survey interviews. The survey questionnaire included modules on migration history, education and employment, religious affiliation and practices, sexual history and behaviour, HIV/AIDS awareness and sociodemographic background. In-depth life history interviews were conducted by the author. These interviews focused primarily on migration histories, sexual behaviour and understandings of HIV/AIDS, but they were open-ended and produced numerous dialogues about religious understandings of sexuality and AIDS.

Participant observation took place over approximately 6 months of fieldwork undertaken in the summers of 2001, 2002 and 2003. Participant observation included spending time with migrants in their homes and their places of work, but also accompanying them to church, observing meetings of their home village associations in the city, and hanging out at bars, restaurants and other night spots that were popular with some of the migrants.

The research assistant lived in a block of flats occupied by young migrants in Aba, and was paid to undertake participant observation with his neighbours and with a dozen other young migrant key informants. Each month he provided detailed field notes about his observations and informal interviews and received feedback with instructions on issues or questions to pursue further.

Results

Christianity in Nigeria

Christianity has been an important direct influence on the Igbo population (as well as other groups) in Nigeria for more than 100 years. Indeed, considerable attention has been paid to the relative receptivity of Igbos to Christianity during the colonial period, both by Western (Ottenberg 1959) and indigenous scholars (Ilogu 1974; Isichei 1976; DomNwachukwu 2000). While Christianity has been a dominant feature of the Igbo cultural landscape for many decades, the recent dramatic rise of Pentecostal and evangelical churches is especially striking.

Prominent themes in the recent literature on Christianity in Africa include the role of Pentecostalism in African peoples' efforts to negotiate globalization and associated social and economic transformations (Gifford 1990; Marshall 1993; Marshall-Fratani 1998), and the intersection of contemporary Christian discourses with accusations of witchcraft and rumours about the occult that similarly grapple with issues of politics, social change, poverty and inequality through the idiom of the supernatural (Meyer 1995, 1998; Smith 2001). These accounts highlight the importance of religion in people's understandings of and responses to social, political and economic processes, and suggest that individual behaviour can only be explained if attention is paid to the meanings people attribute to their actions and the actions of others.

While it is important not to exaggerate the extent to which people's religious beliefs translate into everyday behaviour, it is hard to overstate the impact and pervasiveness of Christian beliefs and practices in the lives of most Igbo people. While perhaps only about a quarter of the total Igbo population (an ethnic group of more than 15 million people) belong to churches that can be correctly characterized as Pentecostal or evangelical, the numbers are growing fast. Belonging to 'born again' churches means not only going regularly to church, but participating in weekly fellowship groups, reading a growing popular literature produced by these churches, watching ubiquitous evangelical TV programmes that air daily (and all day Sunday) in Nigeria, and integrating references to God's 'Word' into the routine discourses of everyday life. Indeed, the dramatic rise of 'born again' Christianity has generated what could arguably be called an entire 'cultural style' (cf. Ferguson 1999).

Though the differences in cultural styles between Pentecostals and other young Christians who belong to older churches are not hard and fast, young people who are 'born again' do affect recognizable styles. Their dress is generally neat and professional, but also less sexually provocative than other modern styles. Their talk incorporates references to Jesus regularly and emphatically. Their behaviours, or at least their behavioural expectations, include abstaining from alcohol use and avoiding 'loose' sexuality.

For the young rural–urban migrants in this study, Christianity influenced by the 'born again' cultural style is central to overall world views and interpretations and responses to the HIV/AIDS epidemic. While slightly less than 30 per cent reported belonging to Pentecostal or evangelical churches, only five young Igbo migrants out of a total of 863 interviewed in Aba and Kano said they were not Christians.

Furthermore, not only were 99 per cent of these young Igbos at least nominally Christian, but 66 per cent in Aba and 72 per cent in Kano identified themselves as 'born again'. The fact that so many young migrants described themselves as 'born again' indicates how pervasive and important the 'born again' identity is among this population. Even among migrants who said they were Roman Catholic (Catholic Church leaders in Nigeria have been the most resistant to adopting the language of being 'born again'), about 70 per cent of migrants described themselves in this way.

Religious interpretations of HIV/AIDS

Before examining the complex ways in which religious understandings of HIV/AIDS affect sexual behaviour and the risk of acquiring HIV in the study population, it is important to briefly describe some of the ways in which these young migrants interpret the epidemic. These interpretive understandings illustrate the cultural context and explain the symbolic frameworks within which the young people make sexual decisions. As indicated earlier, AIDS is commonly understood as a social problem that is the result of immorality. Clearly, the role of churches, particularly 'new breed' churches, in promoting these religious understandings of the aetiology of HIV/AIDS and other social ills has been profound. During fieldwork conducted as part of this investigation, the author attended church services, watched evangelical TV programmes and read Christian literature that equated HIV/AIDS with individual and societal sin.

Moreover, pastors in 'new breed' churches (and in some 'orthodox' churches) preach sermons in which HIV/AIDS is tied to immorality. AIDS is blamed on the failure to live a good Christian life, and protection is promised to those who obey Jesus' teachings. On several occasions, the author heard people who were HIV-positive (and who became 'born again' after learning of their infection) testify about the sinful, immoral lives they had led before 'coming to Christ' – they blamed sin (and the devil) for their infections. In some churches, testimonies included stories of cure through religious healing, which is arguably one of the most dangerous religious messages proffered in relation to HIV/AIDS. While only a few churches offered testimony from people who were 'cured', and while many churches offered support for HIV-infected converts that must be seen as positive in relation to the overall stigma of HIV/AIDS in Nigeria, the larger religious message that HIV/AIDS is the result of immorality and can be prevented by being a good, moral Christian contributes to a social environment in which the disease is highly stigmatized.

The strength of the stigma is illustrated by stories that circulate about the actions of those who contract HIV/AIDS. On several occasions, in both Aba and Kano, versions of a rumour were encountered about someone infected with HIV who escaped from a government hospital and was raping young girls in order to 'carry others with him' (another common rumour is that people who test positive for HIV are quarantined and even secretly killed). The idea that people who have HIV/AIDS might deliberately infect others is widely prevalent in Nigeria (for a similar phenomenon in South Africa see Leclerc-Madlala 1997). The image of an evil person devilishly planning to infect and kill others so that he does not die alone no doubt reflects public fears about AIDS, but it also serves to project risk onto a particularly immoral other. Though there is no evidence to suggest that HIV-positive

Nigerians do, in fact, deliberately infect others, the ubiquity and popular resonance of the rumour reinforce the stigma of HIV/AIDS.

The dominant religious discourse about AIDS is that it is a scourge sent by God to punish a society that has turned its back on religion and morality. When asked at the end of the survey what they thought the ultimate origin of AIDS was, 35 per cent of respondents in Kano and 26 per cent in Aba said that it was 'God's punishment' or that 'only God knows'. Many other responses tied the origin of AIDS to immorality. Numerous young people said explicitly that they believed AIDS was God's punishment for the sins that permeate social life. The words of Nnenna,[2] a 19-year-old migrant in Kano who works in her uncle's small pharmaceutical shop, expressed a view heard frequently from young migrants and from many other Igbos:

> AIDS is a terrible thing. But this place is like Sodom and Gomorrah. Nigerians are being punished for their sins. If people did not have sex here and there, if the society were not so corrupt, there would be no AIDS … Yes, it is God's punishment, but we have brought it on ourselves.

Chima, a 22-year-old male migrant in Aba who sold shoes in the main market, and who belongs to an 'orthodox' Protestant church, discussed AIDS in terms that highlight the influence of the 'born again' view, even among migrants who cannot be formally classified as belonging to 'new breed' churches:

> The fact that there is no medical cure proves that it is only through seeing God that one can prevent AIDS. AIDS is God's way of checking the immoral sexual behaviour that is rampant in Nigeria now. I put my trust in God.

It is within this larger cultural context where HIV/AIDS is clearly interpreted as a consequence of immorality in which young migrants must make their decisions about sexual relationships.

Sin and sexual behaviour

How these dominant religious interpretations of HIV/AIDS and the associated stigma translate into individual sexual decisions and behaviour is complex. Sexual behaviour is clearly influenced by a whole range of factors that are not themselves directly attributable to religious or moral considerations. Nonetheless, the findings from this study suggest that the religious framing of the AIDS epidemic in Nigeria unfolds across at least three distinct patterns of sexual behaviour: abstinence, moral partnering, and denial. Abstinence refers to the segment of the population that refrains from premarital sexual intercourse entirely. Moral partnering refers to those who are sexually active but construct their relationships in the language of monogamy and religion. Many young people actively engage in representing their sexual relationships to themselves and to others as moral. Denial refers to relationships that would be judged by society (and certainly by Christian churches) as obviously immoral, but are somehow rationalized, hidden or denied by the people who participate in them. Of course, these categories are fluid, as people who were once abstinent initiate a sexual relationship and people who were sexually active engage in 'secondary abstinence' (a common goal of young people in Nigeria who convert to 'born again' Christianity), as relationships evolve and are reinterpreted, and as people live in multiple and sometimes contradictory social and sexual worlds. Nonetheless, for analytical purposes, examining how religious understandings play out across these three patterns of sexual behaviour offers important insight into the impact of religion on the epidemic.

Arguably, the most common of the sexual patterns, or at least the one most preferred by young migrants, is moral partnering. About 70 per cent of the migrants surveyed reported that they had had sexual intercourse at some time in their lives, and slightly less than half of the respondents said they were currently in a sexual relationship. The vast majority described their partners as 'boyfriends' or 'girlfriends'. In-depth interviews and participant observation made it clear that the labels 'boyfriend' and 'girlfriend' had positive moral connotations. Indeed, one suspects that respondents would be unlikely to reveal much in survey interviews about relationships they consider immoral. Most significant for understanding the connections between religious understandings of HIV/AIDS and young migrants' sexual decision-making is the association of relationship morality with decreased risk, and the tendency to forego condom use in these 'moral partnerships'. The dynamics of condom use in these sexual relationships is related to other issues besides religious morality, such as expectations about intimacy and cultural values about procreation (Smith 2003). But decisions not to use condoms were clearly related in many migrants' minds to the morality of the relationship.

Less than 40 per cent of migrants currently in sexual relationships at the time of the survey used condoms consistently in those relationships, and migrants who talked about condom use in in-depth interviews suggested that condom use was less necessary in moral partnerships because the risk of contracting HIV was minimal. Nneoma, a 23-year-old hairdresser's apprentice in Kano, put a religious spin on her explanation of why she did not use condoms:

> I met my boyfriend in church. We are both children of God and I know I can trust him. I only have sex with him because I love him and I know that he is only with me. I protect myself from pregnancy [using the pill] but I know he will not give me AIDS.

Numerous conversations with young migrants demonstrated that introducing the possibility of condom use was inhibited by the fact that condoms implied one's own or one's partner's infidelity. Just how protective these 'moral partnerships' were is an open question, but clearly many young people in Nigeria perceived that their risk of contracting HIV was minimized if they and their partners were good Christians. Sexual relationships that fell into the category of 'denial' were the hardest to assess, precisely because they were the most difficult to get migrants to talk about. People talked easily and frequently about the immoral sexual relationships of others, especially nameless others, but informants were much less likely to talk about their own 'immoral' relationships. Yet participant observation made it clear that such relationships were common. In both cities, numerous brothels served large clienteles and included young male migrants as clients and young female migrants as commercial sex workers. In Aba, and especially in Kano, countless young migrant women worked in taverns and restaurants that facilitated sexual connections. These women were not 'prostitutes' per se, but were frequently sexually involved with older men of means. While a few migrants were open about sexual partnering that flouted the Christian-influenced category of moral partnering, most young people preferred to keep these relationships secret.

In terms of the risk of HIV/AIDS, perhaps the most problematic dynamics involve the combination of economic and gender inequality, such that poor young women are pressured to rely on their sexuality to secure resources from men, but denied the power to negotiate safe sex because of sexual double standards (see Schoepf 1993, 1997). In some respects, both these young women and their partners sought to hide from themselves the economic dimensions of these relationships. The words of Onyebuchi, a 24-year-old apprentice learning to repair electrical generators in Kano, were emblematic of how many men felt about the issue:

> If a girl keeps a condom in her room you will feel somehow, you know, like she is a professional.

Even in more obviously economic relationships, moral understandings of sexuality can make it hard for women to negotiate condom use. It was not only young migrant women's involvement in economically motivated sex, or men's participation in these relationships, that fell into the category of denial. Through the rumours, gossip and occasional confessions that were heard commonly during fieldwork, it was clear that many young men (and some, but seemingly fewer, young women) were, in fact, cheating on their 'moral partners'. Some people had (secretly) more than one moral partner. And, commonly, the beginning of one relationship and the end of another relationship overlapped, so at least for a period of time many people violated the supposed trust of their moral partnerships. Popular expectations about what a moral sexual relationship should be, shaped so powerfully in this population by Christian discourses, combined with the messy reality of what people's sexual relationships are really like, created a context in which the risk of HIV/AIDS is difficult for young migrants to confront. Religious interpretations of sex and of AIDS decrease the perceived need for condoms in moral partnerships, but exacerbate the extent to which people must deny the relationships and the risk from relationships that do not fit the moral model.

While religious interpretations of HIV/AIDS and moral judgements about sexual relationships seem clearly to inhibit sexually active young migrants from adequately protecting themselves, the fervent Christianity of the young migrants created, or at least solidified, for some an important arena for individual choice in relation to HIV/AIDS: namely, the possibility of abstinence. Abstinence was the most common response when young migrants were asked how best to prevent AIDS, with 37 per cent in Kano and 44 per cent in Aba stating that it was the best option. More importantly, almost one-third of young migrants reported that they had never had sexual intercourse.[3] Because a significant proportion of young people in any population is abstinent, it is hard to attribute the fact of abstinence to Christianity. But interviews and participant observation leave little doubt that in the minds and words of many young migrants their abstinence was religiously motivated.

Perhaps even more relevant, a large number of young migrants who said they had once had sexual intercourse now proclaimed a renewed abstinence. Uluchi, a 22-year-old migrant in Kano, expressed her decision to embark on a new premarital abstinence (sometimes called secondary virginity) in specifically religious terms, but with a nod to HIV/AIDS that seems to be increasingly common:

> Since I found God I realized that I should save myself for my husband. Sex before marriage is against God. Now that I am off sex I feel closer to God. Besides, you never know what might happen out there, with AIDS and everything.

Abstinence is here imagined not just as a mode of preventing transmission, but as an ethical choice that can combat the unchecked immorality believed to exacerbate the epidemic.

While there is insufficient evidence to prove that the 'born again' cultural style is increasing the prevalence or duration of premarital abstinence among young Igbo migrants in Aba and Kano, given how commonly a significant proportion of young people spoke about the religious virtues of abstinence and the moral underpinnings of HIV/AIDS in the same narratives, it seems worth exploring further whether the 'born again' interpretation of sex and AIDS may be saving some people, even as it puts many at risk.

Discussion

Observing the processes whereby the public health crisis created by HIV/AIDS is understood through an increasingly prevalent 'born again' Christian perspective highlights the dangers of a moralistic view of the disease. But this study also suggests that public health programmes should not ignore the strength of these religious interpretations when trying to address the epidemic in Nigeria. Young migrants' behavioural choices made in relation to moralistic understandings of sexuality and HIV/AIDS pose some obvious dangers in terms of negotiating risk. On the one hand, relationships are legitimized as risk-free and decisions not to use condoms are rationalized; for example, 'Both my partner and I are moral and Christian, therefore we are protected.' On the other hand, behaviour that flouts shared religious moralities is thought about as sin (rather than in terms of health risk) and dealt with through denial. Among young people who are sexually active, religious interpretations of the disease and moral assessments of personal sexual behaviour create obstacles to accurately evaluating risk for both those in 'moral partnerships' and those participating in more stigmatized sexual relationships. Christianity provides explanations for who is at risk and who is not, creating contexts where individuals ignore or deny their own risk.

This study suggests that, for many young Nigerians, risky sexual behaviour is related to the failure to personalize the risk of AIDS. Risk is projected onto variously constructed 'others' in a process that intertwines biological infection, sexual immorality and religious identity. For some young people, social forces and religious values collide in ways that push them toward premarital sexual relationships while at the same time inhibiting condom use. The question is how to respond to the prevalence and power of religious understandings of HIV/AIDS. What are the policy implications of findings like these? To build on the prevailing morality and promote premarital abstinence and marital monogamy as a means of preventing HIV/AIDS ignores the reality that most adolescents have sex, many young people are engaged in premarital sexual relations with multiple partners (Renne 1993; Amazigo et al. 1997; Smith 2000; Arowujolu et al. 2002), and many adults are involved in extramarital relationships (Karanja 1987; Smith 2002). It also appears to contribute to an environment in which sexual behaviour and health risks associated with sexual behaviour are evaluated in moralistic terms that inhibit condom use.

Yet one cannot simply ignore the proportion of the population that is abstinent. Whether those who report abstinence stay virgins until marriage and whether they will remain monogamous once married are difficult questions to answer with certainty, but some young people do seem to heed these strongly promoted moral messages. Studies of Africa's AIDS 'success stories', such as Uganda and Senegal, suggest that delaying sexual debut and partner reduction may be playing major roles in reducing HIV transmission (Green 2001, 2002; Hogle et al. 2002). One need not argue against the promotion of condoms and the treatment of sexually transmitted infections as important interventions in order to acknowledge that abstinence and faithfulness to one partner might have a significant role to play in combating HIV/AIDS.

Evaluating the consequences of public health campaigns that promote abstinence as a means of protection will prove extremely complicated. On the one hand, promoting abstinence in a population where the majority of young people are or have been sexually active risks irrelevance. Even worse, if one assumes that young people will be sexually active, it risks making the negotiation of condom use more difficult by further stigmatizing premarital sexual relations. On the other hand, a large proportion of young migrants do remain abstinent until marriage, for a variety of reasons that include an intertwining of religion, sexual morality and fears about AIDS. The idea that promoting abstinence (and fidelity) is pure fantasy may be wrong with regard to a significant proportion of young Igbos.

In the time since this chapter was first published in 2004, public health programmes in Nigeria have begun to try to harness religious beliefs and institutions in the effort to prevent AIDS. However, such efforts have not been well coordinated across religions and denominations. If societies are as diverse as we claim, surely there must be multiple avenues to AIDS prevention. Without a doubt, one message is not appropriate for all. The intertwining of HIV/AIDS and Christianity in Nigeria illustrates the inadequacy of imposing simplistic explanations and the limitations of one-dimensional intervention strategies that ignore the extent to which religion, health, sexuality and morality intersect in people's everyday lives.

Notes

1 Though Kano is located in predominantly Islamic northern Nigeria and Aba is in south-eastern Nigeria, all of the respondents in this study were Igbo-speakers from the Christian south-east. Igbos are the third largest ethnic group in Nigeria.
2 All names of informants provided in the text are pseudonyms.
3 In surveys and in-depth interviews, respondents were not asked about other forms of sexual penetration, such as anal sex. For many Igbos anal sex is considered an 'abomination' and it is difficult to get people to discuss it candidly. However, colleagues working with young Nigerians in HIV prevention programmes report beginning to come across anecdotal evidence to suggest that anal sex may be becoming more prevalent among young teenagers, and that HIV/AIDS prevention messages in Nigeria may be partly responsible. To date, prevention messages have simply assumed that anal sex is extremely rare in Nigeria; the irony is that by focusing exclusively on vaginal sexual intercourse in their messages, prevention efforts may be encouraging anal sex by ignoring it. Further research is needed on this topic.

References

Achebe, C. 1983. *The Trouble with Nigeria*. London: Heinemann.
Amazigo, U., Silva, N., Kaufman, J. and Obikeze, D. 1997. Sexual activity and contraceptive knowledge and use among in-school adolescents in Nigeria. *International Family Planning Perspectives* 23: 28–33.
Arowujolu, A.O., Ilesanmi, A.O., Roberts, O.A. and Okunola, M.A. 2002. Sexuality, contraceptive choice and AIDS awareness among Nigerian undergraduates. *African Journal of Reproductive Health* 6: 60–70.
Bastian, M. 1993. 'Bloodhounds who have no friends': Witchcraft and locality in the Nigerian popular press. In: J. Comaroff and J. Comaroff (eds) *Modernity and its Malcontents: Ritual and Power in Postcolonial Africa*. Chicago, IL: University of Chicago Press, 129–166.

DomNwachukwu, P. 2000. *Authentic African Christianity: An Inculturation Model for the Igbo*. New York: P. Lang.

Ferguson, J. 1999. *Expectations of Modernity: Myths and Meanings of Urban Life on the Zambian Copperbelt*. Berkeley, CA: University of California Press.

Geschiere, P. 1997. *The Modernity of Witchcraft: Politics and the Occult in Postcolonial Africa*. Charlottesville, VA: University of Virginia Press.

Gifford, P. 1990. Prosperity: A new and foreign element in African Christianity. *Religion* 20: 373–388.

Green, E.C. 2001. *The impact of religious organizations in promoting HIV/AIDS prevention*. Paper presented at Challenges for the Church: AIDS, Malaria and TB. Christian Connections for International Health, Arlington, VA, 25–26 May.

Green, E.C. 2002. *Abstinence, fidelity, and the contribution of religious groups to reducing HIV transmission*. Paper presented at the annual meeting of the American Public Health Association, 11 November.

Hogle, J.A., Green, E.C., Nantulya, V., Stoneburner, R. and Stover, J. 2002. *What Happened in Uganda? Declining HIV Prevalence, Behavior Change and the National Response*. Washington, DC: USAID and TVT/The Synergy Project.

Ilogu, E. 1974. *Christianity and Ibo Culture*. Leiden, the Netherlands: E.J. Brill.

Isichei, E. 1976. *A History of the Igbo People*. New York: St. Martin's Press.

Karanja, W. 1987. 'Outside wives' and 'inside wives' in Nigeria: A study of changing perceptions of marriage. In: D. Parkin and D. Nyamwaya (eds) *Transformations in African Marriage*. Manchester: Manchester University Press, 247–261.

Leclerc-Madlala, S. 1997. Infect one, infect all: Zulu youth response to the AIDS epidemic in South Africa. *Medical Anthropology* 17: 363–380.

Marshall, R. 1993. 'Power in the name of Jesus': Social transformation and Pentecostalism in western Nigeria 'revisited'. In: T.O. Ranger and O. Vaughn (eds) *Legitimacy and the State in Twentieth Century Africa*. London: Macmillan, 213–246.

Marshall-Fratani, R. 1998. Mediating the local and the global in Nigerian Pentecostalism. *Journal of Religion in Africa* 28: 278–313.

Meyer, B. 1995. 'Delivered from the powers of darkness': Confessions of satanic riches in Christian Ghana. *Africa* 65: 236–255.

Meyer, B. 1998. The power of money: Politics, occult forces, and Pentecostalism in Ghana. *African Studies Review* 41: 15–37.

National Intelligence Council. 2002. *The Next Wave of HIV/AIDS: Nigeria, Ethiopia, Russia, India, and China*. Available at: http://csis.org/files/media/csis/pubs/021003_secondwave.pdf [Accessed 7 January 2015].

Nwankwo, A. 1999. *Nigeria: The Stolen Billions*. Enugu, Nigeria: Fourth Dimension Publishing.

Orewa, G. Oka. 1997. *We Are All Guilty: The Nigerian Crisis*. Ibadan, Nigeria: Spectrum Books Limited.

Ottenberg, S. 1959. The Ibo receptivity to change. In W.R. Bascom and M.J. Herskowits (eds) *Continuity and Change in African Cultures*. Chicago, IL: University of Chicago Press.

Renne, E. 1993. Changes in adolescent sexuality and the perception of virginity in a southwestern Nigerian village. *Health Transition Review* 3(suppl.): 121–133.

Renne, E. 2003. *Population and Progress in a Yoruba Town*. Ann Arbor, MI: University of Michigan Press.

Schoepf, B. 1993. Women at risk: Case studies from Zaire. In G. Herdt and S. Lindenbaum (eds) *The Time of AIDS: Social Analysis, Theory, and Method*. Newbury Park: SAGE, 259–286.

Schoepf, B. 1997. AIDS, gender, and sexuality during Africa's economic crisis. In: G. Mikell (ed.) *African Feminism: The Politics of Survival in Sub-Saharan Africa*. Philadelphia, PA: University of Pennsylvania Press, 310–332.

Smith, D.J. 2000. 'These girls today *na war-o*': Premarital sexuality and modern identity in southeastern Nigeria. *Africa Today* 473(4): 98–120.

Smith, D.J. 2001. 'The arrow of God': Pentecostalism, inequality, and the supernatural in south-eastern Nigeria. *Africa* 71: 587–613.

Smith, D.J. 2002. 'Man no be wood': Gender and extramarital sex in contemporary Nigeria. *The Ahfad Journal* 192: 4–23.

Smith, D.J. 2003. Imagining HIV/AIDS: Morality and perceptions of personal risk in Nigeria. *Medical Anthropology* 22: 343–372.

UNAIDS. 2002. *Nigeria: Epidemiological Fact Sheets, 2002 Update.* Available at: www.unaids.org/hivaidsinfo/statistics/fact_sheets/pdfs/Nigeria_en.pdf [Accessed 27 July 2003].

UNAIDS. 2014. *Nigeria.* Available at: www.unaids.org/en/regionscountries/countries/nigeria/ [Accessed 17 April 2014].

Watts, M. 1992. The shock of modernity: Petroleum, protest and fast capitalism in an industrializing society. In: A. Pred and M. Watts (eds) *Reworking Modernity: Capitalisms and Symbolic Discontent.* New Brunswick, NJ: Rutgers University Press, 21–63.

Chapter 18

'Mobile men with money'

The sociocultural and politico-economic context of 'high-risk' behaviour among wealthy businessmen and government officials in urban China

Elanah Uretsky

Introduction

High rates of HIV associated with injection drug use (IDU) have helped categorize China as a country with an injection-driven epidemic. This perhaps offered an accurate description of the situation during the initial stages of China's epidemic when as many as 70 per cent of cases were attributable to IDU, but a vastly different situation is now emerging. In 2003, statistical data on HIV and AIDS in China began to illustrate rapid transition toward a trend of sexual transmission (primarily heterosexual but also including homosexual), and HIV is now primarily spread through sexual contact (Sanderson 2007). Such a shift in the epidemic pattern is raising concern about the potential for HIV to be transmitted among those who are not readily associated with the 'high-risk' behaviours of groups such as injection drug users or sex workers. Chief among these concerns is identification of populations that may act as a conduit between 'high-risk' populations and the population more generally.

Some believe the 100–150 million domestic migrants branded as the 'floating population' (*liudong renkou*)[1] will act as a potential tipping point for the expansion of HIV into the general population as they are exposed to new attitudes toward sex in urban areas and faced with the many psychosocial challenges that have been shown to influence sexual attitudes among migrants around the world (Caldwell *et al.* 1997; Brockerhoff and Biddlecom 1999; Wolffers *et al.* 2002; Anderson *et al.* 2003; Yang and Xia 2006). While the behaviour of some men in this group may give cause for concern, the risk of sexually transmitted HIV in China is spread throughout a complex web of sexual networks that has emerged out of contemporary China's unique sociocultural and politico-economic landscape. Consequently, an effective response to this emerging stage of China's epidemic must recognize how such forces act upon and influence high-risk behaviours.

This chapter examines the sociocultural and politico-economic structures that shape the sexual practices of China's growing class of wealthy urban businessmen and government officials, who are sometimes referred to as 'mobile men with money'.[2] Political and social status protects these men from being included among the marginalized categories of high-risk groups defined by global public health paradigms and, consequently, helps them evade contact with HIV prevention messages. But, as I will explain, the unofficial aspects of the work required for their economic and political success are often associated with practices and behaviours that can potentially expose these men to sexually transmitted infections (STIs) including HIV.

Why pay attention to 'mobile men with money'?

The risk of STIs, including HIV, exists for men at all socio-economic levels who have access to China's complex commercial sex industry.[3] Local popular discourse, cultural practices and observation of the commercial sex industry in China, however, raise greater concern over men with access to wealth. People in China often say:

> *fugui siyin ren bu fengliu zhi wei pin* (A man thinks of sex only after he has succeeded and become wealthy and thus only poor men do not chase women)

A walk through any urban area in modern-day China demonstrates the maintenance of the ideas promoted by this traditional idiomatic expression. The complex politico-economic networks that support economic development are established and maintained in urban karaoke clubs and entertainment establishments that are growing in size, opulence and, consequently, expense. Officially, the women who work in these high-priced establishments provide entertainment as masseuses or partners in song and dance. Informally they can also offer sexual services that comprise a large part of the local sex industry. High demand for their services is supported by men who depend on these activities as a means of establishing the relationships needed to succeed in China's rapidly developing economy. It is no wonder then that Chinese sociologist Pan Suiming (2001) has found that urban Chinese men who hold management positions are ten times more likely than labourers to solicit the services of a sex worker, 'sexual secretary' or minor wife;[4] a ratio that increases to 22:1 in rural areas. And, overall, the men who comprise the top 5 per cent of China's income earners are 33 times more likely than men in the lowest 44 per cent to purchase sex (Pan 2001). This may be partly due to economics but, as I will illustrate, the current politico-economic climate provides extra incentive for men in positions of wealth and power to engage in these types of practices.

It is not simply wealth or even an individual set of behaviours that motivates these men to participate in the myriad forms of entertainment that lead to their high rate of engagement with commercial sex. Rather, such sexual practices stem primarily from a particular set of sociocultural and politico-economic factors that converge within their work-related roles and duties. Economic development in contemporary China is dependent on the success of a new class of entrepreneurs who are now allowed to pursue opportunities in the emergent market economy. Their success, however, is still dependent on the government officials who, under China's socialist bureaucracy, maintain control over the resources, permits and allowances that are crucial for a businessman's participation in the market. The relaxed political controls that have necessarily accompanied market reforms have fostered the re-emergence of many traditional Chinese practices and structured a situation that has helped engender a unique system of patron–clientelism that brings these men together over shared social rituals that include feasting, drinking and female-centred entertainment that is often coupled with sexual services.

Such trends have led some to believe that China's 'mobile men with money' are also well poised to transmit HIV into the general population (du Guerny *et al.* 2003; Pan *et al.* 2006), a suspicion that concurs with the jolts being felt by the public health workers battling the epidemic on the ground. In 2001, one-third of patients hospitalized for AIDS in Beijing had contracted HIV through homosexual contact. At the same time, however, many of the calls to a national AIDS hotline came from men who had solicited services from a sex worker and subsequently learned that such behaviour could expose them to HIV. One of the operators told me that these men, who held positions that conferred high levels of political and social status, were reluctant to approach their local anti-epidemic station[5] for an HIV test and instead were hoping for a remote diagnosis over the phone (which of course was impossible).

During the 18 months I spent researching issues related to HIV and AIDS, masculinity and male sexual culture in China between October 2003 and March 2006, I discovered that people from both the international and domestic communities realized the importance of finding a way to target HIV prevention messages toward the type of hidden men who called into the national AIDS hotline. Several of the Chinese public health workers I met realized that the standard masculine practices used to build networks among business and government partners would imminently affect their local HIV epidemic. They also expressed concern about the wives and regular partners of these men. Local efforts to stem this part of the epidemic, however, are constrained by political sensitivities. The political implication that a government official has engaged in practices deemed immoral for their position can pose a threat to the ruling Communist Party. Additionally, the association of businessmen with HIV/AIDS can threaten important local plans for economic development.

Many foreign observers and representatives of international public health organizations are also aware of the risky behaviours that prompted concern in these local public health workers. The same ritual practices expected of a Chinese partner are also often extended to foreign guests hoping to collaborate with a local host. Foreign guests who are unfamiliar with China, however, often dismiss the drinking and entertainment rituals encountered in these situations as sophomoric. But expatriates who have spent considerable time in China recognize the normality of such behaviours and the risks incurred by the men who regularly engage in related practices. One foreign aid worker I met recounted to me his own concern over the government officials he dealt with on a regular basis. In the rural prefecture where he lived, it was customary, as in other parts of China, to include the provision of sex work in the entertainment of one's guests and, to him, this represented the most major risk of development of an HIV epidemic in this remote corner of the country. The development of the term 'mobile men with money' in late 2004 placed some needed attention on the issue, but the national response is challenged by the global paradigms that structure many international public health programmes.

The same political restrictions and global paradigms that challenge our efforts to target China's wealthy businessmen and government officials with HIV prevention messages also consequently limit our knowledge of the impact of HIV on these men. There are no statistical data that can allow us to assert that men who occupy such positions in China are indeed affected by HIV and are a possible route of transmission to their sexual partners. It is even more difficult to assert that these men themselves are exposed to HIV. After all, while eating, drinking and even karaoke singing are collectively performed rituals, sex is a private act that can be refused without incurring a loss of face. In addition, new trends are arising that bring men together outside the karaoke bar. In Kunming, the capital of Yunnan Province, I saw men getting together on the tennis court. A growing cadre of women entrepreneurs and government officials are also now seeking success within China's political–economic system. And while they are not put at risk of STI or HIV infection by these local practices, many still invite the men who control their success to the entertainment establishments where sexual services are provided. Still, these trends are slow to occur and are most prevalent in large cities. The various men, women and public health workers I spoke to, however, still believe these practices affect the sexual behaviour of the many men seeking success in China.

Methods

This chapter reports on findings from a larger study that examines how contemporary trends of masculinity and male sexual culture in contemporary urban China can expose men to STIs and HIV. Ethnographic research for this project stressed sexual practice over sexual behaviour. As a result, data collection focused primarily on structural factors that cause urban Chinese men to seek sexual experiences outside of marriage and how they negotiate, use and experience sex with various partners rather than on the individual aspects of their behaviour during sexual contact (including questions about rates of condom usage). This led to analysis of the social, cultural and political meanings that help construct sexual behaviour among these men.

Data were collected through participant observation and in-depth interviews that helped me trace the daily lives of urban men who engage in professional networking activities. Participant observation in restaurants, hotels, massage parlours, hair salons, karaoke clubs, saunas and brothels helped me understand the relationship of their related activities to political and economic success in contemporary China. Research conducted in people's homes and their places of work was equally important for the lessons it offered about the sociocultural factors that construct men's lives in urban China, including the struggles encountered between traditional family expectations of marriage and fatherhood, the masculine entitlements offered by traditional Chinese culture, and state expectations and proscriptions that often govern a man's success. In-depth interviews conducted with businessmen, government officials and government workers, entertainment-establishment owners, doctors, nurses, female service providers, sex workers and married women offered further clues about contextual factors that influence a man's decision to seek extramarital sexual relationships.

In addition to ethical review conducted at Columbia University, my institutional affiliation at the time of research, the project was also approved by the Institutional Review Board for Human Subjects Research at Tsinghua University. Participants were recruited through snowball sampling based on a system of referrals and introductions. All participants were informed of my identity as a researcher from the USA and the purpose and activities of the study before giving oral consent.

Both descriptive and analytic impressions from participant observation were recorded as field notes. Fluency in Mandarin Chinese allowed me to conduct interviews directly with research participants. Interviews were taped and transcribed directly into English in the event a participant agreed to audio-taping. Due to the sensitive nature of the research, however, most interviews were recorded in typed field-note format. The large amount of qualitative narrative data collected during participant observation and in-depth interviews was filed and categorized into an indexed system that developed during the course of research. Textual analysis was conducted on this data to understand both popular and official discourse about male sexual culture in China. Common themes that emerged during interviews were categorized together, as were common responses to questions that followed those themes. This initial coding exercise was used to relate certain events to each other through a process of 'textual interrogation' (Dowsett 1996). Analysis also avoided the imposition of categories and classifications from my own cultural background onto the cultural practices I observed. My analysis relies on 'thick description' of local categories in order to preserve the local meanings and cultural practices conveyed during the research process (Asad 1986; Sanjek 1990; Parker 1993; Emerson *et al.* 1995). Finally, the project considered the important historical structures that influence sexual culture and masculinity among middle- and upper-class men in urban China.

Field site

Research for this project was primarily conducted in the city of Ruili, located in Yunnan Province in south-western China adjacent to the Burmese border. The significant role that Ruili plays in the history of China's HIV epidemic as well as its active cross-border trade with Burma make it an ideal location for studying the interaction of male sexual culture and HIV in China. Ruili is a county with an urban centre and surrounding rural areas that depend on agriculture. The county covers 1,020 square kilometres that are situated on a small geographic peninsula surrounded on three sides by Burma and inhabited by 112,000 people of both Han Chinese and ethnic minority background.[6] Approximately 30,000 people officially occupy Ruili's urban centre, but migrant traders from both China and abroad swell the population by an additional 30,000 to 50,000 people.

The first domestic outbreak of HIV in China was detected in 1989 among injection drug users living in Ruili's rural ethnic minority communities. The local epidemic remains one primarily transmitted through IDU, but is increasingly being transmitted through heterosexual contact among the Han population.[7] This transition is partially due to Ruili's economic transformation. Its historically agriculturally based economy is now primarily supported by active trade industries in both legal and illicit goods ranging from jade to timber and heroin. A large contingent of both short-term sojourners and long-term hotel residents who come to Ruili to gamble in an array of casinos located just across the border in Burma also support a lucrative industry of tourism. All the men who work in these industries rely on entertainment, including sex work, as a way of communicating between themselves and the government officials who can facilitate their opportunities. Consequently, the health of the local commercial sex industry relies on the amount of work conducted in the industries that are primarily responsible for supporting Ruili's economy.

Results and discussion

'Work' and its accompanying burdens in the Chinese context

During the initial stages of fieldwork I visited karaoke clubs, massage parlours and saunas in order to understand the structure of the entertainment conducted in these establishments. I also talked to both men and women about the structures that influence the sexual lives of the men who attend such establishments.

Discussion of sex, however, only comprised part of what I heard from these people. Women spoke to me about the effects of incessant episodes of drinking on their husbands' health. Men also spoke of these types of events in conjunction with the accompanying expectations to eat, smoke and participate in entertainment that could include sexual services. These activities were often represented as a burden handed down by their bosses rather than as a choice, desire or luxury.

I soon learned that my enquiries of sexuality were too narrow to understand the sexual behaviour conducted among the wealthy businessmen and government officials I had come to examine because their sexual conduct in these environments did not simply result from an individual pattern of desire and, in fact, represented only the coda to a group of shared masculine ritual practices. Its perfunctory nature for some also made me realize that these activities actually comprised a form of work for these men and not simply entertainment. Low- and mid-level government workers described the consequences that could result if they refused invitations to a banquet or a karaoke club. As one man told me, 'When your boss calls, you have no choice but to drop everything and go for the evening.' In addition to the eating, drinking and smoking, he said, 'You have to do things that are offensive to your own wife (*ni yao duibuqi ni ziji de laopo*).' These activities, which are collectively referred to as *yingchou*, are not only perfunctory, but also dominate the work of the many government workers, government officials and businessmen I met during my research. These initial findings led me to believe that analysis of the cultural practices and politico-economic dynamics that structure work for these men was crucial for understanding their sexual behaviour.

Work or *gongzuo* is a dynamic term in the Chinese context that has a very specific meaning associated with position rather than labour. To 'have work' or 'have a job' (*you gongzuo*) in China implies that you are employed by a state-owned enterprise or work unit (*danwei*) that provides employee entitlements such as housing and health care (Entwistle and Henderson 2000). All other types of work are categorized according to function. For instance, someone who does business is said to *zuo shengyi*, a peasant is said to *laodong* (do labour) and a migrant worker is said to *dagong* (do manual or menial work). All are forms of work, but generally, only work inside a state-owned enterprise is officially called *gongzuo*, a privilege that carries an expectation of Party loyalty demonstrated through adherence to strict moral and political standards.

This institutional framework has led to an ambiguous definition of the activities associated with 'work', which often transcend the expected purview of a given position into a realm dictated by cultural and political expectation. In an environment where a socialist-style patron–client system has intersected with a market-oriented economy, a new politico-economic environment has emerged where many government officials are in positions to control the success sought by various entrepreneurs. Consequently, the official and unofficial activities necessary for establishing trust in a businessman as someone who is both loyal to the Party and to their ensuing interpersonal relationships have become an integral part of the work of both Chinese entrepreneurs and local government officials. Many government officials aspiring for higher positions also rely on these activities to strengthen relationships with the officials who determine their promotion.

After following various businessmen and government officials both inside and outside the karaoke bar, I discovered their days are structured around activities centred outside any formal work environment. A typical workday for many of the men I interviewed begins at 8 o'clock in the morning and often ends at 2 o'clock the next morning. Their busy schedule starts with the invitation of a guest to breakfast. Breakfast is followed by trips to the field to survey (*kaocha*) the particular situation that brought the host and his guest together. For example, the visit of a provincial-level health official on a mission to evaluate local HIV prevention efforts may include perfunctory outings to the homes of some people living with HIV, a local methadone clinic and the local hospital. Similarly, a businessman seeking approval from a government official may invite his guest to visit a factory site or to view the local resources available for conducting business in a particular industry. Showing the guest around these sites demonstrates the host's operational capacity. Successful communication between these men, however, is dependent on a deep level of trust that is established over ritual practice that continues throughout the day and indeed throughout the duration of their professional relationship. The host invites his guest to lunch at 11.30 where they dine on various local delicacies and toast each other with alcohol as a means of demonstrating respect to one another. Lunch is followed by a brief siesta (*xiuxi*) period if time permits and then the official work-related duties resume between 14.30 and 17.30. The host invites his guest to dinner in the evening, which consists of more local delicacies and more toasting between the two partners in order to further demonstrate their mutual respect and appreciation. After dinner, the host invites his guests out for some entertainment, which can include massage (*anmo*), foot reflexology (*xijiao*), hair-washing (*xitou*) or a trip to a local disco and karaoke club. This can often be followed by a midnight meal (*xiaoyan*). In addition, the entertainment can be coupled with sexual services from a service girl, or guests can be offered the services of a brothel-based sex worker who is discreetly solicited to the guest's hotel room. This typical day of hosting and entertainment can define 6 or even 7 days of the workweek for local officials and entrepreneurs.

This cultural scenario, known as *yingchou*, is a necessary minor ritual practice that has been used as a means of establishing and strengthening social relations in China since the Song dynasty (960–1279) (Anon. 1979). The tradition has since evolved into a 'series of scripts and patterned expectations' (Fordham 1995: 154) that help participants develop the emotional feelings (*renqing*) required for building the networks of personal relations (*renji guanxi*) that support contemporary China's unique form of patron–clientelism. For businessmen, *yingchou* is crucial for establishing good relations with the government officials who control the resources, permits and allowances necessary for success in China's developing market economy and often demands more time than their basic operations. The manager of a large and opulent three-storey karaoke club in Beijing told me it took only 3 months to build and furnish the club, but 2 years to go through the process of pleasing the government officials who held the key to the project. Local government officials also participate in *yingchou* activities (often referred to as *jiedai keren* or 'receiving guests') with one another as a means of pleasing superiors who control promotional opportunities. As one former mid-level official told me:

> If you want to be an official and advance up the ladder, you must have personal relations (*renji guanxi*). You cannot advance without these personal relations. And where do personal relations come from? You have to invite them out to eat, for a massage, shoot the breeze with them, solicit prostitutes for them and then they'll see that you're useful. Our country's policies do not permit these things, but our local officials desire them. So slowly, if you give them the impression that you can do these things, you will gradually advance in rank.

Consequently, when reflecting on his subsequent diagnosis with HIV, he blamed his sero-status on his work. This man, who previously spent 5 out of 7 nights of every week engaged in entertainment duties, said to me:

> Our work made us do these things. When a superior (*lingdao*) came down to visit we would go eat with them. Then when we finished eating and finished drinking we would all go out to sing and dance together. And after singing we would go do chaotic things including all the soliciting of prostitutes that comes along with it (*luanqi bazao shenme piaochang de shi ye laile*). That is to say, I know what road I walked to being infected today and I regret it.

Feasting and drinking

As I learned, the sexual relations that were so important to my concern about HIV transmission must be considered within the context of the practices of *yingchou*, which are founded upon rituals of feasting, drinking and entertainment practices that have traditionally been used to structure China's gendered social hierarchy. The feasting and drinking that help lubricate relationships in contemporary China are reminiscent of the proper rituals described for state dinners in the *Book of Rites*, the Confucian text that established standards for social forms, ancient rites and court ceremonies. Proper administration of social ceremony that established hierarchical structure and secured social solidarity dictated the size of the drinking vessel, the spatial positioning or seating of the guests, the order of serving and consuming the drink and food, the number of accompanying dishes and the quantity of drink served to each guest (Smart 2005).

The alcohol consumed at dinners and banquets in contemporary China has also maintained its historical role in establishing the bonds of trust that allow Chinese men to negotiate and cooperate with one another. Like food, alcohol is not consumed individually in China, but is reserved for its use in building and structuring social networks that are founded on culturally prescribed masculine customs of sharing (Heath 1987; Yan 1996). Even within the structure of a social feast, glasses are not simply clinked and then enjoyed individually. The alcohol in those glasses serves an important role in demonstrating respect between men. Each time a cup is raised, the person inviting someone to a drink precedes the request to empty a glass with words of respect, joy and perhaps favour. Someone may thank their counterpart for help in the past, ask them for help in the future, securing success or a better position, or wish them everlasting joy, youth, beauty and health, like government officials whose positions within the Communist Party prohibit them from seeking the wealth and prosperity (*facai*) often conveyed toward counterparts in China. People rehearsed in the art of toasting become quite animated and humorous. Finally, the person who initiates the toast demonstrates their utmost respect by saying to their partner, 'For you, I will empty a cup' (*wo wei ni yao gan yibei*). The partner reciprocates this respect by drinking an equal amount of liquor. The base of trust is finally solidified when the two provide evidence of their empty cups.

Entertainment

Similar feasting and drinking rituals are characteristic of social networking and hierarchical structuring in many modern societies (Mars and Altman 1987), but in China they are accompanied by certain forms of entertainment that are woven into the scripted patterns of *yingchou*. This entertainment, which typically takes place in an establishment that provides female-centred services, has been used to distinguish male social elite in both imperial and modern Chinese society.

In this homosocial society, men who begin establishing a relationship over ritual food and drink have historically extended the process with one that strengthens their trust in each other as members of the same privileged class. During China's late Imperial era (1368–1911), elite male literati validated their status with the attention of talented courtesan women (Hershatter 1997). This tradition was especially popular in eighteenth- and nineteenth-century Shanghai, a cosmopolitan metropolis where educated literati competed with domestic and international traders for attention and status. Female courtesans of this era, trained in poetry, song and dance, entertained wealthy and prestigious men including married officials, artisans and wealthy merchants (Zamperini 1999; Micollier 2004). Courtesans were primarily valued for their talents, but men could also request sexual favours from their favourite entertainers (Xu 1995; Hershatter 1997).

As Shanghai became more commercialized, a new affluent consumer society, which placed more value on a woman's sexual services than her erudition, helped push the roles of courtesan and prostitute closer together (Hershatter 1997; Henriot 2001). Courtesan culture was replaced by a cabaret culture that nurtured a tradition of service girls who accompanied merchants in song and dance. These women primarily worked as companions but also offered 'extra' service for a negotiable fee (Field 1999).

A similar culture has re-emerged in the market-oriented society of post-Mao China. The business entrepreneurs and government officials who comprise contemporary elite male society are once again underscoring and protecting their social status through the consumption of female-centred entertainment activities at saunas, massage parlours, hair-washing salons or disco and karaoke clubs. The modern karaoke club is reminiscent of the cabarets that dotted the landscape of 1920s Shanghai. Similarly, the female masseuses in contemporary China who offer special service[8] for a tip can be harkened back to a custom introduced to Shanghai by Russian émigrés shortly after the 1917 Revolution (Henriot 2001).

For the elite scholar officials of Imperial and Republican era (1911–1949) Shanghai who endured the pressures of scholarship and governance, these leisure activities served a similar role to the masculine cultural practices shared by businessmen in contemporary Japan or Korea (Allison 1994; Cheng 2000). For the elite men of contemporary urban China, however, participation in these activities is a crucial part of their work used to demonstrate the personal respect and Party loyalty that are necessary for professional success.

The cultural and political significance of yingchou

Demonstration of loyalty toward the Communist Party has always been crucial for success in post-revolutionary China. Initially, work output was officially used as a measure to evaluate the 'impersonal loyalties demanded by the modern Leninist party' (Walder 1986: 25). In post-Mao China, however, the criteria seem to have changed to an environment where:

> Nanren bu piao chang, duibuqi dang zhongyang
> Nüren bu zuo ji, duibuqi Zhu Rongji
> (A man who does not solicit prostitutes has insulted the Party central level/A woman who does not work as a prostitute has insulted Zhu Rongji)[9]

The ideas contained in this popular couplet reflect the new system of reward distribution that has emerged in post-Mao China where loyalty is now demonstrated through the practices of yingchou. Development of a market economy has created demand for government-controlled resources from private entrepreneurs who lie outside the trusted network established by demonstrated state loyalty. The government still requires loyalty in exchange for its resources, but the work of these private entrepreneurs, which does not serve the state, must be replaced by an alternative means of demonstration. The traditional cultural practices that have emerged under the relaxed political controls that have accompanied market reform have allowed officials to turn to the personal loyalties characteristic of the traditional authority and patrimonialism that were stressed by Confucian discourse (Walder 1986).

Confucian ideology promoted a system that valued relationships between partners that had an established bond of trust built upon a recognized hierarchy. Constructing these relationships around the strong hierarchical bonds that naturally existed between a ruler and his subjects, a husband and his wife, a father and his son, and an older brother and his younger sibling created an indestructible system of social and bureaucratic order that was dependent on a mutual extension of kinship (Yang 1994). A fifth relationship built upon friendship established loyalties between people of different age groups, social status, educational level and official position who could depend on one another for professional advancement (Kutcher 2000).

The bonds that result from this sociobureaucratic ordering of society serve as the structure for a complex network of personal relations (*renji guanxi*) that govern traditional modes of exchange in China and consequently underscore the structure of patron–client relations in China's contemporary politico-economic system. Chinese people often recount the necessity of *guanxi* for success: a term used to refer to the traditional dyadic relationships that allow people to develop bonds of mutual interest and benefit. 'Once *guanxi* is established between two people, each can ask a favour of the other with the expectation that the debt incurred will be repaid sometime in the future' (Yang 1994: 1). *Guanxi* is traditionally established between people who have long-standing kin or kin-like relationships that grow out of an institutional bond. Standard prerequisites for *guanxi* relations in contemporary China rely on networks of classmates, old friends, army buddies and people who share a common place of origin (*laoxiang*). Like the bonds that ordered the Confucian sociopolitical system, these relationships are imbued with a strong innate sense of human sentiment (*renqing*) that forms an everlasting bond between two people who can turn to each other for favours and assistance.

The inherent conflicts created between the needs of a market-oriented economic system and socialist political system have caused government officials to turn to the personal loyalties engendered by *guanxi* networks in order to facilitate the operation and development of China's market economy. In a politico-economic system fuelled by exchange between the market forces and socialist controls, government officials must interact with businessmen who are required by the market to provide money in exchange for resources. This traditional system of social relations helps them structure a basis of non-monetary exchange that cannot be directly associated with corrupt practices. It is the traditional ideology of *guanxi* that structures this new system and the traditional practice of *yingchou* that allows them to build personal relationships and loyalties with people who lie outside of their formal *guanxi* network. These responsibilities do not end, however, with the establishment of *guanxi*, because social relationships require maintenance.

One of the men in Ruili who worked for a local state-owned company was responsible for sales to a discrete set of local government bureaus. Of course his work entailed a certain amount of *yingchou* to build up necessary *guanxi* with the officials of those bureaus as a way of winning over their business from other private competitors. But I always wondered why he repeatedly went to karaoke clubs and massage parlours after securing these contracts. As he explained to me, gaining their business was only the beginning of their relationship. They are only willing to maintain the relationship with someone who demonstrates their continued trust and loyalty. Such dependence on personal and social networks has resulted in a system where the distribution of power is ultimately dependent on the reproduction and conduct of social relations rather than through the objective measures honoured by the state (Yang 1994).

Conclusion

The epidemiological paradigms that govern many global public health programmes have created a perception that HIV infection is limited to certain high-risk populations. Consideration of the local structural forces that promote high-risk behaviour, however, will help uncover people outside these categories who are also at risk of infection.

While the men I discuss in this chapter are highly mobile, their social and political status precludes them from being targeted by messages aimed at marginalized men of the floating population. Similarly, messages that try to target 'clients of sex workers' evade these men who are engaging in entertainment activities offered by women who work as entertainment service workers. Alternatively, I suggest that an understanding of the role that work plays in their lives and sexual practices can offer important lessons for responding to their risk of STIs, including HIV.

Responding to the epidemic in this context, however, will require us to broaden our definition of the terms 'work' and 'workplace'. Valuable work within the public health and human rights fields has helped us define sex work as work for women. But we have not considered the role that soliciting of sexual services plays in men's work. The political and economic success of many Chinese men is dependent on activities conducted inside myriad entertainment establishments that are often only considered a workplace for women. An understanding of all the work conducted in these spaces will help us design more effective programmes for STI and HIV prevention within this context.

Effective prevention of HIV among these men will also recognize the competing social and political discourses that structure their daily lives and influence public recognition of their risk of HIV. Extramarital relationships with female entertainers, lovers and 'minor' wives are part of masculine entitlement for elite Chinese men. Politically, however, this type of behaviour is proscribed. Such an environment, where elite male entrepreneurs and government officials are caught between the competing discourses of a socialist patron–clientelist system and an incumbent system of cultural values, has incited the rise of an 'economy of desire' (Zhang 2001), where precious commodities and resources are quietly exchanged for corporeal experience.

Several provinces in China have tried to respond to these competing discourses by mandating placement of condoms in hotel rooms and other entertainment establishments where men solicit the services of sex workers. The effectiveness of these policies, however, is dependent on the development of messages that similarly recognize the multiple competing discourses that challenge prevention of HIV among China's wealthy businessmen and government officials who experience sex within this liminal space.

Notes

1 This is an estimate based on demographic analysis. For a more detailed discussion please refer to Zai and Ma (2004).
2 A term developed by the Global Coalition on HIV/AIDS to represent the wealthy Chinese businessmen and government officials who frequently move around as they engage in China's rapid process of economic development.
3 According to sociologist Pan Suiming, China's sex industry comprises seven tiers, ranging from women who exclusively service one man in exchange for material goods to women who provide domestic and sexual services to a group of construction workers in exchange for food and shelter.
4 Chinese men with resources often maintain exclusive sexual relationships with women in exchange for benefits that can include houses, cars and clothes.

5 This nomenclature, which was adopted from the Soviet system, was used to refer to the national system of disease surveillance centres that reached down into every local area. The system has now been renamed the Centre for Disease Control.

6 China's population consists of the Han majority (92 per cent) and 55 ethnic minority communities (8 per cent). Yunnan Province is home to 25 ethnic minority communities. The Dai, the Jingpo, the Lisu, the De'eng and the Achang ethnic minorities comprise 64.5 per cent of Ruili's population.

7 In 2007, 60.4 per cent of new cases of HIV in Dehong Prefecture (the administrative prefecture of Ruili County) were transmitted through sexual contact and only 20.7 per cent were transmitted through IDU.

8 A euphemism used for sexual services.

9 Zhu Rongji served as the Premier of China from 1998 to 2003. He is best known for his pragmatism and insistence on a hard-work ethic as a countermeasure to political corruption within the Party.

References

Allison, A. 1994. *Nightwork: Sexuality, Pleasure, and Corporate Masculinity in a Tokyo Hostess Club.* Chicago, IL: University of Chicago Press.

Anderson, A.F., Qingsi, Z., Hua, X. and Jianfeng, B. 2003. China's floating population and the potential for HIV transmission: A social-behavioural perspective. *AIDS Care* 15: 177–185.

Anon. 1979. *Ci hai [Sea of Words].* Shanghai: Shanghai cishu chubanshe.

Asad, T. 1986. The concept of cultural translation in British social anthropology. In: J. Clifford and G. Marcus (eds) *Writing Culture: The Poetics and Politics of Ethnography.* Berkeley: University of California Press, 141–164.

Brockerhoff, M. and Biddlecom, A.E. 1999. Migration, sexual behaviour and the risk of HIV in Kenya. *International Migration Review* 33: 833–856.

Caldwell, J., Anarfi, J.K. and Caldwell, P. 1997. Mobility, migration, sex, STDs and AIDS: An essay on sub-Saharan Africa and other parallels. In: G. Herdt (ed.) *Sexual Cultures and Migration in the Era of AIDS: Anthropological and Demographic Perspectives.* New York: Oxford University Press, 41–54.

Cheng, S.-L. 2000. Assuming manhood: Prostitution and patriotic passions in Korea. *East Asia: An International Quarterly* 18: 40–78.

Dowsett, G. 1996. *Practicing Desire: Homosexual Sex in the Era of AIDS.* Stanford, CA: Stanford University Press.

du Guerny, J., Hsu, L.-N. and Cao, H. 2003. *Population Movement and HIV/AIDS in the Case of Ruili, Yunnan, China.* Bangkok: UNDP.

Emerson, R.M., Fretz, R.I. and Shaw, L.L. 1995. *Writing Ethnographic Fieldnotes.* Chicago, IL: University of Chicago Press.

Entwistle, B. and Henderson, G. (eds) 2000. *Re-drawing Boundaries: Work, Households, and Gender in China.* Berkeley, CA: University of California Press.

Field, A. 1999. Selling souls in sin city: Shanghai singing and dancing hostesses in print, film and politics, 1920–1949. In: Y. Zhang (ed.) *Cinema and Urban Culture in Shanghai, 1922–1943.* Stanford, CA: Stanford University Press, 99–127.

Fordham, G. 1995. Whiskey, women and song: Men, alcohol and AIDS in northern Thailand. *Australian Journal of Anthropology* 6: 154–177.

Heath, D. 1987. Anthropology and alcohol studies: Current issues. *Annual Review of Anthropology* 16: 99–120.

Henriot, C. 2001 [1997]. *Prostitution and Sexuality in Shanghai.* New York: Cambridge University Press.

Hershatter, G. 1997. *Dangerous Pleasures: Prostitution and Modernity in Twentieth-century Shanghai.* Berkeley, CA: University of California Press.

Kutcher, N. 2000. The fifth relationship: Dangerous friendships in the Confucian context. *American Historical Review* 105: 1615–1629.

Mars, G. and Altman, Y. 1987. Alternative mechanism of distribution in a Soviet economy. In: M. Douglas (ed.) *Constructive Drinking: Perspectives on Drink from Anthropology*. New York: Cambridge University Press, 270–279.

Micollier, E. 2004. Social significance of commercial sex work: Implicitly shaping a sexual culture? In: E. Micollier (ed.) *Sexual Cultures in East Asia: The Social Construction of Sexuality and Sexual Risk in a Time of AIDS*. New York: Routledge Curzon, 3–22.

Pan, S. 2001. *AIDS in China: How much possibility is there in sexual transmitting?* Unpublished paper presented at the First China Conference on AIDS/STDs, Beijing, November.

Pan, S., Huang, Y. and Li, D. 2006. Analyses of the 'problem' of AIDS in China. *Social Sciences in China*, Winter 2006: 27–39.

Parker, R. 1993. Within four walls: Brazilian sexual culture and HIV/AIDS. In: H. Daniel and R. Parker (eds) *Sexuality, Politics, and AIDS in Brazil*. London: Falmer Press.

Sanderson, H. 2007. *Report: Sex Main Cause of HIV in China*. Associated Press, Beijing, 30 November. Available at: www.washingtonpost.com/wp-dyn/content/article/2007/11/29/AR2007112901324. html [Accessed 2 December 2007].

Sanjek, R. 1990. *Fieldnotes: The Makings of Anthropology*. Ithaca, NY: Cornell University Press.

Smart, J. 2005. Cognac, beer, red wine or soft drinks? Hong Kong identity and wedding banquets. In: T. Wilson (ed.) *Drinking Cultures: Alcohol and Identity*. New York: Berg.

Walder, A. 1986. *Communist Neo-traditionalism: Work and Authority in Chinese Industry*. Berkeley, CA: University of California Press.

Wolffers, I., Fernandez, I., Verghis, S. and Vink, M. 2002. Sexual behaviour and vulnerability of migrant workers for HIV infection. *Culture, Health, and Sexuality* 4: 459–473.

Xu, J. 1995. *Jinu Shi* [*The History of Prostitution*]. Shanghai: Shanghai wenyi chuban she.

Yan, Y. 1996. *The Flow of Gifts: Reciprocity and Social Networks in a Chinese Village*. Stanford, CA: Stanford University Press.

Yang, M.M.-H. 1994. *Gifts, Favors and Banquets: The Art of Social Relationships in China*. Ithaca, NY: Cornell University Press.

Yang, X. and Xia, G. 2006. Gender, migration, risky sex and HIV infection in China. *Studies in Family Planning* 37: 241–250.

Zai, L. and Ma, Z. 2004. China's floating population: New evidence from the 2000 census. *Population and Development Review* 30: 467–488.

Zamperini, P. 1999. But I never learned to waltz: The 'real' and imagined education of a courtesan in the late Qing. *Nan Nu* 1: 107–144.

Zhang, E.Y. 2001. Guodui and the state: Constructing entrepreneurial masculinity in two cosmopolitan areas of post-socialist China. In: D. Hodgson (ed.) *Gendered Modernities: Ethnographic Perspectives*. New York: Palgrave, 235–266.

Chapter 19

Race, space, place

Notes on the racialisation and spatialisation of commercial sex work in Dubai, UAE

Pardis Mahdavi

Introduction

The first time I met Ziya, 31, in 2008, she was living with a group of Indonesian and Australian real estate agents in the Jumeirah Beach Residences, a high-end housing complex located in the southern, newer part of Dubai that has emerged as the more affluent part of town. 'Here, I love. JBR very good,' Ziya told me, referring to her current housing situation. 'Me, I'm not liking Bur Dubai. Living on street, living in bus station. Bur Dubai dark, bad. Marina, nice,' she said, contrasting the two very different parts of town she had inhabited since migrating to Dubai in 2007. She walked out to the balcony of her current home to show me the breathtaking view of the Persian Gulf and the accompanying Palm Islands as she settled in to tell her story.

Ziya migrated out of Addis Ababa, Ethiopia, in 2007 after her husband left her with two children and deeply in debt. Having heard from friends that there was an abundance of work in the Middle East and 'a lot of money there', as she said, she decided to migrate to Dubai to pursue domestic work. When she arrived, however, she was placed with a family that was highly abusive towards her. 'They burn my clothes, throw cups at me, very difficult,' she explained. Domestic workers in the Gulf States fall outside the protection of labour laws, and due to the sponsorship system (*kefala*) in the United Arab Emirates (UAE), legal residency in Dubai is dependent on the sponsor-employer (problematically collapsed into the same category) who often retains employees' passports and legal working papers.[1]

When Ziya made the decision to run away from her abusive employers, she not only absconded from her job, but automatically became an illegal alien in doing so. 'I run away, but no passport, no place to go,' she explained, reflecting on a tumultuous time in her life not 6 months earlier. Without her passport (which her former employers still retain), legal working permits or any money, Ziya entered the informal economy, working as a sex worker and sleeping in airport terminals, bus stations or on the streets of Bur Dubai, the older part of town which is now somewhat of a working class neighbourhood populated mostly by migrant workers of South and East Asian origin. Lining the wide streets of the southern part of Dubai and the Marina area, gleaming skyscrapers are often spaced miles apart to allow for breathtaking views of the Gulf, the Palm and the Marina. This urban planning contrasts sharply with the narrow winding streets of Old Dubai in the north, which is home to the neighbourhoods of Deira, Bur Dubai and the Bastakiya (or old fishing village) quarter. When making the drive from south to north on Sheikh Zayed road (the main highway connecting most of the seven emirates), drivers can witness the spaces between buildings narrow incrementally the further north one moves.

After 6 months of living and working on the streets of Bur Dubai, where she faced regular abuse from clients, police and, sometimes, others in the business, Ziya found an informal organisation, supported by locals and expats alike,[2] that provided outreach to street-based sex workers and 'trafficked'[3] persons. The members of this informal group mobilised to provide housing assistance for Ziya while they worked to sort out her legal paperwork so that she could procure a new working visa. When I last spoke with her in September 2009 she had found a job as a nanny for a family in the same building as her temporary home. She laughed as she said, 'I am happy to make money now like this to send home to my family. Next time I go home to Ethiopia, I am happy and proud.'

The first time I met Maryam, a 27-year-old, high-end call girl from Tehran in 2004, she was also living in a modern high-rise skyscraper overlooking Dubai Marina. By the time I left Dubai in 2009, however, Maryam was sleeping in a half-built metro terminal in Bur Dubai (the metro system in Dubai was under construction during the summer of 2009 and had been slated to open the following autumn) and trying her best to avoid the authorities, who had a warrant for her arrest. 'I guess I'm a rags to riches story, but in reverse,' Maryam told me when I talked with her on the phone shortly before my departure from the field that summer. She lamented:

> Remember when we first met? I was making thousands of dollars a night, living the good life. Now look at me. I can't stay here [in Dubai], I am in debt because of my legal cases, and I can't even go back to Iran. Worse yet, no one wants to help me here.

I had initially heard about Maryam through her friends and colleagues in Iran, while conducting field research for a book on sexuality in post-revolution Iran. I had met her friends in Tehran and followed them to Dubai in 2004, where they would make repeated visits to engage in transactional sex. Because women from Iran and Morocco were the two nationalities of sex workers in highest demand in Dubai, these women made up to 12,000 AED (about $3,000) per night. Many of them lived in luxurious apartments paid for by their regular clientele, while others financed their own accommodation in more expensive parts of town with their high salaries. Maryam used the semi-private space of the Internet to attract her customers, and up until 2009 had a steady flow of clients that allowed her to make more money than most of the businessmen I met while in Dubai. She and her friends enjoyed the relative safety provided by the discretionary nature of their work. 'No one is going to find us here, and if they do, they can't prove anything, can't prove we are prostitutes, so it's OK,' Maryam had told me in 2005. When I asked about physical safety, she pointed to a series of cameras in her apartment and indicated that she and her friends had hired a full-time guard who would provide assistance should any problems arise. 'We are living the life,' her friend Sayeh, 25, told me in 2008 when I visited their five bedroom apartment, marvelling at the view and prime real estate location near the Palm Islands.

In 2009, however, all of this changed when the jealous wife of one of Maryam's customers found out about her husband's activities and called the police. Maryam was arrested immediately and spent most of one year's income on legal fees and posting bail. She was permitted to leave her holding cell in early 2009 but was told she could not leave the country while her case was pending. She was charged with the crime of adultery. When another client's wife found out about her, she charged her with a series of crimes ranging from espionage to theft. This time, however, the authorities could not find Maryam. She had lost her apartment when her friends had rented her room out to another young woman from Tehran in her absence and told Maryam not to return home due to unwanted attention she or her clients' wives might bring. Maryam was relegated to working in hotel lobby bars and clubs and occasionally turned to street-based sex work to make ends meet. She began sleeping at the homes of clients or in airport or metro terminals. When she sought out assistance from informal outreach groups, she was turned away.

Why the discrepancy? Why was Maryam turned away, unable to access services and assistance, while Ziya was taken in? The answers to these questions have everything to do with perceptions of female sex workers[4] based on their countries of origin and the spaces in which they work. While women who work in street-based sex work (located at this spectrum of the sex industry because of demand tied to perceived race) are seen as vulnerable and innocent, higher-end sex workers such as Maryam are viewed as predatory, guilty and a threat to the moral fabric of society by those who provide outreach in the form of social support and services. Their perceived complicity in determining their status (one that is assumed rather than based on actual accounts) correlates with the ability to script their subjectivities into programmatic paradigms of 'victimhood'.[5]

The physical spatialisation of female sex work hinges on local and locally produced discourses of 'race' and produces distinct categories and income-generating potential for women engaged in the sex industry in Dubai. Deploying the term 'race' in this context is complex, especially because locals use the word to describe nationality and are not always conscious of the social production of race and racism. In the UAE (and many other Gulf States), where migrants make up a majority of the population, country of migrant origin (labelled 'race' by locals) determines social status and often income earning potential. Although race is socially constructed and not necessarily tied to nationality, country of origin or ethnic group, many of my interlocutors (including clients of sex workers, and locals and expatriates who participate in structuring the discourse on sex work) continued to use the term 'race' to refer to nationality or country of origin of migrant sex workers. For example, women coming from Ethiopia, Sudan, Nigeria and other parts of sub-Saharan Africa were all lumped together by my interlocutors and raced as 'Black'. Therefore, throughout this chapter, I use the term 'race' to mean perceived race (as perceived and constructed in local discourse) to reflect the local vernacular and hierarchical racialisation of labour in the UAE.

The social and physical topography of Dubai is important in marginalising or privileging various groups of sex workers which correlates race, space and place with income-generating potential. I begin with a description of the multidirectional flows of causality between race, space, place and demand. I then discuss how these various groups are inversely spatialised within the discourse on assistance, protection and rights. The findings presented here are based on ethnographic research with transnational migrants conducted in the UAE in 2004, 2008 and 2009. I began this project through my previous work with sex workers in Tehran which facilitated access to women migrating from Iran to Dubai to work in the sex industry in the UAE (Mahdavi 2008). Working with these women provided an entrée for me in speaking with a range of sex workers in Dubai. Furthermore, I also volunteered with a series of informal organisations that provide outreach to women who have been abused or are in need of assistance while in the UAE. My work with these groups provided me with access to providers as well as women in the sex industry. After several years of interviewing female sex workers, I was also able to meet some of their clients. The data presented here are a result of 112 in-depth interviews (with migrant workers in various industries from many different countries), participant observation and long-term correspondence with many of the women I write about. All names and identifying details have been changed to protect the confidentiality of interviewees.

Race, space, place and demand

The racial structures and hierarchy of demand for sex work in Dubai barred Ziya from accessing work in the somewhat safer spaces of high-end brothels, hotel lobby bars or clubs, whereas Maryam had previously enjoyed the luxury of working as a high-end call girl in her own apartment on her own terms. Demand for sex work in Dubai (as in many other parts of the world) is organised hierarchically according to perceived race (tied to nation of migrant origin).[6] This inadvertent racialisation of sex workers both results in, and is a result of, the spatialisation of the sex workers themselves. In recent years, the sex industry in Dubai has grown to include women from the Middle East, Eastern Europe, East Asia and Africa. The increase in sex workers of different nationalities has produced a form of racism embedded in spatialised structures of desire constructing specific locations. In other words, the raced hierarchy of demand both structures and is structured by the locations within the city in which sex workers perform their labour. Women from Iran, Morocco and some parts of Eastern Europe (described as lighter skinned women and labelled as 'White') command the highest price and thus invariably work in the higher paid, more comfortable environments of expensive bars in Jumeirah and Dubai Marina and in luxury apartments in wealthier parts of town. Women from East Asia, the Philippines, India and Pakistan (perceived as 'Brown' women) form a middle tier (based on earnings) and often work in lower-end bars and clubs in Deira or Bur Dubai or else in brothels and massage parlours throughout the city. Finally, women from Africa (specifically sub-Saharan and East Africa – perceived as 'Black') are still conspicuously over-represented in the poorest and most dangerous sectors of the trade, namely in street work. That each group is located in various imagined and physical spaces is a product of their racialisation within the discourse, but is also caused by the construction of hierarchical demand. Causality between race, space, place and demand is thus multidirectional.

The racialised hierarchy of demand for sex workers in the emerging globalised locale of Dubai structures demand through the association of attributes to a particular nationality. Iranian, Moroccan[7] and some Eastern European women are in highest demand, making US$3,000 or more per night, and most often contract work through the semi-private space of the Internet, phone or through informal networks of clients who pass information by word of mouth. When I asked clients of sex workers (informally referred to as 'Johns') about reasons behind the elevation of these particular nationalities to the top of the chain of demand, responses were constructed along the lines of supply/demand, linguistic and cultural compatibility and, in some cases, similarity to pornographic actresses. Some Johns alluded to the fact that the ability to have discreet relationships – the women lived in apartments and could be contacted online – was one of the benefits of engaging in relations with a high-end sex worker. 'I like that they aren't in clubs or on street corners, it makes it seem more classy and less seedy,' said one Iranian man who frequented Maryam's apartment. Many of the most socio-economically privileged men in Dubai come from the Middle East and are of Arab or Iranian descent. For these clients, the ability to relate to the sex workers was also described as essential: 'Believe it or not, I actually want to like the person I'm with,' explained Mohammad, a 33-year-old wealthy Arab-Iranian merchant who frequented a high-end sex work venue in Dubai. 'For me, I like that I can speak in Farsi or Arabic with them, and a lot of my friends feel the same way,' he elaborated, as his friend Karim, 29, nodded in agreement.

Two Moroccan women who work as high-class escorts in Dubai have created their own website entitled 'Sex and the Dubai Hotspot', a blog written in French, Arabic and English (which is a testament to their level of education and status as trilingual), featuring long narratives of encounters with various Johns. Mouna, the 22-year-old author of many postings on this site, told me that

> we make the most money because we can talk dirty to them in Arabic. Who do you think has the most money to spend in town? Right, the guys that want us to talk dirty in Arabic.

Other Johns espoused a supply/demand narrative, reasoning that Moroccan and Iranian women were most in demand because they were most limited in supply. 'There are tons and tons of Asians (meaning East Asian), that's why they aren't the most desired any more,' explained a 40-year-old Romanian client named Vlad. Two British men, Matthew, 41, and Scott, 44, who use web-based escort services, added: 'If I'm in Dubai, I want to be with a Middle Eastern woman; if I'm in East Asia, I will go with an East Asian.' There were some Eastern European women who also worked in high-end brothels or through escort services, and when I asked about the reasons behind their success, they (the women themselves) said that their clients told them they were like the actresses seen in popular pornographic films that were circulating in the region. 'I guess a lot of the porn actresses are blonde,' said Irina, a 24-year-old woman from Poland who had been working as a call girl in Dubai for 4 years:

> That works for me because a lot of the men, Arabs, Iranian, Indian and sometimes Asian [referring to East Asian], will pay me a lot of money. Probably it makes them feel like they are in one of the films.

Irina, Mouna and other women at the top of the pyramid of demand for sex work mostly worked inside lavish apartments in the southern (higher end) part of town, Dubai Marina, Jebel Ali or on the Palm Islands. These women rarely had pimps or agents and worked with other sex workers with whom they shared their residences to manage their clientele. Compared to their counterparts who work on the street, they enjoyed relative privacy and they remained somewhat undetected by the surveillance powers of state authorities, a fact that made them more attractive to their clients.

High-income sex workers and low-wage, street-based sex workers are largely invisible in writings and discussion about sex work in Dubai. Most journalistic and media representations[8] of sex work in the Emirates focus on the 'middle tier' of sex workers (labelled as such because of their income earning potential), namely those who work in hotel lobby bars, nightclubs and massage parlours in the older (northern) part of town. Reliable figures about numbers of sex workers in each category are hard to come by, but the middle range of sex workers are certainly the most visible, which makes it seem as though this type of sex work forms the majority of transactional sex taking place in town. Hotel lobbies in Bur Dubai and Deira play host to a revolving series of nightclubs where one can find sex workers and clients from almost every part of the world every night of the week. Some clubs are known as home to certain nationalities more than others, but the majority of women who work in hotel lobby bars come from East, South-east or South Asian countries. Described by locals as 'Brown' women, sex workers in this range typically earn roughly US$100 to US$1,000 per evening (depending on the season and their location). The clubs tend to be most frequented by expatriates or businessmen from Europe, the USA and, to a lesser extent, the Middle East and South Asia. It appears that these clubs must have some sort of arrangement with the hotel staff or owners to offer relative protection to the women working inside, but such protections and privacy are not extended to cover law enforcement personnel, who occasionally raid clubs, revoke bar licences (as in the case of Cyclone – the club featured in the popular hit movie *Body of Lies* [2008]) and sometimes arrest all of the 'working women' inside, which can ultimately result in their deportation. While some of these women work as sex workers full-time, others are sometimes engaging in sex work on the side (and are employed as mall workers, domestic workers or 'care takers' by day), are working off debts or waiting for legal work permits. Although certainly not all women who migrate to Dubai to work as domestic workers or in other parts of the formal economy also engage in sex work on the side, during my time in the field I met several who did so and at least seven women who had left the formal economy in favour of higher potential wages in the informal economy of sex work.

Women from sub-Saharan Africa make up the majority of street-based sex workers, who sometimes reside and work in the winding alleyways and streets of Bur Dubai in the northern, older part of town. On occasion, these women will venture into hotel lobby bars, but they can face serious backlash from other sex workers or hotel staff at these venues. Kimberly, 25, a part-time hairdresser from Nigeria who engages in sex work on the side, noted that

> people look at me kind of funny when I walk into the hotel lobby bars. It's because of my skin … they don't want me there, and I don't think I can make as much money in a place where I get dirty looks.

Kimberly and some of her friends explained that working on the streets of Bur Dubai was easier than the tense and racially charged atmosphere of the clubs. Although they articulated feeling physically safer working inside the clubs (in that police raids, arrest and abuse were less likely), they noted that working on the street was a risk they were willing to take in order to avoid the regular hostility they felt from hotel employees or sex workers from other backgrounds. Clients of street-based sex workers tend to be lower-wage labourers, and sometimes these women are taken to labour camps to provide sexual services and are given a lump sum. Many of the women working in the informal economy of street-based sex work report regular abuse at the hands of policemen or clients without any avenues of recourse or any social support or safety nets due to the illegal nature of their work coupled with the fact that most have overstayed their visas.

While the racialisation and spatialisation outlined encompasses a majority of the social topography of sex work in Dubai, it should be noted that many female sex workers do in fact cross these categories and spaces. There are cases of White women working as street-based sex workers, Brown women working as high-end call girls and Black women working inside hotel lobbies. Furthermore, while a woman may start at one end of the industry, she can potentially move both up or down the ladder (as was the case with Maryam, who went from working in an apartment in the Marina to living and working on the streets of Bur Dubai). Beyond the physical spatialisation of sex work, however, it is interesting to take note of the racialisation and spatialisation of sex workers in the discourse about trafficking and sex work, as well as the racialisation and spatialisation of the provision of informal social services responding to these issues in the UAE.

Race, gender and the discourse of vulnerability

The way that racism structures the spaces in which various groups participate in sex work stands in sharp contrast with their spatialisation within the discourse on 'victimhood' and 'rights'. Historically and globally, sex work has been racialised and spatialised, but what is particularly interesting and salient in the case of Dubai is that the same localised racism relegating certain groups of women to unsafe, street-based sex work paradoxically enables them to access informal social services and assistance with far more ease.

In Dubai (as in many other parts of the world), sex workers' access to social services hinges on their perceived guilt or complicity in determining their fate.[9] Women who work in street-based sex work or those who are found in lower-end hotel bars or clubs are constructed as 'innocent' non-agents, understood as forced, duped or tricked into sex work by conspiring male pimps or 'traffickers'. This is not limited to Dubai, but a pervasive stereotype amongst members of anti-trafficking organisations around the world who seek to save 'innocent' or 'fallen' women.[10] These sex workers are constructed as 'innocent victims', usually described as trafficked (an assessment relating to their perceived 'innocence' and not related to the particular conditions of their travel and employment process) and in need of 'saving'. This narrative problematically fails to recognise transnational female migrants as active agents working in pursuit of their own objectives, and relies on an artificial dichotomisation of force and choice (Doezema 1998; Saunders 2005).

None of the sex workers with whom I spoke conceptualised themselves as victims (Bernstein and Schaffner 2005). On the contrary, they each narrated a similar set of desires: to earn money, support their families and provide a better life for themselves and their loved ones. Interestingly, however, the rhetoric that casts these women as victims, while refusing their agentive capacity, works to their immediate advantage in that they are painted as innocent, unknowing and non-consenting (thus 'deserving' of support). It is this type of logic that undergirds well-intentioned but uncritical, deeply flawed Euro-American anti-trafficking feminist campaigns to 'save', 'enlighten' or 'civilise' the 'lost' or 'fallen' woman (Chapkis 2003; Soderlund 2005; Parrenas 2010). Unfortunately, in recent years, these campaigns have migrated from Euro-America to other parts of the world, influencing local efforts in places like Dubai to end trafficking through ending prostitution. While this was not always the case in Dubai, in recent years sex workers have come under increased scrutiny due to the elevation and politicisation of the 'trafficking' issue through US Policy such as the Trafficking in Persons Report (TIP) or international policy such as the United Nations Palermo Protocol.[11] The global moral panic that conflates sex work and trafficking has cast a dark shadow on the experiences of sex workers and created a series of stereotypes about women that influence their ability to access social services.

Women who work as higher-end call girls are seen as guilty or predatory and not deserving of the same protection or services as their more 'innocent' and 'vulnerable' counterparts (according to my interviewees). In Dubai, the concept of race that structures the demand for sex workers (which places them in particular locations correlating with certain income-generating potential and risk) adds yet another layer to the false dichotomies of guilty/innocent and force/choice. Women from certain backgrounds (including Iranian, Moroccan and Russian) are perceived as 'guiltier' than their darker skinned counterparts as they are seen as having consented and even strategised for their position. Contrast the cases of Maryam and Ziya. Maryam earned a high income and was able to work and live in Dubai Marina. When she ran into trouble, however, no one would take her in and she was relegated to living on the streets of Bur Dubai. Ziya's circumstance was perhaps the opposite. The racism that structures demand for sex work made it such that she was not able to make more than 120 AED (US$30) per night and was vulnerable to arrest and abuse on a regular basis. After a few months, however, when Ziya decided she could no longer continue in this line of work, she was able to find assistance and support from local groups. Maryam, however, was further marginalised in her time of need because of the perception of Iranian women as guilty or predatory sex workers scheming to destroy happy families.

Paradoxically, the same racism that relegates women like Ziya to the streets of Bur Dubai works in their favour in terms of social service provisions in the UAE. Although the creation of formal government-recognised non-governmental organisations (NGOs) are prohibited in the UAE,[12] many informal groups of co-ethnics, as well as groupings that cross ethnic and national lines, have established in recent years, coalescing around particular issues such as domestic violence. The larger and more successful of such groups, and those that have formed to provide outreach to women in Dubai, typically comprise local Emiratis and Western expats, most frequently women. These women have been influenced by neo-liberal anti-trafficking rhetoric emanating from the Bush era in the USA.[13]

Within their discourses, women coming from sub-Saharan Africa are seen as ignorant, duped or tricked into the dangerous situations in which they find themselves. But it is this stereotype (problematic in its implications and lack of agentive access for these women) that grants street-based Black sex workers access to social services and provisions in the informal civil society networks of Dubai. In contrast, women such as Maryam and her Iranian and Moroccan counterparts are cast as villains who are there to 'corrupt' Emirati society. These women are constructed as guilty and thus deserving of any misfortune that might befall them. This was evident to me when speaking with various groups of informal activists seeking to provide outreach to sex workers who have faced abuse or are in need of assistance. While they had no trouble conceiving of Ethiopian women or other sub-Saharan African women as in need of services, when I asked if they would be willing to assist Maryam, the response quickly turned negative when they heard she was Iranian. The same experience replicated itself when I asked a group of Indian volunteers if they would be willing to work with Eastern European sex workers. These responses were as such not due to a refusal of one ethnic group to help another, but because of the caricatures and stereotypes that have been drawn about sex workers from these particular countries of origin.

Underpinning informal humanitarian interventions lurks a racialised morality that requires some interrogation. Women's bodies are racialised and spatialised in the physical geography of Dubai, while simultaneously racialised in the moral sphere of social service outreach. Street-based sex workers can access services with greater ease; however, this is directed by an underlying saving sentiment similar to efforts written about by Spivak and Abu-Lughod to save Brown (or in this case Black) women from Brown men (Spivak 1996). Though this is a non-Western context, many of those seeking to do the 'saving' are expats from Euro-America or have been trained and influenced by the US approach to trafficking. This 'saving' sentiment, infantilising and condescending in its racialised and moralised approach, directs and restricts the types of solutions and responses that these social service providers are willing and capable of conceiving (Abu-Lughod 1998).

Conclusion

The difficulty is that many of the informal social service providers coalescing around the issue of migrant labourers and abuse are segregated by country of migrant origin. Ethiopians organise to help Ethiopians, Indians to help Indians and so on. Locals are willing to donate money to various causes, but many of the local women in particular feel very strongly about sex workers from certain backgrounds (Middle Eastern and European) and they are adamant about not wanting to support women whom they view as predatory competition. The unevenness in the development of civil society and the attitude that only certain women are deserving of assistance further hierarchically racialises the sex industry in Dubai. While there is a need for social services that are available to all, regardless of employment industry or country of origin, it is also important to encourage various informal groups to begin working together towards a common goal of assisting all migrant workers, regardless of their industry or background, in Dubai.

Furthermore, while groups of non-citizens have been working with locals in Dubai to push for organisations that support the needs of migrants, the issue of trafficking, as it has been constructed by Euro-American moralised and politicised rhetoric, has eclipsed the formation of these groups. Trafficking is currently viewed within a framework of sex work rather than understood as a problem of forced labour and forced migration. The current policies on trafficking (such as the TIP Report or the United Nations Palermo Protocol) seek to address trafficking by policing sex work. That there can be abuses within the sex industry is without question. However, the term 'trafficked' has been articulated and employed to construct the representative experience of women who migrate into the sex industry, while completely neglecting the many women migrating into other industries and the difficulties that they may face. Trafficking seeks to account for migratory experiences characterised by the elements of force, fraud and/or coercion. To be labelled a 'trafficked victim' theoretically entitles one to a particular legal status and its attendant benefits. Born out of an understandable sense of indignation regarding the types of abuse and exploitation that seem all too common in migrant women's worlds, the concept has been expanded beyond reasonable or feasible limits, becoming both conceptually and juristically obtuse, while also being narrowly gendered, sexualised and racialised at the same time. Specifically, the misunderstanding that human trafficking refers only to women who are kidnapped by men and forced into the sex industry has, problematically, become the functional definition of the term. This has altered the way in which trafficking is represented, pursued and prosecuted. The paradigm of human trafficking as it exists today, and, critically, the disjuncture between the legal ambiguity and popular specificity with which trafficking has been defined, offers uncomfortable insight into the complex ways that gender and race permeate popular understandings of victimhood, vulnerability and power.

Notes

1 Dubai is not the only place where the *kefala*, or sponsorship, system governs the rules and experiences of guest workers. In fact, many of the Gulf countries have this same system in place. In these countries, the *kefala* system is problematic in that residence in the country is predicated on the sponsor-employer. Scholars such as Andrew Gardner (2010) have argued successfully that this system imposes a type of structural violence on migrant workers in the Gulf. For domestic workers, the *kefala* system presents particular challenges in that while they are held to the rules of the sponsorship system, they cannot benefit from the protections of said system as their work is relegated

to the 'private realm', and there exists a specific clause in UAE labour laws that notes domestic workers are not protected by labour laws that protect construction or other migrant workers (Embassy of the United Arab Emirates, Washington, DC). Domestic workers in many parts of the world face the dilemma of what scholar Rhacel Parrenas (2001) has termed 'partial citizenship'. However, domestic workers and many other members of the informal economy in the Gulf experience added challenges of not being able to seek out recourse for challenges incurred during their time as domestic workers due to a lack of formal structures in place to protect their rights (for an excellent discussion of domestic work in the Gulf, please see Longva [1999], Gamburd [2000] or Silvey [2004]).

2 Note the population of Dubai consists of only 8 per cent Emiratis or locals (Dubai Statistics Center 2009). The remainder of the population is made up of non-citizens. Of these non-citizens, it is estimated that 70 per cent are unskilled labourers from parts of Asia and Africa, but most commonly South Asia (for more statistics on demographics in the Gulf, see Andrzej Kapiszewski [2001]). Male unskilled workers are typically labelled 'migrants', female unskilled workers are referred to as 'help' or 'care takers', while skilled workers, mostly of Western origin, earn the more melodious term 'expat' according to my interlocutors.

3 I use quotes to indicate the contested nature of a term that has no universal definition; rather, various actors define the term 'trafficked' in ways that are most convenient for their policies, academic discourses or activist procedures. There has been an increasing amount of debate about the definition of 'trafficking', which is most often used to refer to the movement or transport of illegal contraband, specifically arms and drugs. 'Trafficking in people' is defined as the transportation of people across long distances (which may or may not include crossing an international border) through some form of deceit, coercion or force. It is for these reasons and more that it is important not to conflate the often sliding definitions of terms such as 'trafficking', 'migration' or 'labour'. For an in-depth discussion of the strategic deployment of the term 'trafficking' in the Gulf, please see Agustín (2007).

4 Though several interlocutors described the presence of male sex workers in Dubai, I was unable to find any men during my time in the field. Therefore, while I acknowledge the presence of male sex workers in Dubai and the Gulf more broadly speaking, in this chapter I am focusing on women who work in the sex industry.

5 I place 'trafficking victims' in particular in quotations to indicate the arbitrary nature of 'victimhood'. I do not deny that trafficked persons are often subjected to unscrupulous and criminal figures and that migrants, trafficked or not, often are victims of macro and micro instances of violence and exploitation. I am wary, however, of the term victim, because of the unequal power dynamic that is implied. By positioning trafficked women as victims, the attention and power is then shifted to 'rescuers', who set the terms for who gets to 'count' as a victim and what they are understood to be a victim of. For an in-depth explication of the politics of the rescue industry, please see Soderlund (2005).

6 For an in-depth explication of this, please see Mohanty (1991, 1997). In Mohanty's 1997 essay, Mohanty notes that sex work in many parts of the world is racialised hierarchically. In addition, the case of Dubai expands on Mohanty's argument because all labour in Dubai is organised hierarchically (according to nation of migrant origin), as are pay scales. For example, the lowest wage earners in Dubai typically come from Ethiopia and Nigeria and are racialised as 'Black' according to perceived skin colour, followed by unskilled workers perceived as 'Brown' migrating from South Asia. The more pay scales rise, the lighter the skin colour of the employee, thus demonstrating Mohanty's point beyond just the case of sex work.

7 Though it may seem that Iranians and Moroccans should not necessarily be considered White, all of my interlocutors placed them in this category. During my fieldwork, I was told repeatedly that Iranians and Moroccans are favoured over Gulf Arabs because of their reputation for light skin.

8 Examples of this include films such as *Taken* (2008) or *Body of Lies* (2008), journalistic books such as Jim Krane's (2009) *City of Gold: Dubai and the Dream of Capitalism* and two BBC documentaries which are currently being made about commercial sex work in bars in Dubai.

9 For examples of this in other contexts, see Chapkis (1997), Vance and Miller (2004), Bernstein and Schaffner (2005) and Soderlund (2005).

10 For an in-depth discussion of this, please see Vance and Miller (2004), Bernstein and Schaffner (2005) or Cheng (2010).

11 Though colloquially referred to as the United Nations Palermo Protocol, the full title of this act is the 'Protocol to Prevent, Suppress, and Punish Trafficking in Persons' and is housed in the United Nations Office of Drugs and Crime (UNODC).

12 According to Articles 155 and 166 of UAE Federal Law No. 8 of 1980 (known as the 'Labor Law'); Human Rights Watch (2007).

13 The obsessive focus on violence within the sex industry obscures the widespread existence of labour rights abuses against migrants in all industries, and collapses the motivations of female migrants, both those seeking to enter the sex industry as well as those seeking to enter other labour sectors, into a homogeneous tale of victimisation.

References

Abu-Lughod, L. (ed.) 1998. *Remaking Women: Feminism and Modernity in the Middle East.* Princeton, NJ: Princeton University Press.

Agustín, L.M. 2007. *Sex at the Margins: Migration, Labour Markets and the Rescue Industry.* New York: Palgrave Macmillan.

Bernstein, E. and Schaffner, L. (eds) 2005. *Regulating Sex: The Politics of Intimacy and Identity.* New York: Routledge.

Body of Lies. 2008. Directed by Ridley Scott. Burbank, CA: Warner Brothers Pictures.

Chapkis, W. 1997. *Live Sex Act: Women Performing Erotic Labor.* New York: Routledge.

Chapkis, W. 2003. Trafficking, migration and the law: Protecting innocents, punishing immigrants. *Gender and Women* 17(6): 923–937.

Cheng, S. 2010. *On the Move for Love: Migrant Entertainers and the US Military in South Korea.* Philadelphia: University of Pennsylvania Press.

Doezema, J. 1998. Forced to choose: Beyond the free versus forced prostitution dichotomy. In: K. Kempadoo and J. Doezema (eds) *Global Sex Workers: Rights, Resistance and Redefinition.* New York and London: Routledge, 34–51.

Dubai Statistics Center. 2009. *Dubai in Figures, 2009.* Government of Dubai. Available at: www.dsc. gov.ae/en [Accessed 22 March 2010].

Embassy of the United Arab Emirates, Washington, DC. *Labor Rights in the UAE.* Embassy of the United Arab Emirates. Available at: www.uae-embassy.org/uae/human-rights/labor-rights [Accessed 18 March 2010].

Gamburd, W.R. 2000. *The Kitchen Spoon's Handle: Transnationalism and Sri Lanka's Migrant Housemaids.* Cornell, NY: Cornell University Press.

Gardner, A. 2010. *City of Strangers: Gulf Migration and the Indian Community in Bahrain.* Ithaca, NY: ILR Press – an imprint of Cornell University Press.

Human Rights Watch. 2007. *The UAE's Draft Labor Law: Human Rights Watch's Comments and Recommendations.* Available at: www.hrw.org [Accessed 14 March 2010].

Kapiszewski, A. 2001. *Nationals and Expatriates: Population and Labour Dilemmas of the Gulf.* Reading: Garnet.

Krane, J. 2009. *City of Gold: Dubai and the Dream of Capitalism.* New York: St. Martin's Press.

Longva, A.N. 1999. Keeping migrant workers in check: The *kafala* system in the Gulf. *Middle East Report* 29(211): 20–22.

Mahdavi, P. 2008. *Passionate Uprisings: Iran's Sexual Revolution.* Stanford, CA: Stanford University Press.

Mohanty, C.T. 1991. Cartographies of struggle: Third world women and the politics of feminism. In C.T. Mohanty, A. Russo and L. Torres (eds) *Third World Women and the Politics of Feminism.* Bloomington, IL: Indiana University Press, 1–50.

Mohanty, C.T. 1997. Women workers and capitalist scripts: Ideologies of domination, common interests and the politics of solidarity. In: C.T. Mohanty and M.J. Alexander (eds) *Feminist Genealogies, Colonial Legacies, Democratic Futures.* New York: Routledge, 3–30.

Parrenas, R. 2001. *Servants of Globalization: Women, Migration, and Domestic Work*. Stanford: Stanford University Press.

Parrenas, R. 2010. *Migrant mothering in Philippines*. Lecture presented 11 February 2010, at Scripps College, Claremont, CA.

Saunders, P. 2005. Traffic violations: Determining the meaning of violence in sexual trafficking versus sex work. *Journal of Interpersonal Violence* 20(3): 343–360.

Silvey, R. 2004. Power, difference and mobility: Feminist advances in migration studies. *Progress in Human Geography* 28(4): 490–506.

Soderlund, G. 2005. Running from the rescuers: New US crusades against sex trafficking and the rhetoric of abolition. *National Women's Studies Association Journal* 17(3): 64–87.

Spivak, G.C. 1996. Diasporas old and new: Women in the transnational world. *Textual Practice* 10(2): 245–269.

Taken. 2008. Directed by Pierre Morel. Paris: EuropaCorp.

Vance, C. and Miller, A.M. 2004. Sexuality, human rights and health. *Health and Human Rights* 7(2): 5–15.

Index

abstinence: churches' promotion of 46; as means of HIV prevention 29, 57, 241, 243–4; oral sex as type of 31; religious views as reason for 238, 243; teenage magazines on 29
abuse: coping behaviours 213–14; 'gay' as term of 212; sex workers' reluctance to report to police 146; of street-based sex workers 164–5
activism, HIV and the rise in 3
Africa: change in women's status and roles 43; changes to the institution of marriage in 43; criminalisation of consensual male-male sexual activity 158; exchange of material goods as indicator of partner commitment 81; multiple meanings of transactional sex in 82; taboo on talking about sex 49; *see also individual countries*
African-American perspectives *see under* Black
Aggleton, P. 18
Agustín, L. M. 270
AIDS: and community activism 2; dominant religious discourse 241; *see also* HIV/AIDS
AIDS and Reproductive Health Network 3
alcohol: consumption of as demonstration of trust 255; consumption rituals in China 255; *see also* drug/alcohol use
alcohol abuse, homophobia and 216
anal sex: and knowledge regarding HIV transmission 160, 167; male sex workers' experiences 162; receptivity and HIV risk 183; refusal strategies 152–3
anti-retroviral therapy: barriers and facilitators, systematic review of patient reported 221; *see also* post-exposure prophylaxis
asylum seekers: experiences of in Europe 192; *see also* displaced persons
attitudes to sexuality, correlation between exposure to magazines and 25
Australasia, teenage magazines studies 24
Australia: fragmentation of gay community in 100; LGBQ identity construction study 97–110

Belgium and the Netherlands, sexual and gender based violence study 189–203 (*see also* sexual and gender based violence)
bisexuality: challenges of 105–6, 109; invisibility 109; positioning of as illegitimate identity 109
Black gay and bisexual men, negative attitudes towards 73
Black heterosexual men, scarcity of research on gender ideology and sexual risk 65
Black lesbian culture: behavioural continuum 136–7; feminine expression 133; gender debate 133–6; gender expression 126–7; gender sex roles 137; label adoption 130; labels and expectations around partner choices 131; masculine expression 131–2; vs White 133
Black lesbians, gender categorisations 126
Black masculinity ideologies: as compensation for lack of access to financial achievement 75; explicit ideologies and their implications 69–71; gaps in empirical knowledge 65; heterosexuality ideology 70–1, 74; implicit ideologies and their implications 71–3; inability to decline sex ideology 71–2; multiple partners ideology 69–70; women's responsibility for condom use ideology 72–3
'born again' identity, importance of in Nigeria 240
Brazil, HIV prevention program 74
breastfeeding, as HIV transmission vector 59, 61
bridewealth payments 38, 42–3, 81
British Social Attitudes survey 207
brothels, impact of legalisation 155
bullying, and self-destructive behaviour 208
Butler, J. 99

cachaquitos 176, 181
Canada: law enforcement practices 145–6; structure and agency of Vancouver sex workers study 143–55

Chile: HIV prevention and low-income women study 55–62; ratio of men to women living with HIV 55

China: cultural and political significance of *yingchou* 256–7; economic development and rate of engagement with commercial sex 249; first domestic outbreak of HIV in 252; 'high risk' behaviour of wealthy businessman and government officials study 248–58

Chlamydia 26, 28

Christianity: growth of in Nigeria 237, 239–40; impact and pervasiveness on Igbo population 239; influence in Zulu society 41; and *isoka* masculinity 41

commercial sex: and conspicuous consumption 181; factors leading to high rates of engagement with 249; racialisation of 261–71; *see also* sex work

community activism, AIDS and 2

community structures, importance in the response to HIV/AIDS 15

concurrency, in sexual relationships 37, 69, 73, 75, 90–1, 169; *see also under* multiple

condom use: female infidelity and 60; gay men as instigators of 2; gender roles and vulnerability to infection 113; and masculinity ideologies 66; in 'moral partnerships' 242–3; need for interventions to emphasise men's responsibility for 74; overpowering sexual desire and 71, 74; and perceptions of HIV risk 166–8; recognition of as HIV prevention measure 57; as women's responsibility 72, 72–3

condoms: encouraging the use of 46, 161; mandatory placement of in Chinese hotel rooms 258; negotiating the use of *see* safer sex (condoms) negotiation; non-use and wanting to be loved 120; non-use of as affirmation of trust 113; sexual infidelity and 60; teenage magazines on 29; young women's experiences and vulnerability 28, 32

conjugal relationships, reconceptualisation of the complexity of 14

Connell, R. 37

conspicuous consumption: commercial sex and 181; as motivation for transactional sex 82, 84–6, 88

contraception, as women's responsibility 65

contraceptive pill 1, 23

courtesan culture, in Chinese society 255–6

courting, in Zulu society 39

desire in women, missing discourses 33

discrimination: as concrete outcome of stigma 112; male sex work and 164–6; UK legislation 207

displaced persons (asylum seekers; refugees; undocumented migrants) 189, 191, 195, 197, 199–202

domestic violence 18, 59–61, 268

double standard: in Chilean society 56; in magazines for teens and women 24, 31, 33; and media portrayals of sexuality of middle-aged women 25; and negotiation of safe sex 243; virginity and the 24

drug/alcohol use: and HIV risk 164; as risk factor for SGBV 199; *see also* injection drug use; substance abuse

Dubai: female sex work and 'race' discourse 263; informal outreach organisation 262; the place of race and gender in vulnerability discourse 267–8; racialisation of commercial sex study 261–71; racialised hierarchy of demand for sex workers in 264–7, 269; urban planning 261; *see also* UAE

economic crisis, Zimbabwe 83

economic survival, transactional sex in Africa and 80

education, HIV infection and 55

empowerment, requirement for as component of HIV prevention efforts 62

English-language proficiency, importance of in sex work 148

entertainment, and social/business relations in China 255–6

Epprecht, M. 41

essentialist perspectives, social constructionist perspectives vs 98

ethnographic studies, on sexual sub cultures and non-normative sexualities 11

extramarital relations: migrant labour and 41; in South African society 41; in Zulu society 40

female desire, inclusion in teenage magazines 24

Female Masculinity (Halberstam) 132

female sex work: Luise White's work 81; 'race' and income generation 263

female youth culture, and transactional sex 87

femaleness, lesbian culture and the denial of one's 132

femininity, magazines' role in the construction of normative 25

Fine, M. 33

'flesh to flesh' sex 37

fletes 178–83; meaning 176

food, and transactional sex 85–6

Foucault, M. 10, 98

Freud, S. 10

gay pride discourse 108, 216–18
gender: place of in vulnerability discourse 267–8; and risk of SGBV 199
gender blender, meaning 126
gender inequalities in Latin America, and the concepts of machismo and marianismo 55
gender inequality: changing ideologies of 74; impact of on the power to negotiate safe sex 243
gender roles, as barriers to HIV risk reduction among women 61
girls' comics, and the study of sexuality 23
Global South, impact of HIV/AIDS 3
gonorrhoea 26, 28
Gramsci, A. 37
grooming: and social status 87; and transactional sex 86–8
Gulf States: domestic workers' status 261; *see also* UAE

HAART (highly active antiretroviral therapy): mental health and adherence to 222; *see also* antiretroviral therapy
harassment, impact on psychological well-being 208
health, and shame arising from the transgression of social/cultural norms 210
health benefits of sex, women's magazines on the 30
hepatitis B 28
herpes 26, 28
heterosexism: as defining element of masculinity 74; and media portrayals of sexuality of middle-aged women 25
heterosexuality: adherence to in teenage magazines 24; and self-esteem in young boys and girls 121
historical perspectives: changes to the institution of African marriage 43; changing attitudes 1; community level responses to HIV/AIDS 3; epistemology of sexuality research 10–12; *isoka* masculinity 39–49 (*see also isoka* masculinity); private foundations' support for work on HIV/AIDS 3; rapid evolution of sexuality research 9–10; of sex and sexuality 1
HIV: and the categorisation of sexual identity 13; causes of vulnerability to 2; exposure to and adherence to post-exposure medication 221 (*see also* post-exposure prophylaxis); gendered perspective in Chile 55; groundbreaking studies 3; 'mobile men with money' and the transmission of 249–51; ratio of men to women living with in Chile 55; and the rise in activism 3

HIV infection: global statistics 55; rumours about 240
HIV prevention: abstinence as means of 29, 57, 241, 243–4; changing ideologies of masculinity as focus of 74; core focus of theory and research 65; impact of criminalisation on programmes 158; lack of understanding as barrier to 58; limitation of by prejudice and homophobia 159; myths and misconceptions among Chilean women 58; and the needs of men who have sex with men 169; political constraints in China 250; sociocultural factors for low-income Chilean women 59–61; South African strategies 46
HIV risk: alcohol or drug use and 164; and Black masculinity heterosexuality ideology 74; condom use and perceptions of 166–8; and female gender roles 113; masculinity ideologies and 65; and multiple partners 56; and partner's behaviour 59; receptivity in anal sex and 183; spousal abuse and 59–61; stigmatisation and 112; of transgender individuals of colour 112; and work expectations in China 252–4
HIV transmission: Africa vs North America and Europe 37; bisexual men as vectors of in the Black community 70; and Chinese rituals of feasting, drinking and entertainment 255
HIV/AIDS: association with sin 240; common misconceptions 61; community responses 14; escalating rates among Black men and women in the USA 65; immorality narrative 237, 240–1; private foundations' support for work on 3; and the reclaiming of 'queer' identity 98; religious interpretations 240–1, 243; teenage magazines on 28
homelessness: homophobia and the risk of 97; and the transition to adulthood 209
homophobia: and alcohol abuse 216; description of the cumulative effects of 215–16; experiences of 213–15; as form of punishment 99; and LGBQ identity construction 99–100; self-destructive behaviour as an effect of 208, 213; UK legislation against 207
homophobia negotiation strategies: individual responsibility through adult identity 215–16; pride discourse 216–18; problems with 214; routinisation and minimisation 213–14; young people's agency 99–100
homophobic environments 99
homophobic violence, LGBQ Australian experience 97
homosexuality 3, 11–13, 33, 71, 159, 166, 168; inclusion in teenage magazines 24; Kenyan debate 159; treatment of in teenage magazines 32

human rights: lack of as form of violence 192; and residential status 202; SGBV as violation of 189

human sexuality, sociological conceptualisation 98

humanity, SGBV as crime against 189

identity construction: post-structural perspective 98; *see also* LGBQ identity construction

illegal immigrants 146; *see also* displaced persons

immorality narrative, of HIV/AIDS 237, 240–1

inequality: exacerbating factors in Nigeria 238; immorality narrative 237; *see also* gender inequality

infidelity 59–60, 71

information about sex, importance of magazines for providing 25

injection drug use (IDU) 2, 37, 113, 248, 252

International Association for the Study of Sexuality, Culture and Society (IASSCS) 4

the Internet, contacting clients for sex work through 178, 264

intervention: locale-based requirements 12, 169; and men's responsibility for condom use 74; opportunities for with Black heterosexual males 74

isifebe, meaning 38

isoka, meaning 38–40

isoka masculinity: contemporary perspective 42–9; impact of HIV/AIDS on 45; mid-twentieth century perspectives 40–2; nineteenth-century perspectives 39–40; restrictions 41

izibongo (oral praise poetry) 41

karaoke clubs, and Chinese business relations and status 251, 253–4, 256–7

Kenya: criminalisation of same-sex sexual activity 158; HIV prevalence in MSM 158; lack of sexual health services for MSM 159; limited evidence for the relationship between homosexuality, unsafe sex and HIV infection 166

Kenyan male sex workers study 158–70

Kinsey, A. 10

KwaZulu-Natal, multiple partners in historical perspective 37–49 (*see also isoka* masculinity)

Latin America: gender inequalities 55; HIV statistics 55

legal perspectives: impact of law enforcement practices on sex workers 146, 149–50; impact of legalisation of brothels 155; law enforcement practices in Canada 145–6

lesbian and gay activism, focus 2

lesbian culture: androgynous mode of self presentation 125; and the replication of heterosexual norms 133–4; *see also* Black lesbian culture

lesbian gender identity 125–8, 130–1, 133–7

LGBQ identities: limitations 99; negative representations 97

LGBQ identity construction: affirmative 97, 108; and 'coming out' earlier 100; 'coming out' experiences 104; contemporary youth and 100–101; diminishing significance 108; framing lesbian and bisexual identities 105–6; framing lesbian and gay identities 103–5; in homophobic environments 99–100; impact of homophobic attitudes on 97; implications for health and social-care professionals 109; multiple shifting identity frames 106–7; from negative representation to individual affirmation 103–5; problematic frames 105–6; 'queer' identity frame 107; reclaiming of 'queer' 98; reclaiming or redefining 100–101; as source of pride 104, 108 (*see also* gay pride discourse); theorising sexual identities 98–9

LGBT youth: hazards faced by 209; homophobia and self-destructive behaviours 208; and the normative reproduction of heterosexuality in education 209; and the pride/shame binary 209–10, 218; research on suicide and self-harm in 207; suicide attempt rates in North America and New Zealand 208; suicide risk factors 215

lifeworld, Habermasian concept 144

lifeworld of sex workers: media treatment 146–7; need for institutional engagement 154–5; victimhood narrative 147

local categories and classifications, anthropological focus on 12–13

Love Life campaign, South Africa 46, 49

Low Countries, sexual and gender based violence study 189–203 (*see also* sexual and gender based violence)

machismo 55–7, 59, 61

magazines: exposure to and attitudes to sexuality 25; as mediascape for the construction of normative femininity 25; *see also* teenage magazines; women's magazines

Malawi: legislation on male-male sexual activity 158; study of transactional sex among women fish traders 81

male and trans sex work: associated with other economic activities 179; clients 176; contact strategies 176; and economic need, relativity of the concept 181; and geographical mobility 181–2; and lifestyle 181; and the logging industry in Peru 179; means of client contact 178–9; motivations 179–81; Peruvian terminology 176; places and forms of 175–9; social exclusion and 180

male infidelity, as potential risk factor for HIV 59

male sex work: and availability of health facilities 165–6; condom use and perceptions of HIV risk 166–8; context of first sexual encounter and entry into 161–3; and family relationships 165; forced migration and 165; informant network 164; married men as client group 166; meeting locations 163–4; and police harassment 164; practices 164; stigma, discrimination and violence 164–6

male sex workers, strategies for mitigation of stigma 166

male-to-female transgendered persons (MTFs): condom negotiation and HIV prevention 113; domestic gender role preferences 118; experiences of stigma and discrimination 112–13; gender affirming behaviour and HIV risk 113; 'hard life' narrative 116–17; implications of gender roles 113; long-term relationships and HIV risk 119–21; need for partner's acceptance 118–19, 121; and negotiation of condom use 113; stigma and HIV risk 112

Malinowski, B. 90

marianismo 55–7, 59–61

marriage: as implicit consent to sex 30; in South African communities 43; women's magazines on women's responsibility for sex in 29–31

masculinity ideologies: changing, as focus of HIV prevention 74; and HIV risk 65; multiple partnership ideology 73; see also Black masculinity ideologies

massage parlours, and Chinese business relations and status 251, 256–7

masturbation: inclusion in teenage magazines 24; relative silence on in teenage magazines 24

material goods, exchange of as indicator of partner commitment 81

the media: as avenues for understanding of sexuality 23; and confusing messages about HIV 58, 61; portrayal of sexuality among middle-aged women 25; representation of sex workers 146–7; see also teen magazines; women's magazines

medicalisation of sex and sexuality, in teenage and women's magazines 28–9, 32

men who have sex with men: Black men's perceptions of promiscuity 71; HIV prevalence in Kenya and Senegal 158; HIV prevalence in Peru 182; impact of sexual desire on condom use 74; importance of research on communities associated with 14; number of in Kenya's coastal region 159; research attention 15; and sex with women 158

mental health: and barriers to adherence to HAART 222; critical aspects to support following rape 232; LGBT identity and young people's 218; as risk factor for SGBV 199; and sexual identity 207; and the transition to adulthood 209

middle-aged women, lack of investigation into media portrayal of sexuality among 25

migrant labour: and extramarital relations 41; impact on relationship-forming in Zulu society 43; in South Africa 40; see also displaced persons (asylum seekers; refugees; undocumented migrants)

migration, sex work and 181, 183

'mobile men with money,' and the transmission of HIV 249–51

multiple-partnered relationships: benefits for women 46; as Black masculinity ideology 69–70; compensatory narrative 75; and contemporary isoka masculinity 42–9; as distinct African system of sexuality 37; as driver of the HIV pandemic 37; expectations of Chilean men 56; growing asymmetry between men and women's rights 40; hazards 41; HIV risk and 56; normativity of for many Black men 66; respect and admiration for Black men with 70; rising doubts among young men 45; South African men's celebration of 37; transactional sex and 90–1; unmarried women 40; Zulu women 42

Munt, S. R. 209

Nigeria: Christianity and HIV/AIDS-related beliefs and behaviour among rural–urban migrants study 237–45; importance of 'born again' identity 240; legislation on male-male sexual activity 158; oil boom and collapse 238; sense of moral decline in 237

non-normative sexualities, locus of comparison and contrast 11

non-sexual services, transactional sex and 81

oral sex: treatment of in women's magazines 31; as type of abstinence 31

partial citizenship, of domestic workers 270n1

partner commitment, exchange of material goods as indicator of 81

patron–clientelism, Chinese practice 249, 254, 257–8

penetration, and lesbian gender identity 133

penetrative sex, as mark of manliness 41
Pentecostalism, literature on the role of for African peoples 239
Peruvian male and trans sex workers study 173–83; *see also* male and trans sex work
police, sex workers' reluctance to report abuse to 146
polygamy 40–2; machismo and 56
post-exposure prophylaxis (PEP): barriers experienced 224–5; dosage and side-effects 227–8; factors influencing adherence 230–1; fear of blame for rape as barrier to receiving 226–7; forgetfulness and pill taking schedules as barriers to completion 229; impact of poverty and social support on adherence 229–30; impact of psychological responses to rape on adherence 230; and information provision 229; levels of adherence 221; medical advice on adherence 230; period during which PEP should be taken 222; prescription regime 223; side effects as barrier to completion 228; strategies to support adherence 222; Thohoyandou programme's levels of adherence 221–2; victim-blaming and adherence to 231
post-traumatic stress, as barrier to PEP completion 230
poverty: and adherence to post-exposure prophylaxis 229–30; as barrier to PEP completion 225; and HIV infection 55; immorality narrative 237; rates of in Chile study location 56; as risk factor for SGBV 200; and sex work involving men and trans people in Peru 173; and vulnerability to SGBV 189
pregnancy: as HIV transmission vector 59; responsibility for condom use and 72; teenage magazines on 27
premarital virginity, value of in African society 40
prestige, and transactional sex 84–5
pride/shame binary 209–10, 218
promiscuity, perceptions of in Black MSM 71
prophylaxis, South African legislation on the provision of following sexual assault 221
prostitution: female, in Nairobi 81; view of in post-revolutionary China 256

'queer': fluidity of the label 107; vs 'gay' 104; homophobic connotations 100; as political marker 107; reclaiming of 98

race: in discourse of female sex work 263; place of in vulnerability discourse 267–8
racialisation of commercial sex 261–71
rape: barriers experienced to taking prophylaxis following 224–5 (*see also* post-exposure

prophylaxis); fear of stigma following 232; help-seeking and fear of victim-blaming 226–7; impact on mental health and adherence to HAART 222; incidence of in Cape Town 224; marital 225; mental health impact 231; pathways to care 225; South African legislation on prophylaxis provision following 221; stigma as barrier to help seeking 225; *see also* sexual and gender based violence
refugee communities: vulnerability to SGBV 189; *see also* displaced persons
religious perspectives: churches' promotion of abstinence 46 (*see also* abstinence); of HIV/AIDS 240–1, 243; on homosexuality 159; importance of 'born again' identity in Nigeria 240; importance of religion to African peoples 239; sin and sexual behaviour 241–4; and social articulation of sexuality 10
risky behaviours, of Chinese officials and businessmen 249–51

safe sex, sex workers' recognition of the importance of 2
safer sex (condoms) negotiation: double standards and 243; gender inequality and 243; location and 169; moral understandings of sexuality and 243; power imbalances and 164; sex work and 153; and sexual double standards 243
same-sex interactions, focus of anthropological research 11–12
same-sex relationships: parents' minimisation of homophobia directed towards their children 214; public acceptance 207; UK legislation 207
same-sex sexual activity, criminalisation in Kenya 158
same-sex sexuality, representation in popular culture 24
San Francisco, HIV infection in MTFs and FTMs study 112
selfdestructive behaviours, homophobia and 208, 213
self-esteem, impact of homophobia on 208
Senegal, HIV prevalence in MSM 158
sex education, role of teenage magazines 25
sex reassignment surgery, cost of and engagement in risky sex work 112
sex work: agency and 143, 144, 147–9; avoiding arrest 152; and condom use/negotiation 153; contacting clients through the Internet 178, 264; debate about the legality of 143; demand for in Dubai 264; economic perspectives 147–9; false dichotomies 267; as gender

affirmation for MTFs 113; and HIV risk for MTFs 112; importance of English language proficiency 148; literature review of sexual identity and 13–14; locale-based requirements for intervention 169; making choices in employment 151–2; managing client relationships 152, 154; migration and 181, 183; Peruvian studies 173; protection strategies 176; as rational choice 182; reason MTFs turn to 112; and risk of violence 150; slavery narratives 147; transactional sex vs 88; typology proposals 182; venues for 176, 178; women's accounts of structure and agency in 147; work perspective vs oppression perspective 143; *see also* male and trans sex work; male sex work; street-based sex work

sex workers: challenging homogenous representations 154; definition 88; impact of law enforcement practices on 146, 149–50; implications for of regulation 155; 'innocent victims' discourse 267; objectification in news articles 147; racialised hierarchy of demand 264–7, 269; reluctance to report abuse to police 146; representation in the news media 146–7; victimhood rhetoric 267; *see also* lifeworld of sex workers

sexology, the emerging discipline of 10–11

sexual and gender based violence (SGBV): consequences of for displaced persons 198–9; as global public health issue 189; overview of reported cases among displaced persons in the Low Countries 194–7; perceived risk factors for displaced persons 199; perpetrators 189; prevention measures 200–201; and proneness to subsequent victimisation or perpetration of 189; vulnerability of displaced persons to 201; vulnerable groups 189; *see also* rape

sexual behaviour, of businessmen and officials in China 252

sexual culture, understanding 125

sexual diversity, emergence as a social/cultural/historical construction 11

sexual health, historical perspective 3

sexual identity: changes in understanding 13; development models and critiques 99; functions and limitations 98–9; mental health and 207; resource requirements to sustain pride in 218; theorising 98–9

sexual incompatibility, treatment of in women's magazines 32

sexual minorities, marginalisation and stigma 207

sexual networking 37

sexual orientation difficulties, and self-destructive behaviour 208

sexual risk behaviour, and community development and support 15

sexual subcultures: greater research attention 15; importance of research on 14; locus of comparison and contrast 11

sexuality: general agreement on the power of to define who we are as human beings 10; social and cultural dimensions 9; as transmission belt for wider social anxieties 42

sexuality research: diversity, difference and the epistemology of 10–12; emphasis on social organisation of sexual interactions 12; rapid evolution of the field 9–10; sexual cultures, identities and communities 12–15; sexuality and silence 17–18; shift in focus from the natural to the cultural 11; structure and agency 15–16; towards a political economy of the body 15–16

sexuality studies, shaping of the emerging field 11

silence, sexuality and 10, 17–18

social construction, emergence of understanding of sexuality as 12

social constructionist perspectives, vs essentialist perspectives 98

social exclusion, involvement in sex work as consequence of 179

social isolation, and the transition to adulthood 209

social mobility, sex work as means of 180

social movements, research focus 16

social networks: absence of as risk factor in SGBV 192, 198–9; and adherence to post-exposure prophylaxis 229–30; importance of 200, 202

social services: attitudes towards sex workers and access to 267; racialised morality and access to 268; street-based sex work and access to 267–8

South Africa 37, 46, 49, 65, 82, 221–2; barriers to post-exposure prophylaxis completion after rape study 221–32; emergence of an alternative urban masculinity 43; institutionalisation of male doubt 45; Love Life campaign 46, 49; marriage statistics 43; post-rape services provision 221; Thohoyandou Victim Empowerment Programme 221–2; transactional sex in 81–2, 86

spousal abuse, and HIV risk 59–61

stigma: contribution of the religious immorality message to 240; of male sex work 164–6; rumour and 241

stigmatisation: and the concealment of same-sex relationships 74; and HIV risk 112; of sex work involving men and trans people in Peru 173

street-based sex work: and access to informal social services 267–8; avoiding dangers of through use of the Internet 178–9; levels of risk for STI acquisition 183; and violence 164–5, 176
structural violence 16
subaltern patterns, in organisation of gender and sexuality 12
sub-Saharan Africa: percentage of world's population of HIV positive people living in 37; research on sexual concurrency with adult heterosexual men 73
substance abuse: and condom use 72; homophobia and 97, 216; by MTFs 113
sugar daddies: in South Africa 46; Zimbabwean news story 80; Zimbabwean terminology 83; see also transactional sex
suicide, sexual identity as a risk factor for 207, 210, 215
suicide attempts, rates of among LGBT youth in North America and New Zealand 208
survival sex 82, 143
syphilis 26, 28, 41, 50

teenage magazines: on abstinence 29; documentation of ambivalence toward sexuality 24; German-US comparison study 24; on the medicalisation of sex 28–9; paradoxical messages 24; provision of role models 25; on sex, fear and pregnancy 27; on sex, fear and STDs 28; on sex and fear of betrayal 28; sexuality in 27–9; signs of resistance to the dominant discourses 33; treatment of homosexuality 32
tourism: and the demand for commercial sex 179; and demand for sexual services 176; transactional sex and 159
trafficking: defining 270; global moral panic about 267; in the media 147; narrow view of 269; policies on 269; racialised discourse about 266–8
trans and male sex workers study 173–83; see also male and trans sex work
transactional sex: and African systems of interdependence 81; ambiguity of communication and safe sex negotiation 164; assumptions about 81; as business strategy 82; complexity 80; conspicuous consumption as motivation for 82, 84–6, 88; economic anthropological parallel 90; female students' use of 80; food and 85–6; and grooming 86–8; and the importance of non-sexual services 81; literature review of African 81–2; meaning of for the men 89–90; multiple meanings of in Africa 82; and multiple partnerships 90–1; as patron-client relationship 81; and

perceptions of need 86; prestige and 84–5; vs sex work 88; status and 84–5; strategies to avoid reciprocation 88–9; and tourism 159
transgender individuals: HIV rates among 112; see also male and trans sex work; male-to-female transgendered persons
transgressive, meaning 126
travestis 175, 178–83; meaning 176

UAE (United Arab Emirates): ethnographic research with transnational migrants 263; focus of media representations of sex work 265; 'race' discourse 263; sponsorship system 261; see also Dubai
Uganda, legislation on male-male sexual activity 158
ukusoma (thigh sex) 39, 41, 45
ultra femmes 132–3, 136–7
undocumented migrants see displaced persons (asylum seekers; refugees; undocumented migrants)
unemployment: and men's self-esteem 43; in South Africa 43; and the transition to adulthood 209
United Arab Emirates see UAE
United Kingdom: legislation on same-sex relationships 207; LGBT shame avoidance study 207–19
United Nations Palermo Protocol 267, 269
United States: Black lesbian gender and sexual culture study 125–38; the Christian Right 33; HIV risk among MTFs study 112–22; masculinity and HIV sexual risk among Black heterosexual men study 65–75; portrayal of sexuality and sexual health in magazines for teenage and middle-aged women 23–34; research on sexual concurrency with adult heterosexual men 73; three steps of sex 137
unprotected sex, MSM in African settings 158

violence: encountered by sex workers in Peru 176; male sex work and 164–6; minimisation of as homophobia negotiation strategy 214; MTFs' experience 117; perception of asylum situations as form of 192; and psychological well-being 208; sex work and the risk of 150; sex work as form of 143; sexual and gender based violence see sexual and gender based violence; vulnerability of displaced persons to 201
virginity: and the double standard 24; portrayal of in teenage magazines 24; testing 40, 46
vulnerability discourse, place of race and gender in 267–8

Weeks, J. 42, 99
witchcraft, Christianity and accusations of 239
wives, and power in Zulu society 39
women: expectations of Chilean men 56; machismo and discrimination against 56; missing discourses of desire in 33; perception of HIV risk 55–6; ratio of living with HIV in Chile 55; sexuality of middle-aged, lack of investigation into media portrayal 25; tradition of studying the media portrayal of sexualities of 23 (*see also* women's magazines in the US study); vulnerability to HIV infection, factors that increase 55–6; vulnerability to SGBV 189
women fish traders, and transactional sex 81–2

women's independence, and South African masculinity 43
women's magazines: fearmongering in 30; on the health benefits of sex 30; high circulation rates 25; representation of double standard 31; sex in 29–32; on sexual behaviour of teenage children 31; signs of resistance to the dominant discourses 33; on women's responsibility for sex in marriage 29–31
World Health Organization, first expert group meeting on sexual health 2

Zambia, legislation on male-male sexual activity 158
Zimbabwe: economic crisis 83; female students and transactional sex study 80–91

Culture, Health & Sexuality

Culture, Health & Sexuality is a high quality journal publishing internationally relevant, cutting edge research on culture, health and sexuality.

Papers come from a wide range of disciplines – including anthropology, cultural studies, development studies, education, law and human rights, policy studies, psychology, public health, sexual and reproductive health, and sociology.

Key issues focused upon include:

• Culture, sexuality and health, health systems and beliefs, social structures and divisions, and the implications for these for sexual health and wellbeing;

• Sexual and reproductive health – of individuals, communities and populations, including STIs and HIV and sexual/reproductive health problems, along with the positive dimensions of sexual health, including pleasure, reciprocity and sexual fulfilment;

• Sexual and gender inequality and health, including the health and well-being of sexual and gender minorities, sexual and reproductive health and rights, and new forms of sexual expression and desire; and

• Policy and practice dimensions of research on sexuality, culture and health; sexual and gender inequality and health; and sexual and gender violence.

Culture,
Health &
Sexuality

An International Journal for
Research, Intervention and Care

Editor-in-Chief:
Peter Aggleton

Founding Editors:
Susan Kippax
Ramona Plate
Richard Parker
Barbara de Zalduondo

Editor-in-Chief:
Peter Aggleton

Find out more about the journal
at **www.tandfonline.com/tchs**

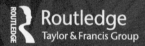

Routledge
Taylor & Francis Group

Printed and bound by CPI Group (UK) Ltd, Croydon, CR0 4YY

18/10/2024

01776250-0002